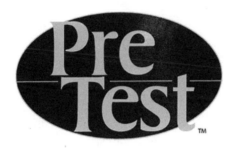

Emergency Medicine

PreTest™ Self-Assessment and Review

Notice

Medicine is an ever-changing science. As new research and clinical experience broaden our knowledge, changes in treatment and drug therapy are required. The authors and the publisher of this work have checked with sources believed to be reliable in their efforts to provide information that is complete and generally in accord with the standards accepted at the time of publication. However, in view of the possibility of human error or changes in medical sciences, neither the authors nor the publisher nor any other party who has been involved in the preparation or publication of this work warrants that the information contained herein is in every respect accurate or complete, and they disclaim all responsibility for any errors or omissions or for the results obtained from use of the information contained in this work. Readers are encouraged to confirm the information contained herein with other sources. For example, and in particular, readers are advised to check the product information sheet included in the package of each drug they plan to administer to be certain that the information contained in this work is accurate and that changes have not been made in the recommended dose or in the contraindications for administration. This recommendation is of particular importance in connection with new or infrequently used drugs.

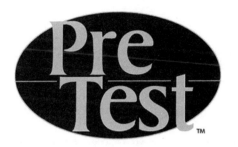

Emergency Medicine
PreTest™ Self-Assessment and Review
First Edition

Adam J. Rosh, MD, MS
Chief Resident
Department of Emergency Medicine
New York University/Bellevue Hospital Center
New York, New York

Stephen H. Menlove, MD
Attending Physician
Department of Emergency Medicine
New York University/Bellevue Hospital Center
New York, New York

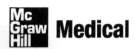

New York   Chicago   San Francisco   Lisbon   London   Madrid   Mexico City
Milan   New Delhi   San Juan   Seoul   Singapore   Sydney   Toronto

Emergency Medicine: PreTest™ Self-Assessment and Review, First Edition

Copyright © 2008 by The McGraw-Hill Companies, Inc. All rights reserved. Printed in the United States of America. Except as permitted under the United States Copyright Act of 1976, no part of this publication may be reproduced or distributed in any form or by any means, or stored in a data base or retrieval system, without the prior written permission of the publisher.

PreTest™ is a trademark of The McGraw-Hill Companies, Inc.

1 2 3 4 5 6 7 8 9 0   DOC/DOC   0 9 8 7

ISBN: 13: 978-0-07-147785-7
MHID: 0-07-147785-3

This book was set in Berkeley by International Typesetting and Composition.
The editors were Catherine A. Johnson and Regina Y. Brown.
The production supervisor was Sherri Souffrance.
Project management was provided by International Typesetting and Composition.
The cover designer was Maria Scharf.
Cover Photo: Doctors intubating a patient.
RR Donnelley was printer and binder.

This book is printed on acid-free paper.

Library of Congress Cataloging-in-Publication Data

Rosh, Adam J.
      Emergency medicine : PreTest self-assessment and review / Adam J. Rosh.—1st ed.
            p. ; cm.
      Includes bibliographical references and index.
      ISBN-13: 978-0-07-147785-7 (pbk. : alk. paper)
      ISBN-10: 0-07-147785-3
      1. Emergency medicine—Examinations, questions, etc.   I. Title.
      [DNLM: 1. Emergencies—Examination Questions.   2. Emergency
      Medicine—Examination Questions. WB 18.2 R818e   2008]
      RC86.9.R67   2008
      616.02′5076—dc22

                                                                  2007026496

A hearty thanks goes out to the dedicated medical professionals of the NYU/Bellevue emergency medicine residency program; my family for their love and support; Catherine Johnson for giving me this opportunity; and my patients who teach me something new each day.

—AJR

Thanks to Stephanie, Max, and Coco for their love and support.

—SHM

Student Reviewers

Michael Curley
University of Wisconsin School of Medicine and Public Health
Class of 2007

David Lazar
Baylor College of Medicine
Class of 2007

Kevin Olsen, MD, Capt, USAF
St. Louis University—Belleville Family Medicine Residency
PGY-2

Contents

Headache

Weakness and Dizziness

Fever

Poisoning and Overdose

Environmental Exposures

Vaginal Bleeding

Eye Pain and Visual Change

Endocrine Emergencies

Psychosocial Disorders

Wound Care

Contributors

Adam Landman, MD, MS, MIS
Resident, Department of Emergency Medicine
Olive View-UCLA Medical Center
Los Angeles, California
Chapters 6, 14

Inna Leybell, MD
Chief Resident, Department of Emergency Medicine
New York University/Bellevue Hospital Center
New York, New York
Chapters 7, 9

Gigi R. Madore, MD
Resident, Department of Emergency Medicine
New York University/Bellevue Hospital Center
New York, New York
Chapters 4, 10

Stephen H. Menlove, MD
Attending Physician
Department of Emergency Medicine
New York University/Bellevue Hospital Center
New York, New York

Jorma B. Mueller, MD
Resident, Department of Emergency Medicine
New York University/Bellevue Hospital Center
New York, New York
Chapters 8, 17

Adam J. Rosh, MD, MS
Chief Resident, Department of Emergency Medicine
New York University/Bellevue Hospital Center
New York, New York
Chapters 1, 3, 5, 11, 15

Maria Vasilyadis, MD
Chief Resident, Department of Emergency Medicine
New York University/Bellevue Hospital Center
New York, New York
Chapters 2, 12, 13, 16

Introduction

Emergency Medicine: PreTest Self Assessment and Review, First Edition, is intended to provide medical students, as well as house officers and physicians, with a convenient tool for assessing and improving their knowledge of medicine. The 500 questions in this book are similar in format and complexity to those included in Step 2 of the United States Medical Licensing Examination (USMLE). They may also be a useful study tool for Step 3.

Each question in this book has a corresponding answer, a reference to a text that provides background to the answer, and a short discussion of various issues raised by the question and its answer. A listing of references for the entire book follows the last chapter.

To simulate the time constraints imposed by the qualifying examinations for which this book is intended as a practice guide, the student or physician should allot about 1 minute for each question. After answering all questions in a chapter, as much time as necessary should be spent in reviewing the explanations for each question at the end of the chapter. Attention should be given to all explanations, even if the examinee answered the question correctly. Those seeking more information on a subject should refer to the reference materials listed or to other standard texts in medicine.

Chest Pain and Cardiac Dysrhythmias

Questions

1. A 59-year-old man presents to the emergency department (ED) complaining of new onset chest pain that radiates to his left arm. He has a history of hypertension, hypercholesterolemia, and a 20-pack-year smoking history. His ECG is remarkable for T-wave inversions in the lateral leads. Which of the following is the most appropriate next step in management?

a. Give the patient two nitroglycerin tablets sublingually and observe if his chest pain resolves
b. Place the patient on a cardiac monitor, administer oxygen, and give aspirin
c. Call the cardiac catherization lab for immediate percutaneous intervention (PCI)
d. Order a chest x-ray, administer aspirin, clopidogrel, and heparin
e. Start a β-blocker immediately

2. A 36-year-old woman presents to the ED with sudden onset of left-sided chest pain and mild shortness of breath that began last night. She was able to fall asleep without difficulty but woke up this morning with persistent pain. The pain is worse when she takes a deep breath. She walked up the stairs at home and became very short of breath, which made her come to the ED. Two weeks ago, she took a 7-hour flight from Europe and since then has left-sided calf pain and swelling. What is the most common electrocardiogram (ECG) finding for this patient's presentation?

a. S1-Q3-T3
b. Atrial fibrillation
c. Right axis deviation
d. Right atrial enlargement
e. Tachycardia or nonspecific ST/T-wave changes

3. A 51-year-old man with a long history of hypertension presents to the ED complaining of 1 week of intermittent chest palpitations. He denies chest pain, shortness of breath, nausea, and vomiting. He recalls feeling similar episodes of palpitations a few months ago but they resolved. His blood pressure is 130/75 mm Hg, heart rate is 130 beats per minute, respiratory rate is 16 breaths per minute, and oxygen saturation is 99% on room air. An ECG is seen below. Which of the following is the most appropriate next step in management?

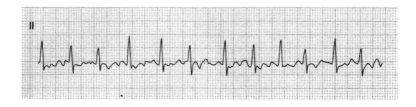

a. Sedate patient for immediate synchronized cardioversion with 100 J
b. Prepare patient for the cardiac catherization lab
c. Administer coumadin
d. Administer amiodarone
e. Administer diltiazem

4. A 51-year-old woman presents to the ED because of a change in behavior at home. She has end-stage renal disease that requires dialysis for the past 3 years. Her daughter states that the patient missed her last two dialysis appointments. The daughter states that the patient has been increasingly confused and disoriented for the past 3 days. On physical examination, the patient is alert and oriented to person only. The remainder of her examination is normal. An initial 12-lead ECG is performed as seen on the next page. Which of the following electrolyte abnormalities best explains these findings?

a. Hypokalemia
b. Hyperkalemia
c. Hypocalcemia
d. Hypercalcemia
e. Hyponatremia

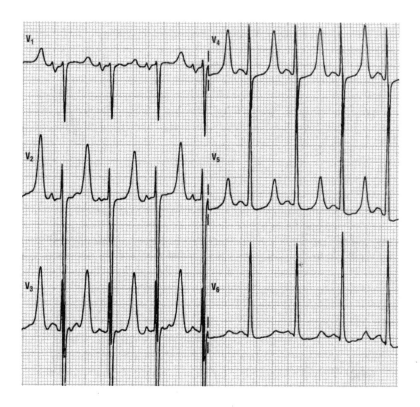

5. A 29-year-old tall, thin man presents to the ED after feeling short of breath for 2 days. In the ED, he is in no acute distress. Heart rate is 81 beats per minute, blood pressure is 115/70 mm Hg, respiratory rate is 16 breaths per minute, and oxygen saturation is 98% on room air. Lung, cardiac, and abdominal exams are normal. An ECG reveals sinus rhythm at a rate of 79. A chest radiograph shows a small right-sided (less than 10% of the hemithorax) spontaneous pneumothorax. A repeat chest x-ray 6 hours later reveals a decreased pneumothorax. Which of the following is the most appropriate next step in management?

a. Discharge the patient with follow up in 24 hours
b. Perform needle decompression in the 2nd intercostal space, midclavicular line
c. Insert a 20-French chest tube into right hemithorax
d. Observe for another 6 hours
e. Admit for pleurodesis

6. A 42-year-old man found vomiting in the street is brought to the ED by emergency medical services (EMS). He has a known history of alcohol abuse with multiple presentations for intoxication. Today, the patient complains of acute onset and persistent chest pain associated with dysphagia and pain upon flexing his neck. His blood pressure is 115/70 mm Hg, heart rate of 101 beats per minute, respiratory rate 18 breaths per minute, and oxygen saturation of 97% on room air. As you listen to his heart, you hear a crunching sound. His abdomen is soft with mild epigastric tenderness. The ECG is sinus tachycardia without ST-T wave abnormalities. On chest x-ray, there is air in the mediastinum. What is the most likely diagnosis?

a. Acute coronary syndrome (ACS)
b. Pancreatitis
c. Alcoholic ketoacidosis
d. Esophageal perforation
e. Aortic dissection

7. A 65-year-old man with a history of chronic hypertension presents to the ED with sudden-onset tearing chest pain that radiates to his jaw. His blood pressure is 205/110 mm Hg, heart rate 90 beats per minute, respiratory rate is 20 breaths per minute, and oxygen saturation is 97% on room air. He appears apprehensive. On cardiac exam you hear a diastolic murmur at the right sternal border. A chest x-ray reveals a widened mediastinum. Which of the following is the preferred study of choice to diagnose this patient's condition?

a. ECG
b. Transthoracic echocardiography
c. Transesophageal echocardiography
d. Computed tomography (CT) scan
e. Magnetic resonance imaging (MRI)

8. A 47-year-old man with a history of hypertension presents to the ED complaining of continuous left sided chest pain that began while snorting cocaine 1 hour ago. The patient states he never experienced chest pain in the past when using cocaine. His blood pressure is 170/90 mm Hg, heart rate is 101 beats per minute, respiratory rate is 18 breaths per minute, and oxygen saturation is 98% on room air. The patient states that the only medication he takes is alprazolam to "calm his nerves." Which of the following medications is contraindicated in this patient?

a. Metoprolol
b. Diltiazem
c. Aspirin
d. Lorazepam
e. Nitroglycerin

9. A 32-year-old woman presents to the ED with a persistent fever of 101°F over the last 3 days. The patient states that she used to work as a convenience store clerk but was fired 2 weeks ago. Since then, she was using IV drugs daily. Cardiac exam reveals a heart murmur. Her abdomen is soft and non-tender but you palpate an enlarged spleen. Chest radiograph reveals multiple patchy infiltrates in both lung fields. Laboratory results reveal WBC 14,000/μL with 91% neutrophils, hematocrit 33%, and platelets 250/μL. Which of the following is the most appropriate next step in management?

a. Obtain four sets of blood cultures, order a transthoracic echocardiogram (TTE), and start antibiotic treatment
b. Order a monospot test and recommend the patient refrain from vigorous activities for 1 month
c. Administer an nonsteroidal anti-inflammatory drug (NSAID) and tell the patient she has pericarditis
d. Administer Isoniazid (INH) and report the patient to the Department of Health
e. Order a Lyme antibody and begin antibiotic therapy

10. A 61-year-old woman was on her way to the grocery store when she started feeling chest pressure in the center of her chest. She became diaphoretic and felt short of breath. She notified EMS who brought her to the ED. On arrival to the ED, her blood pressure is 130/70 mm Hg, heart rate 76 beats per minute, and oxygen saturation of 98% on room air. She is given an aspirin by the nurse and an ECG is performed that is seen below. Which of the following best describes the location of this patient's myocardial infarction (MI)?

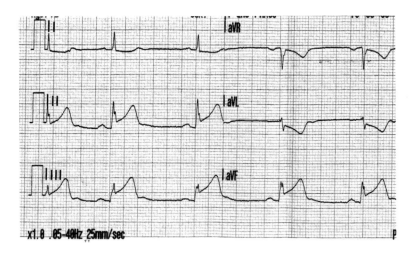

a. Anteroseptal
b. Anterior
c. Lateral
d. Inferior
e. Posterior

11. A 31-year-old man who works for a moving company presents to the ED because he thought he was having a heart attack. He does not smoke and jogs 3 days a week. His father died of a heart attack in his 60s. He describes gradual onset of chest pain that is worse with activity and resolves when he is at rest. His heart rate is 68 beats per minute, blood pressure is 120/70 mm Hg, and respiratory rate is 14 breaths per minute. On exam, his lungs are clear and there is no cardiac murmur. You palpate tenderness over the left sternal border at the third and fourth rib. An ECG reveals sinus rhythm at a rate of 65. A chest radiograph shows no infiltrates or pneumothorax. Which of the following is the most appropriate next step in management?

a. Administer aspirin and send a troponin
b. Administer aspirin, clopidogrel, and heparin and admit for ACS
c. Administer ibuprofen and reassure the patient that he is not having a heart attack
d. Inject corticosteroid into costrochondroid joint to reduce inflammation
e. Observe the patient for 6 hours

12. A 21-year-old woman presents to the ED complaining of lightheaded-ness. Her symptoms appeared 45 minutes ago. She has no other symptoms and is on no medications. She has a medical history of mitral valve prolapse. Her heart rate is 170 beats per minute and blood pressure is 105/55 mm Hg. Physical exam is unremarkable. A 12-lead ECG is performed and shows supraventricular tachycardia (SVT) with a regular rate, shortened PR interval, and a delta wave at the onset of the QRS complex. Based on this information, which of the following is the most likely diagnosis?

a. Sinus tachycardia
b. Ventricular tachycardia
c. Atrial flutter with 3:1 block
d. Atrial fibrillation
e. Wolff-Parkinson-White (WPW) syndrome

13. A 55-year-old man presents to the ED with worsening weakness, muscle cramps, and paresthesias. He states he has had kidney problems in the past. On exam, the patient is alert and oriented. He is diffusely weak. An ECG is seen below. Which of the following is the most important next step in management?

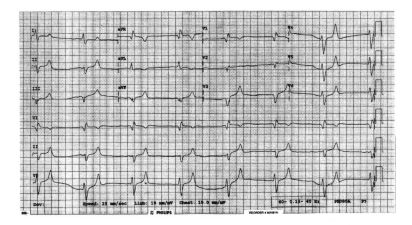

a. Administer calcium gluconate
b. Administer oral potassium binder (Kayexalate)
c. Administer insulin and dextrose
d. Administer sodium bicarbonate
e. Administer nebulized albuterol

14. While eating dinner, a 55-year-old man suddenly feels a piece of steak "get stuck" in his stomach. In the ED, he complains of dysphagia, is drooling, and occasionally retches. On exam, blood pressure is 130/80 mm Hg, heart rate 75 beats per minute, respiratory rate 15 breaths per minute, and oxygen saturation 99% on room air. He appears in no respiratory distress. Chest x-ray is negative for air under the diaphragm. Which of the following is the most appropriate next step in management?

a. Administer 1 mg glucagon intravenously while arranging for endoscopy
b. Administer a meat tenderizer such as papain to soften the food bolus
c. Administer 10 mL syrup of ipecac to induce vomiting and dislodge the food bolus
d. Perform the Heimlich maneuver until the food dislodges
e. Call surgery consult to prepare for laparotomy

15. A 59-year-old man presents to the ED with left-sided chest pain and shortness of breath that began 2 hours prior to arrival. He states the pain is pressure-like and radiates down his left arm. He is diaphoretic. His blood pressure is 160/80 mm Hg, heart rate 86 beats per minute, respiratory rate 15 breaths per minute. ECG reveals 2 mm ST-segment elevation in leads I, aVL, V3–V6. Which of the following is an absolute contraindication to receiving thrombolytic therapy?

a. Systolic blood pressure greater than 180 mm Hg
b. Patient on coumadin and aspirin
c. Total hip replacement 3 months ago
d. Peptic ulcer disease
e. Previous hemorrhagic stroke

16. A 67-year-old woman is brought to the ED by paramedics complaining of dyspnea, fatigue, and palpitations. Her blood pressure is 80/50 mm Hg, heart is 139 beats per minutes, and her respiratory rate is 20 breaths per minute. Her skin is cool and she is diaphoretic. Her lung exam reveals bilateral crackles and she is beginning to have chest pain. ECG shows a narrow complex irregular rhythm with a rate in the 140s. Which of the following is the most appropriate immediate treatment for this patient?

a. Diltiazem
b. Metoprolol
c. Digoxin
d. Coumadin
e. Synchronized cardioversion

17. A 61-year-old woman with a history of congestive heart failure (CHF) is at a family picnic when she starts complaining of shortness of breath. Her daughter brings her to the ED where she is found to have an oxygen saturation of 85% on room air with rales halfway up both of her lung fields. Her blood pressure is 185/90 mm Hg and pulse rate is 101. On exam, she has jugular venous distention (JVD) and lower extremity pitting edema. What is the most rapid method of reducing preload in this patient?

a. Metoprolol
b. Aspirin
c. Oxygen
d. Nitroglycerin
e. Morphine sulfate

18. A 27-year-old man, who is otherwise healthy, presents to the ED with a laceration on his thumb that he sustained while cutting a bagel. You irrigate and repair the wound and are about to discharge the patient when he asks you if he can receive an ECG. It is not busy in the ED so you perform the ECG that is seen below. Which of the following is the most appropriate next step in management?

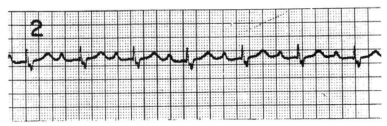

(Reproduced, with permission, from Tintinalli J, Kelen G, and Stapczynski J. Emergency Medicine A Comprehensive Study Guide. *New York, NY: McGraw-Hill, 2004:193)*

a. Admit the patient for placement of a pacemaker
b. Admit the patient for a cardiac catherization
c. Administer aspirin and send cardiac biomarkers
d. Repeat the ECG due to incorrect lead placement
e. Discharge the patient home

19. A 56-year-old woman with a history of ovarian cancer presents to the ED with acute onset of right-sided chest pain, shortness of breath, and dyspnea. Her blood pressure is 131/75 mm Hg, heart rate is 101 beats per minute, respirations are 18 breaths per minute, and oxygen saturation is 97% on room air. You suspect this patient has a pulmonary embolism (PE). Which of the following tests is most likely to be abnormal?

a. Arterial blood gas
b. Oxygen saturation
c. ECG
d. Chest radiograph
e. D-dimer

20. A 61-year-old woman with a history of diabetes and hypertension is brought to the ED by her daughter. The patient states she started feeling short of breath approximately 12 hours ago and then noticed a tingling sensation in the middle of her chest and became diaphoretic. An ECG reveals ST-depression in leads II, III, and aVF. You believe the patient had a non-ST elevation MI. Which of the following cardiac markers begins to rise within 3–6 hours of chest pain onset, peaks at 12–24 hours, and returns to baseline in 7–10 days?

a. Myoglobin
b. Creatinine kinase (CK)
c. Creatinine kinase-MB (CK-MB)
d. Troponin
e. Lactic dehydrogenase (LDH)

21. A 65-year-old man with a history of diabetes and uncontrolled hypertension presents to your ED complaining of crushing chest pain radiating to his back that was worst at onset but continuing until arrival in the ED. An ECG is nondiagnostic and chest x-ray is normal. On physical exam of the patient's pulses you note significant radiofemoral delay. Your hospital does not have access to echocardiography. Which of the following is the diagnostic study of choice?

a. Serial cardiac enzymes
b. Contrast aortography
c. CT of the chest in arterial phase
d. MRI
e. Plain radiographs

22. A 27-year-old man complains of chest palpitations and lightheadedness for the past hour. He has no past medical history and is not taking any medications. He drinks a beer occasionally on the weekend and does not smoke cigarettes. His heart rate is 180 beats per minute, blood pressure 110/65 mm Hg, and oxygen saturation 99% on room air. An ECG reveals a narrow complex tachycardia at a rate of 180 that is regular and without discernable P waves. Which of the following is the most appropriate medication to treat this dysrhythmia?

a. Digoxin
b. Lidocaine
c. Amiodarone
d. Adenosine
e. Bretylium

23. A 59-year-old man presents to the ED with left-sided chest pain and shortness of breath that began 1 hour ago. Initial vital signs are blood pressure 85/45 mm Hg, heart rate 105, respiratory rate 20, and oxygen saturation 94% on room air. An ECG is seen below. Which of the following is the most appropriate definitive treatment?

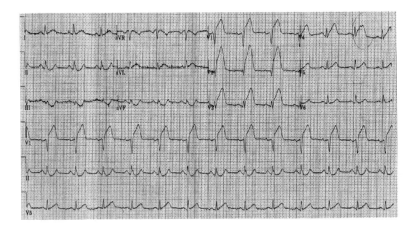

a. Administer metoprolol or diltiazem
b. Electrical cardioversion
c. Administer dobutamine or dopamine
d. Thrombolytic therapy
e. Percutaneous angioplasty

24. A 55-year-old man presents to the ED at 2:00 a.m. with left-sided chest pain that radiates down his left arm. He takes a β-blocker for hypertension, a proton-pump inhibitor for reflux disease, and an antilipid agent for high cholesterol. He also took sildenafil last night for erectile dysfunction. His blood pressure is 130/70 mm Hg and heart rate is 77. Which of the following medication is contraindicated in this patient?

a. Aspirin
b. Unfractionated heparin
c. Nitroglycerin
d. Metoprolol
e. Morphine sulfate

25. A 31-year-old kindergarten teacher presents to the ED complaining of acute onset substernal chest pain that is sharp in nature and radiates to her back. The pain is worse when she is lying down on the stretcher and improves when she sits up. She smokes cigarettes occasionally and was told she has borderline diabetes. She denies any recent surgeries or long travel. Her blood pressure is 145/85 mm Hg, heart rate is 99 beats per minute, respiratory rate is 18 breaths per minute and temperature is 100.6°F. Examination of her chest reveals clear lungs and a friction rub. Her abdomen is soft and her legs are not swollen. Chest radiography and echocardiography are unremarkable. Her ECG is shown below. Which of the following is the most appropriate next step in management?

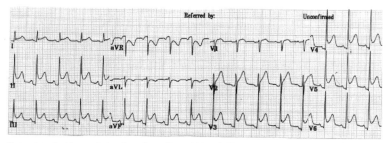

(Reproduced, with permission, from Fuster V. et al. Hurst's The Heart. New York, NY: McGraw-Hill, 2004: 304)

a. Anticoagulate and CT scan to evaluate for a PE
b. Prescribe a NSAID and discharge the patient
c. Aspirin, heparin, clopidogrel, and admit for ACS
d. Administer thrombolytics if the pain persists
e. Prescribe antibiotics and discharge the patient

26. A 71-year-old man is playing cards with some friends when he starts to feel a pain in the left side of his chest. His fingers in the left hand become numb and he feels short of breath. His wife calls the ambulance and he is brought to the hospital. In the ED, an ECG is performed. Which of the following best describes the order of ECG changes seen in a MI?

a. Hyperacute T wave, ST segment elevation, Q wave
b. Q wave, ST segment elevation, hyperacute T wave
c. Hyperacute T wave, Q wave, ST segment elevation
d. ST segment elevation, Q wave, hyperacute T wave
e. ST segment elevation, hyperacute T wave, Q wave

27. A 63-year-old insurance agent is brought to the ED by paramedics for shortness of breath and a respiratory rate of 31 breaths per minute. The patient denies chest pain, fever, vomiting, or diarrhea. His wife says he ran out of his water-pill 1 week ago. His blood pressure is 185/90 mm Hg, heart rate 101 beats per minute, oxygen saturation 90% on room air, and temperature 98.9°F. There are crackles midway up both lung fields and 2+ pitting edema midway up his legs. An ECG shows sinus tachycardia. The patient is sitting up and able to speak to you. After placing the patient on a monitor and inserting an IV, which of the following is the most appropriate next step in management?

a. Obtain blood cultures, complete blood cell (CBC) count, and start antibiotic therapy
b. Order a statim (STAT) portable chest x-ray
c. Administer oxygen via nasal cannula and have the patient chew an aspirin
d. Administer oxygen via nonrebreather, furosemide, nitroglycerin, and consider noninvasive respiratory therapy
e. Rapid sequence endotracheal intubation

28. A 16-year-old boy is brought to the ED after collapsing during a basketball game. His blood pressure is 80/palp. His father died from a "heart-condition" at a young age. He is placed on a monitor and you see the rhythm below. Which of the following choices best describes this rhythm?

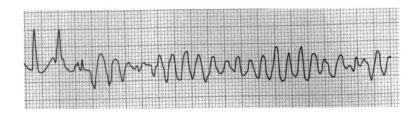

a. Ventricular fibrillation
b. Atrial fibrillation
c. Wolf-Parkinson-White
d. Supraventricular tachycardia
e. Torsade de pointes

29. Which of the following patients has the lowest clinical probability for the diagnosis of a PE?

a. A 21-year-old woman two days after a cesarean delivery
b. A 55-year-old woman on estrogen replacement therapy who underwent a total hip replacement procedure 3 days ago
c. A 39-year-old man who smokes cigarettes occasionally who underwent an uncomplicated appendectomy 1 month ago
d. A 62-year-old man with pancreatic cancer
e. A 45-year-old man with factor V Leiden deficiency

30. A 75-year-old man goes out to shovel snow from his driveway. After 5 minutes of shoveling, he feels short of breath, chest pain, and then passes out. He awakens minutes later to his wife shaking him. In the ED, he denies chest pain or dyspnea. His blood pressure is 160/85 mm Hg, heart rate 71 beats per minute, and oxygen saturation 97% on room air. On exam, you hear a harsh systolic ejection murmur. ECG reveals a sinus rhythm with left ventricular hypertrophy. Which of the following is the most likely diagnosis?

a. Asystolic cardiac arrest
b. Brugada syndrome
c. Subclavian steal syndrome
d. PE
e. Aortic stenosis

31. A 33-year-old lawyer, who smokes a pack of cigarettes daily, was sitting at home reading the newspaper when he felt acute onset shortness of breath and chest pain that was worse with inspiration. He remembers a similar pain 2 years ago that lasted over 1 week. In the ED his heart rate is 101, blood pressure is 125/70 mm Hg, respiratory rate is 20 breaths per minute, and oxygen saturation is 98% on room air. A chest x-ray is performed and is seen below. Which of the following is the most likely diagnosis?

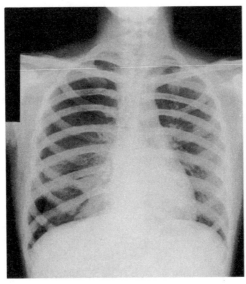

(Reproduced, with permission, from Doherty GM, Way LW. Current Surgical Diagnosis & Treatment. New York, NY: McGraw-Hill, 2006: 349)

a. Lobar pneumonia
b. Pneumomediastinum
c. Pneumothorax
d. Pericardial tamponade
e. CHF

32. A 62-year-old woman presents to the ED with substernal chest pain that radiates to her left shoulder, shortness of breath, and general weakness. Her blood pressure is 155/80 mm Hg, heart rate 92 beats per minute, and respiratory rate 16 breaths per minute. You suspect that she is having an acute MI. Which of the following therapeutic agents has shown to independently reduce mortality in the setting of an acute MI?

a. Nitroglycerin
b. Aspirin
c. Unfractionated heparin
d. Lidocaine
e. Diltiazem

33. A 22-year-old college student went to the health clinic complaining of a fever over the last 5 days, fatigue, myalgias, and a bout of vomiting and diarrhea. The clinic doctor diagnosed him with acute gastroenteritis and told him to drink more fluids. Three days later, the student presents to the ED complaining of substernal chest pain that is constant. He also feels short of breath. His temperature is 100.9°F, heart rate is 119 beats per minute, blood pressure is 120/75 mm Hg, and respiratory rate is 18 breaths per minute. An ECG is performed that shows sinus tachycardia. A chest radiograph is unremarkable. Laboratory test are normal except for a slightly elevated WBC. Which of the following is the most common cause of this patient's diagnosis?

a. *Streptococcus viridans*
b. *Staphylococcus aureus*
c. Coxsackie B virus
d. Atherosclerotic disease
e. Cocaine abuse

34. A 51-year-old woman presents to the ED after 5 consecutive days of crushing substernal chest pressure that woke her up from sleep in the morning. The pain resolves spontaneously after 20–30 minutes. She is an avid rock climber and jogs 5 miles daily. She has never smoked a cigarette and has no family history of coronary disease. In the ED, she experiences another episode of chest pain. An ECG reveals ST-segment elevations and cardiac biomarkers are negative. The pain is relieved with sublingual nitroglycerin. She is admitted to the hospital and diagnostic testing reveals minimal coronary atherosclerotic disease. Which of the following is the most appropriate medication to treat this patient's condition?

a. Aspirin
b. Calcium channel blocker
c. β-Blocker
d. H₂-Blocker
e. Proton pump inhibitor

35. A 23-year-old woman who is an elementary school teacher is brought to the ED after syncopizing in her classroom while teaching. Prior to passing out, she describes feeling lightheaded and dizzy and next remembers being in the ambulance. There was no evidence of seizure activity. She has no medical problems and does not take any medications. Her father died of a "heart problem" at age 32 years. She does not smoke or use drugs. Blood pressure is 120/70 mm Hg, pulse rate is 71, respiratory rate is 14, and oxygen saturation is 100% on room air. Her physical exam and laboratory results are all normal. A rhythm strip is seen below. Which of the following is the most likely diagnosis?

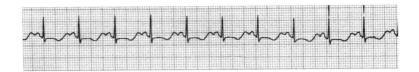

a. Hypovolemia
b. Long QT syndrome
c. Hyperkalemia
d. Complete heart block
e. ACS

36. A 37-year-old man presents to the ED stating that for the past 24 hours he has been experiencing left-sided anterior chest pain. The pain began suddenly while he was in bed watching television. He has never had a pain like this before. He describes the pain as being sharp and worsening when he lies down. He has some hesitation taking very deep breaths because this also causes pain. Last week he recalls having a cough with flu-like symptoms. There is no pain while palpating the chest wall. You appreciate a rub on cardiac exam. The lungs are clear to auscultation and there is no chest wall tenderness. A chest radiograph is within normal limits. Which of the following is the most likely cause of the patient's chest pain?

a. Musculoskeletal chest pain
b. Angina
c. Aortic dissection
d. Pericarditis
e. Community acquired pneumonia

37. A 64-year-old man with a long-standing history of hypertension presents to the ED with sudden-onset excruciating chest pain that was worst at its onset and is now mildly improved. The pain radiates into his back. Two years ago he underwent a percutaneous angioplasty. His blood pressure is 200/90 mm Hg in his right arm and 160/60 mm Hg in his right leg. Physical exam reveals a murmur with variable intensity that is consistent with aortic insufficiency. A chest radiograph shows an enlarged aortic knob. Which of the following is the most likely diagnosis?

a. Aortic dissection
b. Abdominal aortic aneurysm
c. Tension pneumothorax
d. Gastroesophageal reflux disease (GERD)
e. Pulmonary embolism (PE)

38. A 55-year-old man presents to the ED with chest pain and shortness of breath. His blood pressure is 170/80 mm Hg, heart rate is 89 beats per minute, and oxygen saturation is 90% on room air. Physical exam reveals crackles mid way up both lung fields and a new holosystolic murmur that is loudest at the apex and radiates to the left axilla. ECG reveals ST elevations in the inferior leads. Chest radiograph shows pulmonary edema with a normal sized cardiac silhouette. Which of the following is the most likely cause of the cardiac murmur?

a. Critical aortic stenosis
b. Papillary muscle rupture
c. Pericardial effusion
d. CHF
e. Aortic dissection

39. An 82-year-old woman is brought to the ED by her daughter for worsening fatigue, dizziness, and lightheadedness. The patient denies chest pain or shortness of breath. She has not started any new medications. Her blood pressure is 140/70 mm Hg, heart rate 37 beats per minute and respiratory rate 15 breaths per minute. An IV is started and blood is drawn. An ECG is seen below. Which of the following is the most appropriate next step in management?

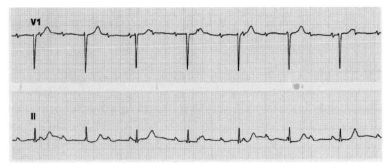

(Reproduced, with permission, from Fuster V. et al. Hurst's The Heart. New York, NY: McGraw-Hill, 2004: 904)

a. Bed rest for the next 48 hours and follow up with her primary care physician
b. Check her hemogram, guaiac her stool for occult blood, and order a transfusion if she is anemic
c. Order a CT scan to rule out a cerebral vascular event
d. Administer aspirin, order a set of cardiac enzymes, and admit
e. Place on a cardiac monitor, place external pacing pads on the patient, admit to the cardiac care unit (CCU)

40. A 22-year-old man presents to the ED with a history consistent with an acute MI. His ECG reveals ST-elevations and his cardiac biomarkers are positive. He smoked a few cigarettes in High School but has since quit. He drinks alcohol when hanging out with his friends. His grandfather died of a heart attack at 80 years old. The patient does not have hypertension or diabetes mellitus and takes no prescription medications. A recent cholesterol check revealed normal levels of total cholesterol, low-density lipoprotein (LDL), and high-density lipoprotein (HDL). Which of the following is the most likely explanation for why he has developed an MI at this age?

a. Cigarette smoking in High School
b. Family history of heart attack at age 80 years
c. Incorrectly placed leads on the ECG
d. Undisclosed cocaine use
e. Alcohol use

41. A 38-year-old woman with a history of sickle cell disease presents to the ED complaining of 2 days of right-sided chest pain that is worse on inspiration. She had a fever yesterday to 100.9°F. She feels short of breath and has a cough productive of yellow sputum. She denies leg swelling, hemoptysis, or vomiting. Her vital signs are blood pressure 120/65 mm Hg, pulse 96 beats per minute, respiratory rate 18 breaths per minute, and oxygen saturation 94% on room air. Physical exam is remarkable for crackles in her lower right lung field. There is no jugular venous distension, calf swelling, or lower extremity edema. Chest x-ray reveals a new infiltrate in the right lower lobe. Which of the following is the most appropriate next step in management?

a. Supplemental oxygen, IV hydration, analgesia, and antibiotics
b. Aspirin, nitroglycerin, clopidogrel, and heparin
c. D-dimer, V/Q scan, and heparin
d. Nebulized albuterol, prednisone, and antibiotics
e. Omeprazole and endoscopy

42. A 61-year-old woman with metastatic breast cancer presents to the ED with chest pain, cough, and shortness of breath. She states these symptoms began 1 week ago and progressively worsened. She denies fever or chills. On exam, you notice jugular venous distension. Her blood pressure is 105/70 mm Hg and heart rate is 98 beats per minute. A chest radiograph is seen below. Which of the following ECG finding is associated with this presentation?

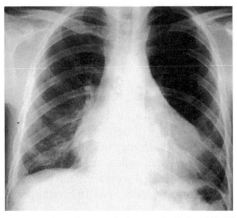

(Reproduced, with permission, from Cheitlin MD, Sokolow M, McIlroy MB. Clinical Cardiology. New York, NY: McGraw-Hill, 1996: 641)

a. Low voltage complexes
b. ST segment elevation
c. ST segment depression
d. T wave inversion
e. Peaked T waves

43. A 68-year-old woman with recently diagnosed uterine cancer is brought to the ED by her daughter. The patient complains of acute onset right-sided chest pain that is sharp in character and worse with inspiration. Her blood pressure is 135/85 mm Hg, heart rate 107 beats per minute, respiratory rate 20 breaths per minute, and oxygen saturation 97% on room air. Physical exam reveals a swollen and tender right calf. ECG is sinus tachycardia. Which of the following is the most appropriate next step in management?

a. Start heparin therapy prior to diagnostic study
b. Administer thrombolytics

c. Order a ventilation-perfusion scan
d. Order a CT angiogram
e. Obtain a transthoracic echocardiogram

44. A 57-year-old man complains of chest palpitations and lightheadedness for the past hour. Five years ago he underwent a cardiac catherization with coronary artery stent placement. His smokes 1/2-pack of cigarettes daily and drinks a glass of wine at dinner. His heart rate is 140 beats per minute, blood pressure 115/70 mm Hg, and oxygen saturation 99% on room air. An ECG reveals a wide complex tachycardia at a rate of 140 that is regular in rhythm. An ECG from 6 months ago shows a sinus rhythm at a rate of 80. Which of the following is the most appropriate medication to treat this dysrhythmia?

a. Digoxin
b. Diltiazem
c. Amiodarone
d. Adenosine
e. Bretylium

45. A 55-year-old man with hypertension and a 1-pack per day smoking history presents to the ED complaining of three episodes of severe heavy chest pain this morning that radiated to his left shoulder. In the past, he experienced chest discomfort after walking 20 minutes that resolved with rest. The episodes of chest pain this morning occurred while he was reading the newspaper. His blood pressure is 155/80 mm Hg, heart rate 76 beats per minute, respiratory rate 15 breaths per minute. He does not have chest pain in the ED. An ECG reveals sinus rhythm with a rate of 72. A troponin I is negative. Which of the following best describes this patient's diagnosis?

a. Variant angina
b. Stable angina
c. Unstable angina
d. Non-ST elevation MI
e. ST elevation MI

46. A 58-year-old man is brought to the ED for a syncopal episode at dinner. His wife states that he was well until suddenly slumping in the chair and losing consciousness for a minute. The patient recalls having some chest discomfort and shortness of breath prior to the episode. His rhythm strip obtained by EMS is shown below.

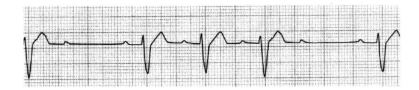

Which of the following best describes these findings?
a. Mobitz type I
b. Mobitz type II
c. First-degree AV block
d. Atrial flutter
e. Ventricular tachycardia

47. As you are examining the patient above, he starts to complain of chest discomfort and shortness of breath and has a syncopal episode again. His ECG is shown below. Which of the following is the most appropriate next step in management?

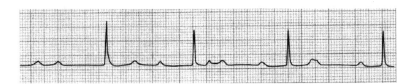

a. Call cardiology consult
b. Cardiovert the patient
c. Administer metoprolol
d. Administer adenosine
e. Apply transcutaneous pacemaker

Chest Pain and Cardiac Dysrhythmias

Answers

1. The answer is b. (*Rosen, pp 1039–1044.*) The patient's presentation is classic for an ACS. He has *multiple risk factors* with T-wave abnormalities on his ECG. The most appropriate initial management includes *placing the patient on a cardiac monitor* to detect dysrhythmias, establish intravenous access, provide supplemental *oxygen*, and administer *aspirin*. If the patient is having active chest pain in the ED, sublingual *nitroglycerin* or *morphine* should be administered until the pain resolves. This decreases wall tension and myocardial oxygen demand. A common mnemonic used is that MONA (morphine, oxygen, nitroglycerin, aspirin) greets chest pain patients at the door.

(a) Although nitroglycerin is one of the early agents used in ACS, it is prudent to first rule out a right ventricular infarct, which if present, may lead to hypotension. **(c)** Percutaneous intervention (PCI) is warranted if the patient's ECG showed ST-segment elevation. **(d)** The patient will require a chest x-ray and most likely receive clopidogrel and heparin; however this is done only after being on a monitor with oxygen and chewing an aspirin. **(e)** β-Blockers are usually added for tachycardia, hypertension, and persistent pain and only given once the patient is evaluated for contraindications. Relative contraindications to the use of β-blockers include asthma or chronic obstructive lung disease, CHF, and third-trimester pregnancy.

2. The answer is e. (*Feied, 2006.*) The patient most likely has a *pulmonary thromboembolism (PE)* that embolized from a thrombus in her left calf. The diagnosis of a PE is usually made with a CT angiogram, echocardiogram, or a ventilation-perfusion scan. The most common ECG abnormalities in the setting of PE are *tachycardia and nonspecific ST-T wave abnormalities*. Any other ECG abnormality may appear with equal likelihood, but none are sensitive or specific for PE. If ECG abnormalities are present, they may be suggestive of PE, but the absence of ECG abnormalities has no significant predictive value. Moreover, 25% of patients with proven PE have ECGs that are unchanged from their baseline state.

(**a, b, c, d**) The finding of S1-Q3-T3 is nonspecific and insensitive in the absence of clinical suspicion for PE. The classic findings of right heart strain and acute cor pulmonale are tall, peaked P waves in lead II (P pulmonale), right axis deviation, right bundle-branch block, a S1-Q3-T3 pattern, or atrial fibrillation. Unfortunately, only 20% of patients with proven PE have any of these classic ECG abnormalities.

3. The answer is e. (*Rosen, pp 1083–1085.*) Atrial fibrillation (AF) is a rhythm disturbance of the atria that results in irregular, chaotic, ventricular waveforms. This chaotic activity can lead to reduced cardiac output from a loss of coordinated atrial contractions and a rapid ventricular rate, both of which may limit diastolic filling and stroke volume of the ventricles. Atrial fibrillation may be chronic or paroxysmal, lasting minutes to days. On the ECG, fibrillatory waves are seen and accompanied by an irregular QRS pattern. The main ED treatment for atrial fibrillation is *rate control.* This can be accomplished by many agents, but the agent most commonly used is diltiazem, a calcium channel blocker with excellent AV nodal blocking effects.
(**a**) If the patient was unstable, he should be immediately cardioverted. However, this patient is stable and asymptomatic; therefore, the goal in the ED is rate control. (**b**) Catherization would be correct if the patient exhibited ST segment elevations on the ECG. (**c**) If the patient is in atrial fibrillation for greater than 48 hours, then he needs to be anticoagulated prior to cardioversion. Coumadin, along with heparin, are agents used for anticoagulation. In general, a patient with stable atrial fibrillation undergoes an echocardiogram to evaluate for thrombus. If there is a thrombus present, patients are placed on coumadin for 2–3 weeks and cardioversion takes place when their INR is therapeutic. If no clot is seen on echocardiogram, then heparin is administered and cardioversion can take place immediately. (**d**) Amiodarone is also used for rate control in atrial fibrillation; however, it is not a first line agent and is recommended to be used selectively in patients with a low left ventricular ejection fraction.

4. The answer is b. (*Rosen, pp 1727–1731.*) Patients with end-stage renal disease, who require dialysis, are prone to electrolyte disturbances. This patient's clinical picture is consistent with *hyperkalemia.* The ECG can provide valuable clues to the presence of hyperkalemia. As potassium levels rise, *peaked T waves* are the first characteristic manifestation. Further rises are associated with progressive ECG changes, including *loss of P waves and* *widening of the QRS complex.* Eventually the tracing assumes a *sine-wave pattern,* followed by ventricular fibrillation or asystole.

(**a**) ECG manifestations of hypokalemia include flattening of T waves, ST-segment depression, and U waves. (**c**) Hypocalcemia manifests as QT prolongation, whereas hypercalcemia (**d**), manifests as shortening of the QT interval. (**e**) There are no classic ECG findings with hyponatremia.

5. The answer is a. *(Rosen, pp 1000–1004.)* The patient presents with a *primary spontaneous pneumothorax (PTX),* which occurs in individuals without clinically apparent lung disease. Whereas, secondary spontaneous pneumothorax occurs in individuals with underlying lung disease, especially chronic obstructive pulmonary disease (COPD). For otherwise healthy, young patients with a small primary spontaneous PTX (less than 20% of the hemithorax), observation alone may be appropriate. The intrinsic reabsorption rate is approximately 1–2% a day, and accelerated with the administration of 100% oxygen. Many physicians *observe these patients for 6 hours* and then *repeat the chest x-ray.* If the repeat chest x-ray shows no increase in the size of the PTX, the patient can be *discharged with follow up in 24 hours.* Air travel and underwater diving (changes in atmospheric pressure) must be avoided until the PTX completely resolves.

(**b**) Needle decompression is a temporizing maneuver for patients with suspected tension PTX. (**c**) Tube thoracostomy is used in secondary spontaneous PTX, trauma PTX, and PTX > 20% of the hemithorax. (**d**) Unless there is a change in his status, the patient does not need to be observed for another 6 hours. (**e**) A pleurodesis is an operative intervention to prevent recurrence of PTX. It is performed on patients with underlying lung disease.

6. The answer is d. *(Rosen, pp 1236–1237.)* *Esophageal perforation* is potentially life-threatening conditions that can result from any valsalva-like maneuver, including childbirth, cough, and heavy lifting. Alcoholics are at risk due to their frequent vomiting. The most common cause of esophageal perforation is from iatrogenic causes such as a complication from upper endoscopy. The classic physical exam finding is *mediastinal or cervical emphysema.* This is noted on palpation of the chest wall or by a *crunching sound heard on auscultation, also known as Hamman's sign.*

(**a**) The patient has no ST-T wave abnormalities on ECG. The history and physical exam are not consistent with ACS. (**b**) Alcoholics have a high incidence of pancreatitis and can present with epigastric tenderness, however they usually don't have mediastinal air on radiography. (**c**) Alcohol ketoacidosis usually occurs in a heavy alcohol user who has temporarily stopped drinking and eating. Aortic dissection (e) usually occurs in patients with chronic hypertension or connective tissue disorders. They should not have Hamman's sign.

7. The answer is c. (*Rosen, pp 1171–1174.*) The patient's clinical picture of chronic hypertension, acute onset tearing chest pain, diastolic murmur of aortic insufficiency, and chest x-ray with a widened mediastinum is consistent with an *aortic dissection*. The preferred study of choice is a *transesophageal echocardiogram (TEE),* which is highly sensitive (98%). It can be quickly performed at the bedside and does not require radiation or contrast.

(a) ECG changes that are consistent with an aortic dissection are ischemic changes, low voltage complexes, and electrical alternans. However, this is suggestive but not diagnostic. (b) A transthoracic echocardiogram (TTE) is limited in diagnosing aortic dissections because wave transmission is hindered by the overlying sternum. It can be useful to see pericardial fluid as a result of proximal dissection. (d) A CT scan is an excellent study with sensitivities that approach TEEs. It is the study of choice if a TEE is not readily available. However, it requires that the patient leave the ED and receive IV contrast. (e) An MRI has high sensitivity and specificity and has the benefit of identifying an intimal tear. However, the study requires that the patient leave the ED for an extended period of time. Currently, it is most useful for patients with chronic dissections.

8. The answer is a. (*Tintinalli, p 1077.*) Patients with chest pain in the setting of cocaine use should be evaluated for possible myocardial ischemia. Patients suspected of ACS should be managed accordingly with oxygen, nitrates, morphine, aspirin, and benzodiazepines. However, *β-adrenergic antagonist* therapy is *absolutely contraindicated.* If β-adrenergic receptors are antagonized, α-adrenergic receptors are left unopposed and available for increased stimulation by cocaine. This may worsen coronary and peripheral vasoconstriction, hypertension, and possibly ischemia. Therefore, benzodiazepines, which decrease central sympathetic outflow, are the cornerstone in treatment to relieve cocaine related chest pain.

(b) Diltiazem, a calcium channel blocker, can be used in patients with cocaine related chest pain. It is used to lower heart rate. (c) Aspirin should be administered to all patients with chest pain, unless there is a contraindication. In patients with cocaine related chest pain who also seize, aspirin may be held until a CT scan is performed to rule out an intracranial bleed. (d) Lorazepam, a benzodiazepine, is an excellent medication to use in cocaine related chest pain as it reduces their sympathetic drive leading to a reduction in blood pressure and heart rate. (e) Nitroglycerin should be administered to these patients if they have chest pain. Nitrates dilate the coronary arteries, increasing blood flow to the myocardium.

9. The answer is a. (*Tintinalli, pp 1893–1940.*) The incidence of *endocarditis in the intravenous drug user (IVDU)* is estimated to be 40 times that of the general population. Unlike the general population, endocarditis in IVDUs is typically *right-sided* with the majority of cases involving the *tricuspid valve*. Patients with IVDU-related endocarditis usually have no evidence of prior valve damage. Patients may present with fever, cardiac murmur, cough, pleuritic chest pain, and hemoptysis. Right-sided murmurs, which vary with respiration, are typically pathologic and more specific for the diagnosis. In patients with right-sided endocarditis and septic pulmonary emboli, pulmonary complaints, infiltrates on chest radiographs, and moderate hypoxia have been described in greater than 33% of patients, and may mislead the physician to identify the lung as the primary source of infection. *Blood cultures* will be positive in more than 98% of IVDU-related endocarditis patients if *3–5 sets* are obtained. Diagnosis generally requires microbial isolation from a blood culture or to demonstrate typical lesions on echocardiography. *TTE* is the most sensitive imaging modality for demonstrating vegetations and tricuspid valve involvement in IVDU-related endocarditis. Initial antibiotic treatment should be directed against *S. aureus* and *Streptococcus spp.*

(b) Mononucleosis presents with fever, sore throat, and lymphadenopathy. Patients may also have an enlarged spleen, which is more prone to trauma. However, mononucleosis does not cause a heart murmur or patchy infiltrates on chest radiograph. (c) Pericarditis can present with fever and chest pain and NSAIDs are used for treatment. However, it does not cause valvular abnormalities leading to a murmur and pulmonary infiltrates. (d) Tuberculosis generally does not present with chest pain or cardiac murmur. (e) In Lyme disease, patients frequently have a bulls-eye rash called erythema migrans. Although Lyme disease does not lead to valvular abnormalities, patients may present with cardiac conduction abnormalities.

10. The answer is d. *(Rosen, p 1021.)* The standard 12-lead ECG is the single best test to identify patients with acute myocardial infarction (AMI) upon presentation in the ED. It is important to identify the anatomic location of an AMI to estimate the amount of endangered myocardium. The right coronary artery (RCA) supplies the AV node and inferior wall of the left ventricle in 90% of patients. *Inferior wall MIs are characterized by ST elevation in at least two of the inferior leads (II, III, aVF).* Reciprocal ST changes (i.e., ST depression) in the anterior precordial leads (V1–V4) in the setting of an inferior wall AMI, predict a larger infarct distribution, an increased severity of underlying CAD, more severe pump failure, and increased mortality. In general, the more elevated the ST segments and the more ST segments that are elevated, the more extensive the injury.

(**a**) The anteroseptal wall of the heart is supplied by the left anterior descending coronary artery (LAD). An AMI is identified by ST elevation in leads V1, V2, and V3. (**b**) The anterior wall of the heart is also supplied by the LAD and an infarct exhibits ST elevations in leads V2, V3, and V4. (**c**) The lateral wall of the heart is supplied by the left circumflex coronary artery (LCA) and an infarct exhibits ST elevations in leads I, aVL, V5, and V6. (**e**) A posterior MI refers to the posterior wall of the left ventricle. It occurs in 15–20% of all MIs and usually in conjunction with inferior or lateral infarction. The figure below summarizes the distribution.

I Lateral	aVR	V$_1$ Septal	V$_4$ Anterior
II Inferior	aVL High Lateral	V$_2$ Septal	V$_5$ Lateral
III Inferior	aVF Inferior	V$_3$ Anterior	V$_6$ Lateral

Inf   II III aVF   Sep V₁ V₂
Lat   I aVL V₅ V₆
Ant   V₃ V₄

11. The answer is c. *(Flowers, 2005.)* The patient has *costochondritis,* an inflammatory process of the costochondral or costosternal joints that causes *localized pain and tenderness.* Any of the seven costochondral junctions may be affected, and more than one site is affected in 90% of cases. The second to fifth costochondral junctions most commonly are involved. In contrast to myocardial ischemia or infarction, costochondritis is a benign cause of chest pain and is an important consideration in the differential diagnosis. Yet, 5–7% of patients with cardiac ischemia have chest wall tenderness. The onset is often insidious. Chest wall pain with a history of repeated minor trauma or unaccustomed activity (e.g., painting, moving furniture) is common. The goal of therapy is to reduce inflammation. *NSAIDs* are typically prescribed.

(a) The patient has no cardiac risk factors and his ECG and chest radiograph are normal. **(b)** This is a regime for ACS. **(d)** This is not a first line therapy. Corticosteroid injection may lead to bone degradation. **(e)** The patient does not need to be observed.

12. The answer is e. *(Tintinalli, pp 198–199.)* WPW syndrome is caused by an *accessory electrical pathway (bundle of Kent)* between the atria and ventricles, which predisposes the individual to reenter tachycardias (supraventricular tachycardia). The classic ECG findings include a *short PR interval, widened QRS interval,* and a *delta wave* at the beginning of the QRS which causes a slurred upstroke of the complex.

(a) Sinus tachycardia typically does not exceed 160 beats per minute. **(b)** Ventricular tachycardia may be difficult to distinguish from WPW. In a young patient with classic ECG findings, however, WPW is more likely. **(c)** Atrial flutter will have flutter waves that take on a saw-tooth pattern. **(d)** Atrial fibrillation is an irregular rhythm.

13. The answer is a. *(Rosen, pp 1727–1731.)* The patient has *life-threatening hyperkalemia.* His ECG shows a wide QRS complex and no p-waves. At any moment the patient's rhythm can go into ventricular fibrillation or asystole. Although all of the answer choices are used to treat hyperkalemia, this patient requires immediate administration of calcium because he has an unstable cardiac rhythm. *Calcium (gluconate or chloride)* antagonizes potassium and briefly stabilizes the cardiac membrane. However, calcium will not lower the potassium level; in order to promote transcellular shifts and removal from the body, other measures are required.

(b) Sodium polystyrene sulfonate (Kayexalate) is a definitive treatment for hyperkalemia because it removes potassium from the body. However, the process is not immediate, taking between 30 minutes and 2 hours to take effect. The other definitive treatment for hyperkalemia is dialysis. (c) Administration of insulin causes cellular uptake of potassium. (d) Sodium bicarbonate also produces a shift of potassium into cells. It is less efficacious than insulin or albuterol. (e) Albuterol, a β_2-agonist, also causes potassium to move into cells.

14. The answer is a. (*Rosen, pp 1234–1236.*) The patient most likely has a *partial or complete obstruction in his lower esophagus* secondary to the steak he ate. This usually occurs near the *gastroesophageal junction*. Administration of *glucagon* may cause enough *relaxation of the esophageal smooth muscle* to allow passage of the bolus in approximately 50% of patients. Its relaxant affect is limited to smooth muscle and therefore can only be used for impactions in the lower esophagus. If glucagon does not work, definitive management is with *endoscopy*.

Meat tenderizer (b), once used for this situation, is now contraindicated secondary to the possibility of perforation due to its proteolytic affect on an inflamed esophageal mucosa. Syrup of ipecac (c) is used rarely in situations of toxic ingestions. Also, vomiting should be avoided in our patient to avoid risk of esophageal perforation. The Heimlich maneuver (d) can be a lifesaving procedure but is not necessary in this patient who is not in respiratory distress. Respiratory compromise may occur when a foreign body lodges in the oropharynx, proximal esophagus, or is large enough that it impinges on the trachea. Laparotomy (e) is not indicated for esophageal perforations.

15. The answer is e. (*Tintinalli, pp 352–353.*) Thrombolytic therapy (clot-busters) can be administered to patients having an acute ST-elevation MI that is within 6–12 hours from symptom onset. Contraindications to fibrinolytic therapy are those that increase the risk of hemorrhage. The most catastrophic complication is intracranial hemorrhage. Absolute contraindications include:

- Previous hemorrhagic stroke
- Known intracranial neoplasm
- Active internal bleeding (excluding menses)
- Suspected aortic dissection or pericarditis

(a) SBP > 180 mm Hg is a relative contraindication. However, if thrombolytics are going to be administered and the patient's SBP is > 180 mm Hg, antihypertensive medication can be administered to lower the SBP to below 180 mm Hg. (b) Anticoagulation is a relative contraindication. Many patients who suffer from an ST-elevation MI are on aspirin and other antiplatelet and anticoagulant therapies. (c) Major surgery less than 3 weeks prior to administration of thrombolytics is a relative contraindication. (d) Active peptic ulcer disease is a relative contraindication.

16. The answer is e. (*Rosen, pp 1084–1085.*) This patient is hypotensive and exhibits signs and symptoms of heart failure (dyspnea, fatigue, respiratory crackles, and chest pain) and is in atrial fibrillation (irregular, narrow complex). Any patient with *unstable vital signs* with a tachydysrhythmia should receive a dose of sedation and undergo *synchronized cardioversion* starting at 100 J.

(a) Diltiazem, a calcium channel blocker, is used as a rate control agent for patients in atrial fibrillation. If the patient was not hypotensive or exhibiting signs of heart failure, diltiazem is used to slow the ventricular response. (b) Metoprolol is sometimes used to control ventricular rate in atrial fibrillation, however, it is contraindicated in patients with heart failure. In addition, it has a greater negative inotropic affect than calcium channel blockers (CCBs), thereby causing hypotension more often. (c) Digitalis is another option to control the ventricular response in atrial fibrillation; however its relatively slow onset precludes it from use in the acute setting. (d) Coumadin is an anticoagulant that is administered to a select group of patients in chronic atrial fibrillation to prevent thrombus formation. It is also used to anticoagulate stable patients who have been in atrial fibrillation for longer than 48 hours and are going to be pharmacologically or electrically cardioverted. Cardioversion of atrial fibrillation (if longer than 48 hours) carries the risk of thromboembolism.

17. The answer is d. (*Rosen, p 1122.*) This patient has *decompensated heart failure (CHF) with pulmonary edema. Nitroglycerin* is the most effective and most rapid means of *reducing preload* in a patient with CHF. Nitrates decrease myocardial preload and, to a lesser extent afterload. Nitrates increase venous capacitance, including venous pooling, which decreases preload and myocardial oxygen demand. It is most beneficial when the patient who presents with CHF is also hypertensive. It is administered sublingually, intravenously, or transdermally.

(a) Metoprolol, a β-blocker is contraindicated in acute decompensated heart failure. (b) Aspirin should be administered if the heart failure is thought to be secondary to ischemia. However, aspirin has no effect on preload reduction. (c) This patient is hypoxic with an oxygen saturation of 85% and requires supplemental oxygen. In the acute setting this patient should be placed on a nonrebreather with 100% oxygen flowing through the mask. (e) Morphine sulfate reduces pulmonary congestion through a central sympatholytic effect that causes peripheral vasodilation. This decreases central venous return and reduces preload. However, morphine sulfate is a respiratory depressant and may lead to hypoventilation. It does not act as rapidly or as effectively as nitroglycerin in preload reduction.

18. The answer is e. (*Rosen, p 1069.*) The patient's ECG shows a sinus rhythm at a rate of 70 with *first-degree heart block*. First-degree heart block is defined as prolonged conduction of atrial impulses without the loss of any impulse. On an ECG this translates to a *PR interval greater than 200 msec* with a narrow QRS complex. First-degree heart block is often a normal variant without clinical significance, occurring in 1–2% of healthy young adults. This variant requires no specific treatment.

(a) A pacemaker is considered in patients with a second-degree type II AV block or third-degree complete heart block. (b) A cardiac catherization is performed for patients with ST-elevation MI or other coronary disease. (c) Aspirin and cardiac biomarkers are sent for patients thought to have ACS. (d) The ECG leads are placed correctly on the patient.

19. The answer is e. (*Tintinalli, pp 386–391. Rosen, pp 1210–1224.*) *D-dimer* is a degradation product produced by plasmin-mediated proteolysis of cross-linked fibrin. There are two types of D-dimer assays. Those with greatest sensitivity are the enzyme-linked immunosorbent assays and the turbidimetric assays. Because of their high negative predictive value, D-dimer levels are typically used to *rule out the diagnosis of PE.* In conjunction with a low pretest probability, a negative D-dimer is predictive of not having a PE. Therefore, in this patient with a high probability of PE (dyspnea, chest pain, tachycardia, malignancy), it is likely that the D-dimer will be abnormal.

(a) Arterial blood gas has a very low predictive value in a typical population of patients in whom PE is suspected because they typically have some pulmonary pathology that affects pulmonary gas exchange more than a PE does. Most patients with a PE have a normal PaO_2. (b) Oxygen saturation is rarely depressed and not very useful in the work up of PE. **(c)** The most common ECG findings are tachycardia and nonspecific ST/T-wave abnormalities. Occasionally, signs of right heart strain are noted. **(d)** Chest radiographs are also usually normal. Twenty-four to seventy-two hours after a PE, atelectasis or a focal infiltrate may be seen. Radiographic findings classically associated with PE are Hamptom's hump (triangular pleural-based infiltrate) and Westermark's sign (dilation of pulmonary vessels proximal to PE with collapse of distal vessels).

20. The answer is d. (*Tintinalli, p 347.*) Serum cardiac markers are used to confirm or exclude myocardial cell death, and are considered the gold standard for the diagnosis of MI. There are many markers currently used; the most sensitive and specific markers are *troponin I and T*. A rise in these levels, as seen below, is diagnostic for an AMI. Troponin levels *rise within 3–6 hours of chest pain onset, peak at 12–24 hours,* and *remain elevated for 7–10 days.*

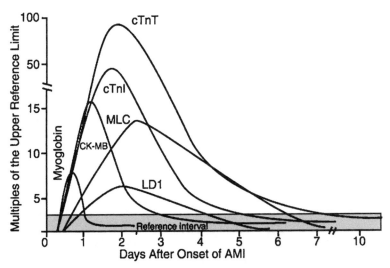

(Reproduced, with permission, from Tintinalli J, Kelen G, and Stapczynski J. Emergency Medicine A Comprehensive Study Guide. *New York, NY: McGraw-Hill, 2004: 337)*

(a) Myoglobin is found in both skeletal and cardiac muscle and released into the bloodstream when there is muscle cell death. It tends to rise within 1–2 hours of injury, peaks in 4–6 hours, and returns to baseline in 24 hours. **(b)** Creatinine kinase is an enzyme found in skeletal and cardiac muscle. Following AMI, increases in serum CK are detectable within 3–8 hours with a peak at 12–24 hours after injury, and normalizes within 3–4 days. (c) CK-MB is an isoenzyme found in cardiac muscle and released into the bloodstream upon cell death. It rises 4–6 hours after AMI, peaks in 12–36 hours, and returns to normal within 3–4 days. (e) Lactic dehydrogenase is an enzyme found in muscle and rises 12 hours after AMI, peaks at 24–48 hours, and returns to normal at 10–14 days.

21. The answer is c. *(Rosen, pp 1171–1176.)* The diagnosis in question is an acute *aortic dissection*. The diagnosis should be considered in patients with poorly controlled hypertension with crushing chest pain that classically radiates to the back. Delay of pulses is a supporting finding on physical exam. *Computed tomography with arterial phase contrast* is highly sensitive and specific for diagnosing dissection. The ideal study is transesophageal echocardiography, which is not always available.

(a) Cardiac enzymes are useful for determining the presence and extent of damage due to MI but are not useful in diagnosing dissection. (b) A contrast aortogram was the traditional gold standard but the advent of newer technologies has shown it to be less sensitive. (d) An MRI has high sensitivity and specificity and has the benefit of identifying an intimal tear. However, the study requires that the patient leave the ED for an extended period of time. Currently, it is most useful for patients with chronic dissections. (e) Plain films have little role in confirming a diagnosis of aortic dissection. On PA and lateral, plain radiographs with a widened mediastinum (>8 cm) supports the diagnosis but is not definitive. Eighty percent of patients with an acute dissection will have an abnormal chest radiograph but 12% with have an entirely normal film.

22. The answer is d. *(Tintinalli, p 1079.)* *Narrow-complex tachycardias* are defined as rhythms with a QRS complex duration less than 120 msec and a ventricular rate greater than 100 beats per min. Although virtually all narrow-complex tachydysrhythmias originate from a focus above the ventricles, the term supraventricular tachycardia (SVT) is conventionally used to denote those rhythms aside from sinus tachycardia, atrial tachycardia, atrial fibrillation, and atrial flutter. *Adenosine,* an ultrashort acting AV-nodal blocking agent, is typically used to treat SVTs. Because it is so fast-acting, it must be delivered through a large vein (i.e., antecubital fossa) in a rapid intravenous bolus. In addition to adenosine, *maneuvers that increase vagal tone* have been shown to slow conduction through the AV node. Some of these maneuvers include carotid sinus massage, valsalva maneuver, and facial immersion in cold water.

(a) Although digoxin is occasionally used to slow the rate in SVTs, it has a long onset of action and potential hazard in patients with accessory tracts (b and c). Lidocaine and amiodarone are agents used to treat wide-complex or ventricular tachycardias. (e) Bretylium is no longer available in the United States due to its poor safety profile.

23. The answer is e. *(Rosen, pp 1011–1049.)* This ECG depicts an *acute anterior wall myocardial infarction (AMI) with ST elevations in leads V1–V4.* The patient is also hypotensive secondary to *cardiogenic shock.* The preferred treatment for an ST elevation MI (STEMI) is primary percutaneous intervention (e.g., angioplasty, coronary stent). It has shown to improve long-term mortality over thrombolytic therapy.

(a) β-Blockers and CCBs are contraindicated in patients who are hypotensive. (b) The patient does not have a dysrhythmia and therefore should not be cardioverted. (c) Dobutamine and dopamine are agents used in cardiogenic shock. Although they should be administered to raise the blood pressure, they are not definitive treatments.

24. The answer is c. *(Tintinalli, p 356.)* *Sildenafil (Viagra)* is a selective cyclic guanosine monophosphate (GMP) inhibitor that results in smooth muscle relaxation and vasodilation by the release of nitric oxide. It is used in men for erectile dysfunction. It is *contraindicated to administer nitroglycerin* to individuals who have taken sildenafil in the previous 24 hours. The combination of nitroglycerin and sildenafil can lead to hypotension and death. If nitrates are coadministered with sildenafil, the patient should be closely monitored for hypotension. Fluid resuscitation and pressor agents may be needed to restore blood pressure.

(a) Aspirin is contraindicated in individuals with an anaphylactic allergy or active bleed. (b) Heparin is contraindicated in individuals with heparin-induced-thrombocytopenia, and those who are actively bleeding. (d) Metoprolol is contraindicated in hypotensive individuals. (e) Morphine sulfate is contraindicated in patients with respiratory depression.

25. The answer is b. *(Rosen, pp 1130–1133.)* The classic presentation of *pericarditis* includes *chest pain, a pericardial friction rub, and ECG abnormalities.* A prodrome of fever and myalgias may occur. Pericarditis chest pain is usually substernal and varies with respiration. It is classically sharp or pleuritic in character. It is typically *relieved by sitting forward and worsened by lying down or swallowing.* The physical exam hallmark of acute pericarditis is the *pericardial friction rub.* The earliest ECG changes are seen in the first few hours to days of illness and include *diffuse ST segment elevation* seen in leads I, II, III, aVL, aVF, and V2–V6. Most patients with acute pericarditis will have concurrent *PR-segment depression.* The mainstay of treatment includes supportive care with *anti-inflammatory* medications (i.e., NSAIDs). The use of corticosteroids is controversial. An echocardiogram should be performed to rule out a pericardial effusion and tamponade.

(a) PE can present with substernal chest pain that is sharp in nature and worse with inspiration. However, the patient doesn't exhibit any risk factors for a PE (c and d). It is very important to be able to differentiate an acute MI from acute pericarditis because thrombolytic therapy is contraindicated in pericarditis as it may precipitate hemorrhagic tamponade. Unlike the ECG in an acute MI, the ST elevations in early pericarditis are concave upward rather than convex upward. Subsequent tracings do not evolve through a typical MI pattern and Q waves do not appear. (e) Antibiotics are not routinely used to treat pericarditis.

26. The answer is a. *(Rosen, pp 1019–1020.)* The earliest ECG finding resulting from an AMI is the *hyperacute T wave,* which may appear minutes after the interruption of blood flow. The hyperacute T wave, which is short-lived, evolves to progressive *elevation of ST segments.* In general, *Q waves* represent established myocardial necrosis and usually develop within 8–12 hours after a ST elevation MI, yet they may be noted as early as 1–2 hours after the onset of complete coronary occlusion.

27. The answer is d. *(Rosen, pp 1120–1128.)* The patient has acute *CHF exacerbation* with *acute pulmonary edema (APE).* Although not always apparent at presentation, it is important to find the cause of the exacerbation. This patient has been noncompliant with his medications. Treatment begins with the airways, breathing, circulations (ABCs) and initial stabilization is aimed at maintaining airway control and adequate ventilation. Preload and afterload reduction is integral with *nitroglycerin* being the agent of choice provided the patient is not hypotensive. Volume reduction with *diuretics* is also critical to lower blood pressure and cardiac filling pressures. *Noninvasive airway techniques (e.g., bilevel positive airways pressure [BiPAP], continuous positive airway pressure [CPAP])* also aid in improving oxygen exchange, reduce the work of breathing, decrease left ventricular preload and after-load by raising intrathoracic pressure, in the compromised but not agonal APE patients. (a) It is important to first address the ABCs. If infection is thought to be the cause, then obtaining a CBC, blood cultures and starting antibiotics should be performed after stabilization. (b) A chest x-ray is valuable, but initial stabilization takes priority. (c) Oxygen via nasal cannula is not suffi-cient for this patient who is hypoxic and tachypneic. If you are suspicious for ACS causing the CHF exacerbation, then aspirin should be adminis-tered. (e) At this time, the patient does not require invasive airway control. If medication and noninvasive techniques fail and the patient's hypoxia worsens, then endotracheal intubation may be necessary.

28. The answer is e. (*Rosen, p 1096.*) Torsade de pointes ("twisting of the points"), is a life-threatening uncommon variant of ventricular tachycardia (VT). The ventricular rate can range from 150 to 250 beats per minute. It may occur secondary to medications that prolong the QT-interval such as some antipsychotics. It is also caused by electrolyte disturbances and con-genital prolonged-QT syndrome. This form typically presents in childhood or early adulthood and is precipitated by catecholamine excess such as exercise or medications. (a) Ventricular fibrillation is disorganized electrical activity causing no effective contraction of the ventricles. A pulse or blood pressure never is present with ventricular fibrillation. (b) Atrial fibrillation occurs when there is disorganized atrial activity that leads to the lack of P-waves on an ECG. In general, the QRS complex is narrow unless there is a bypass tract or bundle branch block. (c) WPW syndrome is caused by an accessory electrical pathway (bundle of Kent) between the atria and ventricles, which predisposes the individual to reentry tachycardias. (d) Supraventricular tachycardias occur secondary to a reentry circuit. Patients typically exhibit a narrow complex tachycardia on ECG.

29. The answer is c. (*Tintinalli, pp 386–391.*) Risk factors for venous thromboembolism were first described by Virchow's triad: *hypercoagulability, stasis, endothelial injury.* Hypercoagulability can be broadly classified into malignancy-related or nonmalignancy-related. Malignancies of primary adenocarcinoma or brain malignancy are the most likely to cause throm-bosis. Some causes of nonmalignancy-related thrombosis are estrogen use, pregnancy, antiphospholipid syndromes, factor V Leiden mutation, and protein C and S deficiencies. Immobility such as paralysis, debilitating diseases, or recent surgery or trauma also place patients at risk.

30. The answer is e. (*Rosen, p 1155.*) The *classic triad of aortic stenosis is dyspnea, chest pain, and exertional syncope.* Syncope is a result of either inadequate cerebral perfusion or occasional dysrhythmias. The classic auscultory finding is a *harsh systolic ejection murmur* that is best heard in the second right intercostal space with radiation to the carotid arteries. Syncope in the setting of a new systolic murmur always should raise the suspicion for aortic stenosis as the etiology. The ECG usually reveals *left ventricular hypertrophy.*

(**a**) Asystole denotes the lack of electrical activity of the heart. Individuals usually don't recover from an asystolic cardiac arrest. (**b**) Brugada syndrome is due to an autosomal dominant trait resulting in total loss of function of the cardiac sodium channel or in acceleration of recovery from sodium channel activation. It leads to syncope and may cause sudden cardiac death secondary to a polymorphic ventricular tachycardia. It is associated with a distinctive ECG pattern of downsloping ST segment elevation in leads V1–V3 with a right bundle branch block pattern. (**c**) The subclavian steal syndrome is a rare but important cause of syncope. The syndrome results from occlusion of the proximal subclavian artery and the development of retrograde flow to the subclavian artery from the vertebral artery. (**d**) A PE that causes syncope usually causes the individual to have unstable vital signs secondary to obstruction of a major vessel.

31. The answer is c. (*Rosen, pp 1000–1004.*) The patient's clinical presentation is consistent with a PTX. Primary spontaneous PTX seems to result from rupture of a subpleural bleb, usually in the upper lobe. The two most common risk factors are *smoking* and *changes in atmospheric pressure.* Symptoms of primary spontaneous PTX typically begin suddenly while at rest. Ipsilateral *chest pain* and *dyspnea* are the most common symptoms. A mild tachycardia is the most common physical finding. With a large PTX, *decreased or absent breath sounds* with hyperresonance to percussion may be present. Recurrences are common with studies reporting a range of rates between 16% and 50%.

(**a**) The radiograph shows no evidence of opacification. (**b**) There is no evidence of air in the mediastinum. (**d**) Tamponade is not a radiographic diagnosis. Indirect evidence of tamponade includes a large cardiac silhouette. (**e**) Radiographic CHF typically presents with an enlarged cardiac silhouette, pulmonary congestion, cephalization, and effusion.

32. The answer is b. *(Rosen, pp 1042–1044.)* Aspirin is an antiplatelet agent that should be administered early to all patients suspected of having an ACS, unless there is a contraindication. The ISIS-2 trial provides the strongest evidence that aspirin *independently reduces the mortality* of patients with AMI. **(a)** Nitroglycerin provides benefit to patients with ACS by reducing preload and dilating coronary arteries. However, there is no mortality benefit with its use. **(c)** Unfractionated heparin acts indirectly to inhibit thrombin, preventing the conversion of fibrinogen to fibrin. Thus, inhibiting clot propagation. Heparin has not shown to have a mortality benefit. **(d)** Routine use of lidocaine as prophylaxis for ventricular arrhythmias in patients who have experienced an AMI has been shown to increase mortality rates. **(e)** Use of CCBs in the acute setting has come into question, with some trials showing increased adverse effects.

33. The answer is c. *(Rosen, pp 1138–1139.)* The patient has *myocarditis.* The *enteroviruses,* especially the *Coxsackie B* virus, predominate as causative agents in the United States. Coxsackie B virus usually causes infection during the summer months. Some other causes of myocarditis include adenovirus, influenza, HIV, *Mycoplasma, Trypanosoma cruzi,* and steroid abuse. *Flu-like complaints,* such as fatigue, myalgias, nausea, vomiting, diarrhea, and fever, are usually the earliest symptoms and signs of myocarditis. *Tachycardia is common and can be disproportionate to the patient's temperature.* This may be the only clue that something more serious than a simple viral illness exists. Approximately 12% of patients also complain of chest pain. Cardiac enzymes may be elevated and the CBC and erythrocyte sedimentation rate (ESR) are nonspecific.

(a) *Streptococcus viridans* is a common cause of acute bacterial endocarditis, an infection of a cardiac valve. **(b)** *Staphylococcus aureus* is not known to cause myocarditis. **(d)** Myocarditis can masquerade as an acute MI because patients with either may have severe chest pain, ECG changes, elevated cardiac enzymes, and heart failure. Patients with myocarditis are usually young and have few risk factors for coronary artery disease. **(e)** Cocaine use can cause chest pain and tachycardia. It does not lead to flu-like symptoms.

34. The answer is b. *(Selwyn A, 2005.)* The patient's clinical presentation is consistent with *Prinzmetal's or variant angina.* This condition is caused by focal *coronary artery vasospasm.* It *occurs at rest* and exhibits a *circadian pattern,* with most episodes occurring in the early hours of the morning. The pain commonly is severe. Distinguishing unstable angina related to coronary atherosclerosis from variant angina may be difficult and requires special investigations, including coronary angiography. Patients may also exhibit ST elevations on their ECGs. Nitrates and CCBs are the mainstays of medical therapy for variant angina. Nitroglycerin effectively treats episodes of angina and myocardial ischemia within minutes of administration, and the long-acting nitrate preparations reduce the frequency of recurrent events. CCBs effectively prevent coronary vasospasm and variant angina, and they should be administered in preference to β-blockers.

(a) Aspirin is an antiplatelet agent that helps reduce progression of plaque formation in the coronary arteries. Aspirin won't treat the vasospasm that is responsible for variant angina. (c) β-blockers can be beneficial in patients with fixed coronary artery stenosis and exertional angina. However, for variant angina, nonselective β-blockers may be detrimental in some patients because blockade of the β-receptors, which mediate vasodilation, allows unopposed α-receptor–mediated coronary vasoconstriction to occur, thus possibly causing an actual worsening of symptoms (d and e). H_2-Blockers and proton pump inhibitors (PPIs) are used to treat acid reflux symptoms.

35. The answer is b. (*Zareba W, 2005.*) *Long QT syndrome (LQTS)* is a congenital disorder characterized by a *prolongation of the QT interval* on ECG and a propensity to *ventricular tachydysrhythmias*, which may lead to *syncope, cardiac arrest, or sudden death* in otherwise healthy individuals. The QT interval on the ECG, measured from the beginning of the QRS complex to the end of the T wave, represents the duration of activation and recovery of the ventricular myocardium. In general, heart rate corrected QTc values above 440 msec are considered abnormal. LQTS has been recognized as the *Romano-Ward syndrome* (familial occurrence with autosomal dominant inheritance, QT prolongation, and ventricular tachydysrhythmias) or the *Jervell and Lang-Nielsen syndrome* (familial occurrence with autosomal recessive inheritance, congenital deafness, QT prolongation, and ventricular arrhythmias). Patients with LQTS usually are diagnosed after a cardiac event (e.g., syncope, cardiac arrest) already has occurred. In some situations, LQTS is diagnosed after sudden death in family members. Some individuals are diagnosed with LQTS based on an ECG showing QT prolongation. β-Blockers are drugs of choice for patients with LQTS. The protective effect of β-blockers is related to their adrenergic blockade diminishing the risk of cardiac arrhythmias.

Implantation of cardioverter-defibrillators appears to be the most effective therapy for high-risk patients.

(a) Hypovolemia from dehydration or blood loss is a cause of syncope. There is no indication of this in the patient. (c) Hyperkalemia manifests itself with peaked T waves, a sine wave pattern, and ultimately ventricular fibrillation or asystole. (d) Complete heart block is characterized by the absent conduction of all atrial impulses resulting in complete electrical and mechanical AV dissociation. (e) ACS typically presents in older individuals with chest pain.

36. The answer is d. *(Tintinalli, p 345.)* The pain of *acute pericarditis* is typically described as severe, sharp, and constant. It is usually substernal with radiation to the back, neck, or shoulders, and worsens with lying supine and with inspiration. Classically, it is relieved with leaning forward. A *pericardial friction rub* is a key finding on physical exam. The ECG may reveal diffuse ST-segment elevations, T wave inversions, and PR segment depression. Acute pericarditis may be preceded by a viral syndrome.

(a) Musculoskeletal chest pain may occur secondary to costochondritis. Patients typically exhibit reproducible chest pain upon palpation of the chest wall. (b) Anginal symptoms include chest pressure, heaviness, tightness, fullness, or squeezing. Sometimes it is described as sharp or stabbing. It usually occurs substernally or in the left chest and may radiate to the left arm, neck, or jaw. The patient may experience chest wall tenderness. Exercise, stress, or a cold environment classically precipitates angina pectoris. (c) Aortic dissection classically presents with tearing chest pain that radiates to the back and is worst at the onset. Patients usually have a history of long-standing hypertension. Cardiac exam may reveal a murmur of aortic insufficiency. (e) Pneumonia can present with sharp, pleuritic chest pain. Patients typically have a cough and fever. Chest radiograph usually reveals an opacification.

37. The answer is a. *(Wiesenfarth J, 2005.)* An *aortic dissection* occurs when there is a tear in the aortic intima which exposes the underlying tissue layers. Subsequently, the driving force of blood splits the aortic media into two layers creating the dissection. Certain diseases, such as *Marfan's*, weaken the media making it prone to dissection. However, the most common cause is *long-standing hypertension* and *atherosclerosis*. Chest pain is the most common presenting symptom in patients with an aortic dissection. The pain usually is described as ripping or tearing and sudden in onset.

Hypertension is usually present; hypotension is an ominous finding. A pressure differential in the upper or lowers extremities of greater than 20 mm Hg should increase the suspicion of aortic dissection. Patients may present with a new bruit consistent with aortic insufficiency.

(b) An aortic aneurysm is a localized dilation of the aorta. It can develop in any segment of the aorta, but most commonly involves the infrarenal portion. Patients with a ruptured abdominal aortic aneurysm (AAA) are typically older who present with back pain and hypotension. (c) A tension pneumothorax is a life-threatening condition caused by air within the pleural space that is under pressure and displaces mediastinal structures leading to hemodynamic compromise. Patients are hypotensive rather then hypertensive. (d) GERD usually presents with epigastric discomfort although pain may radiate into the chest. It is commonly worse after a meal. (e) A PE may present with sudden onset of pleuritic chest pain. It is usually associated with shortness of breath and tachypnea.

38. The answer is b. (*Rosen, pp 1154–1155.*) The patient's presentation is consistent with *acute mitral valve regurgitation* due to a *ruptured papillary muscle* in the setting of an AMI. Patients usually present with *pulmonary edema in the setting of an AMI.* Chest x-ray characteristically reveals pulmonary edema with a normal heart size. The characteristic murmur of mitral regurgitation is a *holosystolic murmur that is loudest at the apex.*

(a) Critical aortic stenosis produces a loud systolic murmur that is best heard at the second right intercostal space and radiates to the carotids. (c) The classic finding of a pericardial effusion is a pericardial friction rub. (d) CHF does not cause a murmur but rather an extra heart sound (S3) from fluid overload. (e) Aortic dissection is associated with a murmur of aortic insufficiency.

39. The answer is e. (*Roberts & Hedges, pp 283–285.*) The patient's ECG reveals *third-degree complete heart block.* This may occur secondary to MI, drug intoxication, infection, or infiltrative diseases. Individuals with second-degree type 2 or third-degree complete heart block are considered unstable. *External pacing pads* should be placed on them, followed by a transvenous pacer if their blood pressure is unstable. They may require a permanent pacemaker for irreversible complete heart block.

(a) Clearly this patient is unstable and should not be discharged home. (b) Anemia can cause dizziness and lightheadedness. These items should be checked during her hospital stay. However, her cardiac status takes priority. (c) Stabilizing the heart block takes precedence over a CT scan. (d) The patient should receive an aspirin and have cardiac biomarkers obtained, however, the ABCs must be followed and the patient's rhythm is currently unstable.

40. The answer is d. *(Burnette LB, 2006.)* Often young people are afraid to disclose a history of drug use. *Cocaine* is well-known to cause *AMI in young*, otherwise health individuals. Patients with cocaine-related MI often have fixed atherosclerotic lesions. Although these lesions may themselves be of clinical significance, cocaine-induced elevations in pulse and blood pressure increase myocardial work. The additional metabolic requirements that result may convert an asymptomatic obstruction into one of clinical significance.

(a) Isolated smoking in this young individual would not lead to coronary artery disease and an acute MI. The patient has no other cardiac risk factors. (b) If his grandfather or father had a heart attack at age 40 or younger, there would be concern about his family history. A heart attack in a related family member at age 80 is not a risk factor. (c) The patient's cardiac biomarkers are also positive and consistent with the ECG. (e) Alcohol use at this age will not lead to an AMI.

41. The answer is a. *(Tintinalli, p 892.) Acute chest syndrome,* a complication of *sickle-cell disease,* usually presents with *chest pain, fever, hypoxia, and a new pulmonary infiltrate on chest x-ray.* Treatment of acute chest syndrome involves supplemental oxygen, IV hydration, and analgesia. Because it is difficult to determine whether acute chest syndrome has an infectious or noninfectious cause, empiric antibiotics are usually started.

(b) This combination is used to treat ACS. (c) This is relevant for patients suspected of having a PE. (d) These medications are used for a COPD exacerbation. (e) Omeprazole and endoscopy are used for patients with GERD.

42. The answer is a. *(Rosen, pp 1135–1136.)* The patient presents with a *pericardial effusion* probably secondary to her metastatic breast cancer. Pericardial effusion is often asymptomatic but with accumulating fluid can cause chest pain, shortness of breath, cough, and fever. Ultimately, it can lead to cardiac tamponade, which develops in up to 10% of all cancer patients. The ECG classically shows *low voltage complexes* and, rarely, *electrical alternans.* Treatment of pericardial effusion and tamponade is pericardiocentesis to remove the fluid.

(b) ST elevation is seen in acute MI, pericarditis, and early repolarization. (c) ST depression is seen in cardiac ischemia, and reciprocal changes in acute MI. (d) T wave inversion is seen in cardiac ischemia. (e) Peaked T waves are associated with hyperkalemia.

43. The answer is a. *(Tintinalli, pp 386–391.)* In the absence of a contraindication and a pretest probability that exceeds 50%, *empiric heparin therapy should be administered.* The patient has a high pretest probability for a **PE** (malignancy, tachycardia, tachypnea, suspected DVT, pleuritic chest pain, dyspnea). Although heparin has no intrinsic fibrinolytic affect, it has an immediate affect on thrombin inhibition, thus *preventing extension of the PE.*

(b) Thrombolytics are reserved for patients who are hemodynamically unstable. (c, d, e) Any of these diagnostic studies should be performed to confirm the diagnosis of PE. Because significant time may elapse until the study is performed, and there is a risk that the clot will propagate, anticoagulant therapy should be initiated.

44. The answer is c. *(Rosen, pp 1092–1096.)* This patient has a *ventricular tachycardia* defined by a *QRS complex greater than 120 msec* and a *rate greater than 100 beats per minute.* Ventricular tachycardia is the result of a dysrhythmia originating within or below the termination of the His bundle. Most patients with ventricular tachycardia have underlying heart disease. Treatment begins with assessing whether or not the patient is stable. If the patient shows signs of instability such as hypotension or altered mental status, then cardioversion should be performed. However, if the patient is stable, medications can be administered to treat the dysrhythmia. *Amiodarone,* a class III antidysrhythmic that has pharmacologic characteristics of all four classes, is considered a first-line agent in treating ventricular dysrhythmias.

(a) Digoxin, a cardiac glycoside, has positive inotropic effects on the heart and slows conduction through the AV-node. It should not be used to treat ventricular dysrhythmias. (b) Diltiazem, a calcium channel blocker, acts on the AV-node to slow cardiac conduction and will not treat ventricular tachycardia. In addition, it can lead to hypotension in patients with ventricular tachycardia secondary to its peripheral dilatory affects. (d) Adenosine, an ultrashort acting AV-nodal blocking agent, is typically used to treat supraventricular tachycardias. (e) Bretylium is no longer available in the United States due to its poor safety profile.

45. The answer is c. (*Rosen, pp 1011–1015.*) The patient exhibits *unstable angina*, which is defined as *new-onset angina, angina occurring at rest lasting longer than 20 minutes, or angina deviating from a patient's normal pattern.* Unstable angina is considered the harbinger of an AMI and, therefore, should be evaluated and treated aggressively. Unstable angina is one of the three diagnoses that make up ACS, the other two being stable angina and AMI (ST or non-ST elevation). Patients may be pain free and have negative cardiac biomarkers with unstable angina. In general, unstable angina is treated with oxygen, aspirin, clopidogrel, low molecular weight or unfractionated heparin, and further risk stratification in the hospital.

(a) Variant or Prinzmetal's angina is caused by coronary artery vasospasm at rest with minimal coronary artery disease. It is sometimes relieved by exercise or nitroglycerin. It is generally treated with CCBs. Patients with Prinzmetal's angina may have ST elevations on their ECG that is indistinguishable from an acute MI. (b) Stable angina is described as transient episodic chest discomfort resulting from myocardial ischemia. The discomfort is typically predictable and reproducible, with the frequency of attacks constant over time. The discomfort is thought to be due to fixed, stenotic atherosclerotic plaques that narrow a blood vessel lumen and reduce coronary blood flow (d and e). Non-ST elevation MI (NSTEMI) and ST elevation MI (STEMI) results from myocardial necrosis with release of cardiac biomarkers (i.e., troponin).

46. The answer is b. (*Tintinalli, p 194.*) The rhythm strip shows *second-degree AV block type II or Mobitz type II*. Mobitz II presents with a prolonged PR interval (PR > 0.2 seconds) and random dropped beats (P wave without QRS complex). This heart block reflects serious cardiac pathology and may be seen with an anterior wall MI, which is what happened to this patient.

Mobitz type I (a) (also called Wenckebach phenomenon) shows progressive prolongation of PR interval with each beat until AV conduction is lost causing a dropped beat. First-degree AV block (c) presents with prolonged PR interval (PR > 0.2 seconds) without loss of AV conduction. This block is asymptomatic. Atrial flutter (d) is a tachydysrhythmia with rapid atrial beat and variable AV block. It has a characteristic "saw tooth" appearance of atrial flutter waves. Ventricular tachycardia (e) is a rapid ventricular rhythm, often associated with hemodynamic compromise.

47. The answer is e. (*Tintinalli, p 194.*) The rhythm strip findings are consistent with *third-degree AV block*, also called *complete heart block*. It is characterized by absent conduction through the AV node resulting in dissociation of atrial and ventricular rhythms. The ECG shows independent P waves and QRS complexes. Mobitz type II often progresses to third-degree heart block as seen in this case. The immediate step in managing complete heart block is applying a *transcutaneous pacemaker* for ventricular pacing as a temporizing measure. However, patients need *implantable ventricular pacemakers* for definitive management. In addition, the underlying cause of the block needs to be addressed.

Consulting cardiology (**a**) is a good choice as they will implant a permanent pacemaker and manage any underlying cardiac disease. However, the patient must first be stabilized. Cardioversion (**b**) is used to treat unstable patients with reentrant arrhythmias, such as atrial fibrillation. It is not helpful in a setting of conduction abnormality such as heart block. Metoprolol (**c**), a *β*-blocker, and adenosine (**d**), are contraindicated in complete heart block. These agents prolong AV nodal conduction.

Shortness of Breath

Questions

48. A 55-year-old woman with a past medical history of diabetes walks into the emergency department (ED) stating that her tongue and lips feel like they are swollen. During the history, she tells you that her doctor just started her on a new blood pressure (BP) medication. Her only other medication is a baby aspirin. Her vitals at triage are: blood pressure 130/70 mm Hg, heart rate (HR) 85 beats per minute, respiratory rate (RR) 16 breaths per minute, oxygen saturation 99% on room air, and temperature 98.7°F. On physical exam, you detect mild lip and tongue swelling. Over the next hour, you notice that not only are her tongue and lips getting more swollen, but her face is starting to swell, too. What is the most likely inciting agent?

a. Metoprolol
b. Furosemide
c. Aspirin
d. Lisinopril
e. Diltiazem

49. A 45-year-old woman presents to the ED immediately after landing at the airport from a transatlantic flight. She states that a few moments after landing she felt short of breath and felt pain in her chest when she took a deep breath. Her only medications are oral contraceptive pills and levothyroxine. She is a social drinker and smokes cigarettes occasionally. Her BP is 130/75 mm Hg, HR is 98 beats per minute, temperature is 98.9°F, RR is 20 breaths per minute, and oxygen saturation is 97% on room air. You send her for a duplex ultrasound of her legs, which is positive for a deep vein thrombosis. What is the most appropriate management for this patient?

a. Place patient on a monitor, provide supplemental oxygen, and administer unfractionated heparin
b. Place patient on a monitor, order a chest computed tomography (CT) scan to confirm a pulmonary embolism (PE), then administer unfractionated heparin
c. Place patient on a monitor and administer an aspirin
d. Instruct the patient to walk around the ED so that she remains mobile and does not exacerbate thrombus formation
e. Place the patient on a monitor, provide supplemental oxygen, and administer warfarin

50. A 54-year-old undomiciled woman presents to the ED with severe cough, general malaise, and subjective fevers for the last week. She also describes coughing up "chicken livers" during this time and reports that her symptoms are getting progressively worse. Her initial vitals include a HR of 100 beats per minute, a BP of 145/66 mm Hg, and a RR of 16 breaths per minute with an oxygen saturation of 95% on room air. She states that she has a history of alcohol abuse but denies taking any medications or illicit drugs. A chest radiograph shows a lobar pneumonia. Given this patient's clinical presentation, which of the following etiologies is this patient at risk for contracting?

a. *Streptococcus pneumoniae*
b. *Klebsiella pneumoniae*
c. *Mycoplasma pneumoniae*
d. *Legionella pneumoniae*
e. *Haemophilus pneumoniae*

51. An 18-year-old tall, thin male presents to the ED with acute onset of respiratory distress while at rest. The patient reports sitting at his desk when he felt a sharp pain on the right side of his chest that worsened with inspiration. He reports to be otherwise healthy and denies any illicit drug use or recent travel. His initial vitals include a HR of 100 beats per minute, a BP of 120/60 mm Hg, and a RR of 14 breaths per minute with an oxygen saturation of 97% on room air. On physical examination, you note decreased breath sounds on the right side. Which of the following tests should be performed next?

a. Electrocardiogram (ECG)
b. Chest x-ray
c. Complete blood panel
d. Toxicological drug screen
e. Upright abdominal x-ray

52. An 11-year-old girl is brought to the ED with acute onset of respiratory distress. She recently emigrated from Africa. Her initial vitals include a HR of 115 beats per minute, a BP of 110/60 mm Hg, and a RR of 20 breaths per minute with an oxygen saturation of 88% on room air. She is also febrile to 101.5°F. Her mother tells you that she had a sore throat that began 2 days prior and that she was to see her pediatrician this week for her vaccinations. Given this patient's history and presentation, which of the following should be of particular concern?

a. Epiglottitis
b. Retropharyngeal abscess
c. Pharyngitis
d. Ludwig's angina
e. Tonsillitis

53. A 30-year-old woman presents to the ED after reportedly passing out in her apartment. The patient recalls walking from the bed to the bedroom closet and next remembering that she was on the floor. She states that she was short of breath and had to crawl over to the phone to call for help. Upon presentation, the patient's vitals include a HR of 109 beats per minute, a RR of 20 breaths per minute and an oxygen saturation of 95% on room air. Her ECG indicates right heart strain. The patient states that she traveled to Moscow 1 month prior, occasionally smokes but denies any illicit drug use. Upon arrival back to the United States, the patient developed a persistent cough associated with dyspnea. She was seen by a Pulmonologist who diagnosed her with bronchitis and prescribed an inhaler. However over the oncoming weeks, the patient's symptoms progressed to the point that she could not ambulate outside of her apartment in the days prior to the event. Given this patient's history and presentation, what is the most likely etiology for her symptoms?

a. Pneumonia
b. Neurocardiogenic syncope
c. Aortic dissection
d. PE
e. Subarachnoid hemorrhage

54. A 24-year-old woman is brought to the ED after being found on a nearby street hunched over and in mild respiratory distress. Upon arrival, she is tachypneic at 20 breaths per minute with an oxygen saturation of 97% on face mask oxygen administration. Upon physical examination, the patient appears to be in mild distress with supraclavicular retractions. Scattered wheezing is heard throughout bilateral lung fields. Which of the following medications should be administered first?

a. β_2-Agonist nebulizer treatment
b. Magnesium sulfate
c. Epinephrine
d. Corticosteroids
e. Anticholinergic nebulizer treatment

55. An 81-year-old woman presents to the ED with acute onset of shortness of breath shortly before arrival. She refuses to answer other questions but repeatedly states that she is feeling short of breath. Her initial vitals include a HR of 89 beats per minute, a BP of 168/76 mm Hg, and a RR of 18 breaths per minute with an oxygen saturation of 89% on room air. A portable chest x-ray appears normal. Her physical examination is unremarkable, except for a systolic ejection murmur. After obtaining intravenous access, placing the patient on oxygen and a monitor, which of the following procedures should be performed first?

a. Basic metabolic panel
b. D-dimer
c. Rectal temperature
d. Repeat chest x-ray
e. ECG

56. A 30-year-old man is brought to the ED by emergency medical service (EMS) in respiratory distress. His initial vitals include a HR of 109 beats per minute, a BP of 180/90 mm Hg, and a RR of 20 breaths per minute with an oxygen saturation of 92% on room air. A chest x-ray shows a bilateral diffuse infiltrative process. A subsequent toxicologic screen is positive. Which of the following agents is most likely responsible for this patient's presentation?

a. Cannabis
b. Opioid
c. Crack cocaine
d. Methamphetamine
e. Alcohol

57. A 26-year-old woman presents to the ED with acute onset of dyspnea after falling down a few steps. The patient denies any loss of consciousness and just reports feeling short of breath. Her initial chest x-ray appears normal; however she continues to be symptomatic with stable vital signs. Which of the following procedures should be performed next?

a. Repeat upright chest x-ray
b. Inspiratory and expiratory chest radiographs
c. Chest CT scan
d. Chest thoracostomy
e. Chest thoracotomy

58. A 16-year-old boy is brought to the ED by his mother who reports that he has progressive lower extremity weakness over the last day and is now experiencing difficulty breathing. His initial vitals include a respiratory rate of 10 breaths per minute with an oxygen saturation of 92% on room air. Upon physical examination, you note decreased bilateral patellar reflexes. He states that he had an upper respiratory infection 1 week ago, which self-resolved. Given this patient's history and physical examination, which of the following agents is useful in treating the cause of his respiratory distress?

a. β_2-agonist nebulized treatment
b. Aspirin
c. Acetaminophen
d. Intravenous flumazenil
e. Intravenous immunoglobin G

59. A 32-year-old firefighter presents to the ED in acute respiratory distress. He was taken to the ED shortly after extinguishing a large fire in a warehouse. His initial vitals include a HR of 90 beats per minute, a BP of 120/55 mm Hg, and a RR of 18 breaths per minute with an oxygen saturation of 98% on 2 L nasal cannula. An ECG shows a first-degree heart block. Upon physical examination, there are diffuse rhonchi bilaterally. The patient is covered in soot and the hairs in his nares are singed. Given this clinical presentation, which of the following may be responsible for this patient's respiratory distress?

a. Asthma
b. Foreign body aspiration
c. Thermal burns
d. Pneumothorax
e. Myocardial infarction (MI)

60. A 76-year-old man presents to the ED in acute respiratory distress, gasping for breath while on face mask. Paramedics state that he was found on a bench outside of his apartment in respiratory distress. Initial vitals include a HR of 90 beats per minute, a BP of 170/90 mm Hg, and a RR of 33 breaths per minute with an oxygen saturation of 90%. Upon physical examination, the patient is coughing up pink, frothy sputum, has rales two-thirds of the way up in both lung fields and has pitting edema of his lower extremities. A chest x-ray is consistent with pulmonary edema. After obtaining intravenous access and placing the patient on a monitor, which of the following medical interventions is most appropriate?

a. Morphine sulfate only
b. Nitroglycerin only
c. Nitroglycerin and a loop diuretic
d. Aspirin
e. Loop diuretic only

61. A 67-year-old man is brought to the ED in respiratory distress. His initial vitals include a HR of 112 beats per minute, a BP of 145/88 mm Hg, and a RR of 18 breaths per minute with an oxygen saturation of 92% on room air. He is also febrile to 102°F. After obtaining intravenous access, placing the patient on a monitor and administering oxygen via nasal cannula, a chest radiograph is performed and shows patchy alveolar infiltrates with consolidation in the lower lobes. On review of systems, the patient tells you that he had 5–6 watery bowel movements a day for the last 2 days with a few bouts of emesis. Which of the following infectious etiology is most likely present in this clinical scenario?

a. *Streptococcus pneumoniae*
b. *Haemophilus influenzae*
c. *Mycoplasma pneumoniae*
d. *Chlamydia pneumoniae*
e. *Legionella pneumophila*

62. A 3-month-old boy is brought to the ED by his mother who reports that the infant has been breathing with extra effort for the last 2 days. She reports that the child has had rhinorrhea and a cough. Upon physical examination, the infant has audible wheezing with diffuse rhonchi upon chest auscultation. He also has intercostal retractions and nasal flaring. A chest radiograph shows bilateral diffuse infiltrates. Given this patient's history and physical examination, which of the following is the most likely etiology of his symptoms?

a. Respiratory syncytial virus
b. Chronic obstructive pulmonary disease (COPD)
c. Asthma
d. Rotavirus
e. Parvovirus B19

63. A 23-year-old woman presents to the ED with palpitations and dyspnea that began last night. Her initial vitals include a HR of 110 beats per minute, a BP of 105/60 mm Hg, a RR of 23 breaths per minute, and an oxygen saturation of 93% on room air. The patient states that she recently returned from a cross-country road trip with her friend and is otherwise healthy, except for a recent upper respiratory infection. She is currently on oral contraceptives and occasionally smokes cigarettes. Upon physical examination, the patient states that she has chest pain upon deep inspiration; however her lung sounds are clear to auscultation. A chest radiograph is normal. Given this patient's symptoms and physical examination, which of the following is the most likely etiology of her clinical presentation?

a. Pneumothorax
b. Tension pneumothorax
c. PE
d. Asthma
e. Pleural effusion

64. A 58-year-old man presents to the ED with progressive dyspnea over the course of 1 week. Upon arrival, he is able to speak in full sentences and states that he stopped taking all of his medications recently. Initial vitals include a HR of 92 beats per minute, a BP of 180/100 mm Hg, and a RR of 16 breaths per minute with an oxygen saturation of 94% on room air. Upon physical examination, the patient has bibasilar crackles, jugular venous distention, and pedal edema. Which of the following medication regimens was the patient most likely on?

a. Loop diuretic only
b. Aspirin only
c. Loop diuretic and β-blocker
d. Calcium-channel blocker
e. Loop diuretic, β-blocker, and ACE inhibitor

65. A 4-month-old girl is brought in by her mother to the ED with respiratory distress. The mother reports that her daughter developed trouble breathing after she had fed her some homemade honey earlier in the day. Physical examination reveals a limp baby with diminished breath sounds bilaterally. Given the history of this patient, which of the following is most likely responsible for this patient's symptoms?

a. Dehydration
b. Botulism
c. Pneumonia
d. Respiratory syncytial virus
e. Epiglottitis

66. A 32-year-old woman presents to the ED with a 1 month history of general malaise, mild cough, and subjective fevers. She states that she is HIV positive and her last CD4 count taken 6 months prior was 220. She is not on antiretroviral therapy or other medications. Initial vitals include a HR of 88 beats per minute, a BP of 130/60 mm Hg, and a RR of 12 breaths per minute with an oxygen saturation of 91% on room air. Her chest radiograph shows diffuse, patchy infiltrates bilaterally. Subsequent labs are unremarkable except for an elevated lactate dehydrogenase level. Given this patient's history and physical examination, which of the following is the most likely organism responsible for her clinical presentation?

a. *Staphylococcus aureus*
b. *Mycoplasma pneumoniae*
c. *Pneumocystis carinii*
d. *Legionella pneumoniae*
e. *Haemophilus pneumoniae*

67. A 56-year-old presents to the ED in respiratory distress. His initial vitals include a HR of 56 beats per minute, a BP of 120/58 mm Hg, a RR of 16 breaths per minute, and an oxygen saturation of 90% on room air. An ECG is performed which shows ST-segment elevations in the inferior leads. Upon physical examination, the patient's chest is clear to auscultation with a regular, slow heart rate. Given the clinical presentation, which of the following is the most likely reason for this patient's respiratory distress?

a. Anterolateral wall MI
b. Inferior wall MI
c. Pericarditis
d. Pneumothorax
e. Hypokalemia

68. A 27-year-old woman presents to the ED complaining of an intensely pruritic rash all over her body, abdominal cramping, and chest tightness. She states that 1 hour ago she was at dinner and accidentally ate some shrimp. She has a known anaphylactic allergy to shrimp. Her BP is 115/75 mm Hg, HR is 95 beats per minute, temperature is 98.9°F, RR is 20 breaths per minute, and oxygen saturation is 97% on room air. She appears anxious, her skin is flush, and has urticarial lesions. Auscultation of her lungs reveals scattered wheezes with decreased air entry. Which of the following is the most appropriate next step in management?

a. Administer oxygen via nonrebreather, place a large-bore IV, begin intravenous (IV) fluids, and administer methylprednisolone intravenously

b. Administer oxygen via nonrebreather, place a large-bore IV, begin IV fluids, and administer methylprednisolone and diphenhydramine intravenously

c. Administer oxygen via nonrebreather, place a large-bore IV, begin IV fluids, administer methylprednisolone and diphenhydramine intravenously, and give subcutaneous epinephrine

d. Administer oxygen via nonrebreather, place a large-bore IV, begin IV fluids, and start aerosolized albuterol

e. Administer oxygen via nonrebreather, place a large-bore IV, begin IV fluids, and start aerosolized epinephrine

69. An 82-year-old woman becomes acutely short of breath while at rest on the rehabilitation unit. She is brought into the ED with an oxygen saturation of 86% on room air and in acute respiratory distress. Her initial ECG is within normal limits and unchanged from a recent previous exam. Her initial chest x-ray is also negative. Upon chest auscultation, there are equal bilateral breath sounds with some scattered rhonchi. Her nurse tells you that 2 days ago she underwent internal fixation of a right femur fracture and has been on anticoagulant therapy. Given the history and presentation of this patient, what is the most likely etiology of her symptoms?

a. PE
b. Acute MI
c. Fat embolism
d. Pneumothorax
e. Rib fracture

70. A 4-year-old boy is brought to the ED after an acute onset of respiratory distress. His mother reports that the child was alone in his playroom when she found him struggling to breathe. Upon arrival, the child has audible wheezing and stridor. He is afebrile with an oxygen saturation of 95% on room air. Given this child's presentation, which of the following is the most likely etiology of his symptoms?

a. Croup
b. Pneumothorax
c. Bacterial tracheitis
d. Foreign body aspiration
e. Pneumonia

71. A 72-year-old man presents to the ED in with worsening shortness of breath. His initial vitals include a HR of 86 beats per minute, BP of 145/50 mm Hg, and RR of 18 breaths per minute with an oxygen saturation of 90% on room air. Upon physical examination, the patient appears to be in mild distress and is breathing with pursed lips. Breath sounds are distant but you hear scattered wheezes and a prolonged expiratory phase. An ECG is normal. Given this patient's history and physical examination, which of the following conditions does this patient most likely have?

a. Chronic bronchitis
b. Asthma
c. Emphysema
d. Congestive heart failure (CHF)
e. Pneumothorax

72. A 71-year old woman presents to the ED after a reported mechanical fall 1 day ago. Her initial vitals include a HR of 55 beats per minute, a BP of 110/60 mm Hg, a RR of 12 breaths per minute, and an oxygen saturation of 95% on room air. The patient does not appear to be taking deep breaths. Her physical examination is significant for decreased breath sounds bilaterally and tenderness to palpation along the right side of her chest. After initial stabilization, which of the following is the diagnostic test of choice for this patient's condition?

a. Chest x-ray
b. Chest CT scan
c. ECG
d. Rib radiographs
e. Thoracentesis

73. A 29-year-old woman presents to the ED for hyperventilation. Her initial vitals include a RR of 28 breaths per minute with an oxygen saturation of 100% on room air. She states that she cannot breathe and that her hands and feet are cramping up. She denies any trauma, past medical history, or illicit drug use. Chest auscultation reveals clear breath sounds bilaterally. A subsequent chest x-ray is normal. Upon, reevaluation the patient reports that she is breathing better. Her vitals include a RR of 12 breaths per minute with an oxygen saturation of 100% on room air. Which of the following conditions is most likely the etiology of this patient's symptoms?

a. Pneumothorax
b. Hemopneumothorax
c. Pleural effusion
d. Anxiety attack
e. Asthma exacerbation

74. A 42-year-old man presents to the ED via ambulance after activating EMS for dyspnea. He is currently on an oxygen face mask and was administered one nebulized treatment of a β_2-agonist by the paramedics. His initial vitals include a RR of 16 breaths per minute with an oxygen saturation of 96%. The patient appears to be in mild distress with some intercostal retractions. Upon chest auscultation, there are minimal wheezes localized over bilateral lower lung fields. The patient's symptoms completely resolve after two more nebulizer treatments. Which of the following medications, in addition to a rescue β_2-agonist inhaler, should be prescribed for outpatient use?

a. Magnesium sulfate
b. Epi-Pen
c. Corticosteroids
d. β-Blocker
e. Calcium-channel blocker

75. A 22-year-old woman is brought to ED by paramedics who state that they found the patient hunched over on a park bench barely breathing. The patient is arousable only to painful stimuli. Her initial vitals include a HR of 78 beats per minute, a BP of 125/58 mm Hg, and a respiratory rate of 6 breaths per minute with an oxygen saturation of 94% on 2 L nasal cannula. Upon physical examination, the patient has clear breath sounds bilaterally and no signs of trauma. You note pinpoint pupils bilaterally.

Which of the following agents may be used in reversing this patient's presentation?

a. Oxygen
b. Flumazenil
c. Anticholinergic inhaler treatment
d. β_2-Agonist nebulized treatment
e. Naloxone

76. A 33-year-old man presents to the ED in respiratory distress. His initial vitals include a HR of 102 beats per minute, a BP of 90/60 mm Hg, a RR of 21 breaths per minute with an oxygen saturation of 95% on 2 L nasal cannula. He denies any illicit drug use and continues to complain of right anterior chest pain. An electrocardiogram is shown below. Given this ECG, which of the following etiologies should be further investigated in this patient?

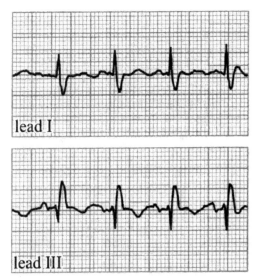

(Reproduced, with permission, from Stead LG, Stead SM, Kaufman MS. First Aid for the Emergency Medicine Clerkship. New York, NY: McGraw-Hill, 2002:118.)

a. Pneumonia
b. Tension pneumothorax
c. Pericarditis
d. PE
e. Pleural effusion

77. A 43-year-old undomiciled man is brought to the ED after being found intoxicated on the street. He is currently arousable and expresses a request to be left alone. Initial vitals include a HR of 74 beats per minute, a BP of 140/80 mm Hg, and a RR of 10 breaths per minute with an oxygen saturation of 94% on room air. His rectal temperature is 101.2°F. A chest radiograph shows a density in the right middle lobe with surrounding infiltrates. Given this clinical presentation, what initial antibiotic coverage is most appropriate for this patient?

a. Broad-spectrum with anaerobic coverage
b. Antiviral therapy
c. Antifungal therapy
d. Pneumocystis carinii pneumonia (PCP) prophylaxis
e. Gram-negative coverage

78. A 42-year-old man presents to the ED with labored breathing that worsened over the course of the day. He reports having recent dental work 4 days ago and has been persistently febrile since despite being on oral antibiotics. Today he noticed some tongue swelling in addition to his respiratory symptoms. The patient's initial vitals include a HR of 98 beats per minute, a BP of 140/80 mm Hg, a RR of 14 breaths per minute, an oxygen saturation of 96% on room air, and a temperature of 101°F. On exam, his mouth and neck are swollen, his breath is malodorous, and you note that he is having difficulty handling his oral secretions. Which of the following is the most important initial step in the management of this patient?

a. Obtaining a chest x-ray
b. Obtaining IV access
c. Securing the airway
d. Giving intravenous antibiotics
e. Giving intravenous steroids

79. A 32-year-old man is brought into the ED by EMS with fever, shortness of breath, and stridor. The patient was treated yesterday in the ED for a viral syndrome. His BP is 90/50 mm Hg, HR is 110 beats per minute, temperature is 101.2°F, and his RR is 28 breaths per minute. A chest radiograph reveals a widened mediastinum. The patient is endotracheally intubated, given a 2 L bolus of normal saline, and started on antibiotics. His BP improves to 110/70 mm Hg and he is transferred to the intensive care unit (ICU). You see a friend that accompanied the patient to the hospital and ask him some questions. You find out the patient is a drum maker and recently returned from Africa with animal hides. What is the most likely organism that is responsible for the patient's presentation?

a. Streptococcus pneumoniae
b. Corynebacterium diphtheriae
c. Coxiella burnetii
d. Haemophilis influenzae
e. Bacillus anthracis

80. A 22-year-old man is brought to the ED after being involved in a motorcycle crash. His initial vitals include a HR of 88 beats per minute, a BP of 125/55 mm Hg, and a RR of 18 breaths per minute with an oxygen saturation of 94% on face mask oxygen. The patient is able to speak in complete sentences and tells you that he has a history of mild intermittent asthma for which he occasionally uses an inhaler. He reports losing consciousness after being hit by a car from behind. Upon physical examination, you hear decreased breath sounds on the left with no palpable chest crepitus. A stat portable chest x-ray shows only a left pleural effusion. Given this patient's presentation, which of the following is most likely responsible for this patient's signs?

a. Pneumothorax
b. Ruptured bladder
c. Pelvic fracture
d. Hemothorax
e. Pulmonary edema

81. A 62-year-old man presents to the ED with gradual dyspnea over the last few weeks. He reports that he is a daily smoker and has not seen a physician in years. Upon physical examination, there are decreased breath sounds on the right as compared to the left. A chest radiograph indicates blunting of the right costophrenic angle with a fluid line. A thoracentesis is performed. Given this patients' history, which of the following is the most likely analysis of the effusion?

a. Transudative effusion
b. Exudative effusion
c. Transudative and exudative effusion
d. Lactate dehydrogenase <200 U
e. Fluid-to-blood protein ratio <0.5

82. A 40-year-old man with a history of untreated human immunodeficiency virus (HIV) for 8 years comes into the ED complaining of cough, fever, and malaise for 3 days. He is tachypneic and diaphoretic. Chest radiograph reveals bilateral infiltrates that are atypical in appearance. Arterial blood gas analysis is significant for a PaO_2 of 62 on room air. His chest radiograph is seen below. Which of the following is the most appropriate initial management?

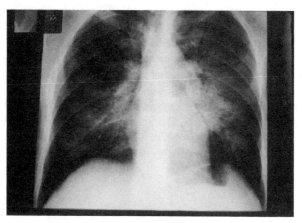

(Reproduced, with permission, from Knoop KJ, Stack LB, Storrow AB. Atlas of Emergency Medicine. New York, NY: McGraw-Hill, 2002: 666.)

a. Corticosteroid treatment prior to definitive antibiotic therapy
b. Immediate treatment with intravenous trimethoprim/sulfamethoxazole (TMP/SMX)
c. Brief delay of antibiotics until a rapid sputum gram stain can be obtained
d. Nebulizer treatment even if the patient is not wheezing
e. Racemic epinephrine if the patient is in respiratory distress

83. A 9-year-old boy is brought in to the ED by his father who noticed a change in his son's voice over the course of the day. The child is sitting on a stretcher with his neck slightly hyperextended, is drooling from the left side of his mouth, and complains of neck pain. His father reports that the child had upper respiratory symptoms the week prior. Upon chest auscultation, the child's lungs are clear. His posterior oropharynx is erythematous without any visible fluctuant masses. His initial vitals are within normal limits except for an oxygen saturation of 95% on room air and a temperature of 102.5°F. Given this patient's history and physical examination, which of the following conditions is most likely causing his symptoms?

a. Epiglottitis
b. Retropharyngeal abscess
c. Peritonsillar abscess
d. Ludwig's angina
e. Pharyngitis

84. A 49-year-old woman presents to the ED with difficulty breathing after a morning jog. Her initial vitals include a HR of 60 beats per minute, a BP of 120/55 mm Hg, and a RR of 20 breaths per minute with an oxygen saturation of 94% on room air. Upon physical examination, the patient appears to be in mild distress with audible wheezing. She is able to speak in partial sentences and states that she occasionally uses an inhaler. Given this patient's history and physical examination, which of the following measures should be taken next?

a. Peak expiratory flow
b. Chest radiograph
c. β-Naturietic peptide level
d. Rectal temperature
e. Arterial blood gas

85. A 62-year-old man presents to the ED in acute respiratory distress. Initial vitals include a HR of 100 beats per minute, a BP of 140/80 mm Hg, and a RR of 22 breaths per minute with an oxygen saturation of 90% on room air. A chest radiograph is taken. Upon physical examination, the patient is breathing through pursed lips and appears to be in moderate distress. Upon chest auscultation, there are bilateral wheezes with a prolonged expiratory phase. The patient reports a long smoking history. Given this patient's history and physical examination, which of the following is expected to be seen on the chest radiograph?

a. Right middle lobe pneumonia
b. Pneumothorax
c. Hyperinflated lung fields with decreased vascular markings
d. Pleural effusion
e. Pulmonary edema

Shortness of Breath

Answers

48. The answer is d. (*Lippincott's Pharmacology, p 187.*) The patient has *angioedema*, a rare, but significant side affect of *angiotensin-converting enzyme inhibitors (ACE-I)*. This type of angioedema is usually limited to the *lips, tongue, and face.* If pharyngeal or laryngeal structures become involved, or there is significant tongue swelling, the patient may begin to *compromise their airway* and emergent intubation or surgical cricothyroidotmy needs to be performed. ACE-I induced angioedema can occur after short or long-term use of the medication. None of the other medications listed cause angioedema. The medication should be immediately discontinued.

49. The answer is a. (*Rosen, pp 1226–1228.*) The patient has a confirmed *venous thrombosis* and has symptoms consistent with a *pulmonary thromboembolism.* Data now shows that almost every deep venous thrombosis (DVT) embolizes to some extent. The presence of a PE in this patient can be presumed by a confirmed DVT with pulmonary symptoms. All patients need to be on a monitor and should receive supplemental *oxygen* despite normal oxygen saturation. Oxygen acts as a pulmonary vasodilator. *Heparin* is the first-line therapy in this patient and should be administered promptly. Failure to achieve a therapeutic partial thromboplastin time (PTT) value within the first 24 hours leads to a 23% incidence of new embolism.

(b) A chest CT scan is not urgently needed since a DVT is already confirmed by duplex ultrasound and should not delay administration of anticoagulation. **(c)** Aspirin is not effective in preventing propagation of a DVT. The patient needs an anticoagulant, not just an antiplatelet agent. **(d)** Although immobility can lead to increased thrombus, a patient with a diagnosed DVT should be monitored in bed receiving anticoagulation. **(e)** Warfarin should never be started without concomitant administration of heparin. After the INR is at a therapeutic level (2–3), heparin can be stopped and warfarin can be taken alone. Warfarin initially causes a temporary hypercoagulable state because the anticoagulants, protein C and S (inhibited by warfarin) have shorter half-lives compared with the procoagulant vitamin K-dependent proteins that warfarin also inhibits.

50. The answer is b. *(Rosen, pp 986–998.)* Undomiciled, *alcoholic patients* are at particular risk of contracting *Klebsiella pneumoniae*. Classically it presents with a productive cough with *currant jelly sputum*, fever, general malaise, and an overall toxic looking appearance. A dense lobar infiltrate with a bulging fissure appearance on a chest radiograph is often described.

Streptococcus pneumoniae **(a)** is the most common etiology in community-acquired pneumonia among adults. *Mycoplasma pneumoniae* **(c)** is a common cause of community-acquired pneumonia in patients under the age of 40. Legionella **(d)** is an intracellular organism that lives in aquatic environments and is not transmitted person-to-person. *H. influenzae* **(e)** is common among patients with COPD, alcoholism, malnutrition, or malignancy. It is a pleomorphic gram-negative rod that can be encapsulated and identified as various serotypes, with type b as the most common one causing bacteremia.

51. The answer is b. *(Rosen, pp 388–391, 1000–1005.)* A *spontaneous pneumothorax* typically presents with ipsilateral, *pleuritic chest pain,* and dyspnea while at rest. Physical findings tend to correlate with the degree of symptoms. Mild tachycardia, decreased breath sounds to auscultation or hyperresonance to percussion are the most common findings. It typically occurs in healthy young men of taller than average stature without a precipitating factor. Mitral valve prolapse and Marfan's syndrome are also associated with pneumothoraces. The most common condition associated with secondary spontaneous pneumothorax is COPD. Although suggested by this patient's symptoms, the diagnosis of pneumothorax is generally made with a chest radiograph. The classic sign is the appearance of a thin, visceral pleural line lying parallel to the chest wall, separated by a radiolucent band that is devoid of lung markings. If clinical suspicion is high with a negative initial chest x-ray, inspiratory and expiratory films, or a lateral decubitus film may be taken to evaluate for lung collapse.

An ECG **(a)** may be performed at a later time to investigate this patient's symptoms, but given the high likelihood of pneumothorax, a chest radiograph should be done first. An upright abdominal x-ray **(e)** can evaluate for abdominal perforation. A complete blood panel **(c)** and a toxicologic screen **(d)** may be performed if the radiograph does not show a pneumothorax.

52. The answer is a. *(Rosen, pp 2249–2250.)* *Epiglottitis* is a life-threatening inflammatory condition of the epiglottis, aryepiglottic, and paraglottic folds. The etiology is usually infectious, with *H. influenzae* type b as the most common etiology prior to the introduction of the *H. influenzae* type b vaccination. Most cases now appear in *adults* and *nonimmunized children*. Signs and symptoms include a prodromal period of 1–2 days, high fever, dysphagia, secretion pooling, and dyspnea. Patients usually sit in an erect or tripod position to improve their symptoms. Radiographs of the neck may show the classic *thumbprint sign* of an enlarged, inflamed epiglottis, although a CT scan of the neck may delineate the condition further. Often times, patients are not stable enough to leave the ED and need continuous monitoring in case of airway compromise. Direct laryngoscopy is contraindicated because it may induce laryngospasm. It is important to have fiber-optic and surgical airway capacity. Intravenous antibiotics and steroids are indicated to help in treating the infection and decreasing swelling.

(**b**) Retropharyngeal abscesses present in patients with difficulty breathing, fever, severe throat pain, stridor, drooling, tender cervical lymph nodes, and an overall toxic appearance. A simple pharyngitis (**c**) may present with erythema or exudate of the tonsils, dysphagia, fever, and cough but will not present with airway compromise. Ludwig's angina (**d**) is an infection of the submandibular space. (**e**) Tonsillitis is usually a benign self-limited viral infection that may be complicated by abscess formation leading to a peritonsillar abscess.

53. The answer is d. (*Rosen, pp 172–178.*) The differential for *syncope* is very broad; however it is the job of the Emergency Medicine physician to rule out the most life-threatening causes after first stabilizing the patient. This patient is currently stable, but has the propensity to decompensate given the severity of her symptoms. In the history there are details that lead you to suspect *pulmonary embolus*: recent travel, progressive dyspnea despite inhaler treatment, and an unusual debilitation in her ambulatory status. Objectively her ECG shows right heart strain, which is due to a heart that is beating against an essentially blocked pulmonary vasculature, back-flowing, and resulting in right ventricular enlargement. She is both tachycardic and hypoxic, both cardinal signs of cardiovascular distress. To aid in the diagnosis, a chest CT with contrast or a ventilation-perfusion (V-Q) scan must be performed.

Infectious etiologies, such as pneumonia (**a**) are generally of gradual onset which may progress to sepsis and shock without treatment. However, patients with these presentations generally do not recover from the point of syncope or shock on their own without medical intervention. Neurocardiogenic syncope (**b**) or vasovagal stimulation occurs when a patient strains, is emotionally afflicted or in pain. It is generally situational, acute, and completely resolves on its own. Patients present with normal vital signs with improvement in symptoms when placed in the supine position. A prodrome of lightheadedness, diaphoresis, nausea, or blurry vision is common. Aortic dissection (**c**) is associated with tearing chest or abdominal pain, history of hypertension or some other condition predisposing to vascular tears such as Marfan's syndrome. Subarachnoid hemorrhage (**e**) classically presents with a thunderclap headache with patients complaining of the "worst headache of their life." Symptoms may be mild including photophobia, neck pain, or the patient may be unresponsive upon arrival.

54. The answer is a. *(Rosen, pp 938–956.)* This patient is suffering from an *acute asthma attack.* This is a reversible bronchospasm initiated by a variety of environmental factors that produce a narrowing of the bronchial airways and inflammation. The first-line treatment in order to open the airways includes a *β_2-agonist,* which acts to decrease bronchospasm of the smooth muscle.

Magnesium sulfate (**b**) is also thought to act in a similar manner, but should be initiated in refractory cases of asthma. Epinephrine (**c**) decreases bronchospasm, but given its clinical side effects should only be given in those patients deemed to be in severe respiratory distress. Corticosteroids (**d**) are an effective measure for decreasing the late inflammatory changes involved in asthma. Anticholinergics (**e**) are effective in patients with COPD and are also administered in combination with a β_2-agonist to patients with an acute asthma exacerbation. However, it should never be given alone to treat asthma.

55. The answer is e. *(Rosen, pp 1011–1052.)* All patients with chest pain and shortness of breath should receive an *ECG.* It is a quick, noninvasive test that often provides substantive information. An ECG will show that this patient is having a large anterolateral wall MI affecting much of her left ventricle, a reason for her heart murmur. An ECG must be performed in those crucial first moments so that the proper care may be administered. This example reminds us of the importance of keeping the differential diagnosis broad in patients that present with respiratory distress. The other procedures may be done in a timely manner, but do not necessarily need to be performed next.

56. The answer is c. *(Rosen, pp 2119–2124.)* The crystallized free base of cocaine is known as "crack cocaine." This form, smoked through a pipe, produces a highly lipid soluble vapor that allows for rapid transport from the lungs to the brain for a quicker high than regular cocaine that is snorted or injected. Due to this mechanism, the substance can be concentrated in high amounts in the lung parenchyma causing an *infiltrative inflammatory process* and *pneumonitis* referred to as "crack lung." This can subsequently result in respiratory failure.

Cannabis **(a)** used in conjunction with inhaled β_2-agonists may result in bleb formation and subsequent pneumothorax, but not pneumonitis. Opioids **(b)**, methamphetamine **(d)** and alcohol **(e)** may have pulmonary effects through secondary mechanisms but are not primarily responsible for this type of presentation.

57. The answer is b. *(Rosen, pp 388–391, 1000–1005.) Inspiratory and expiratory radiographs* allow better visualization of the lung pleura and may help better elucidate the presence of a pneumothorax not initially visualized on the chest radiograph.

A repeat chest x-ray **(a)** may be performed; however it will be low-yield if the original was performed correctly. A chest CT scan **(c)** may be done, but after the proper films are performed. Chest thoracostomy **(d)** involves placing a tube inside the pleural cavity to evacuate the intrapleural air and may be performed if the patient continues to decompensate and the suspicion for a pneumothorax remains high. Chest thoracotomy **(e)** involves opening the chest cavity and is reserved for the severest cases of cardiovascular collapse.

58. The answer is e. *(Rosen, pp 1508–1509.)* This patient is suffering from *Guillain-Barré syndrome (GBS)*, an autoimmune demyelinating polyneuropathy. The majority of patients seek treatment for days to weeks after recovering from a respiratory or gastrointestinal (GI) illness. They present to the ED with progressive, *symmetric weakness* of the distal and proximal musculature. Symptoms are worse in the lower extremities. Upon physical examination, *loss of deep tendon reflexes* and diminished sensory findings may be found. GBS affects individuals of all age groups, but is mainly seen in adolescents and younger adults. Variants may be mainly sensory or present as ophthalmoplegia and ataxia (Miller-Fischer variant). Nearly one-third require respiratory support as the syndrome progresses proximally affecting the phrenic nerves that innervate the diaphragm. Cerebrospinal fluid analysis may demonstrate the characteristic picture of *elevated protein* with a normal or near-normal white blood cell count. This finding is highly specific in the setting of GBS. Magnetic resonance imaging

(MRI) may show selective enhancement of the spinal nerve roots, but is not diagnostic. Electrophysiologic and pulmonary function testing is useful in assessing the extent of involvement. Alveolar hypoventilation should also be assessed by an arterial blood gas. Preparation for a definitive airway should be made. Treatment involves *immunoglobulin* therapy to combat the autoimmune response.

(a) β_2-Agonist nebulized treatment is used for patients with reactive airway disease. (b) Aspirin is an antipyretic agent that is linked with Reye's syndrome, a rare but serious illness that can affect the blood, liver, and brain of children and teenagers recovering from a viral infection. (c) Acetaminophen is also an antipyretic that has a good safety profile in children. (d) Flumazenil is a benzodiazepine receptor antagonist.

59. The answer is c. *(Rosen, pp 801–813.)* The *singed nares* seen in this patient should clue you in to the possibility of severe *thermal burns*. Although there is minimal external involvement, damage from the heat may extend deep into the pulmonary system through inspiration. This results in a severe inflammatory reaction causing a *pneumonitis*.

Although you should always consider a foreign-body aspiration (b) in the differential diagnosis of respiratory distress, it is not consistent with the history. Asthma (a) and pneumothorax (d) do not explain this patient's symptoms given the clinical scenario. The ECG (e) shows a first degree heart block which is not indicative for an MI and may be seen in an otherwise healthy person.

60. The answer is c. *(Rosen, pp 1113–1114.)* *Pulmonary edema* can be divided into cardiogenic and noncardiogenic. Cardiogenic varieties are commonly seen in the ED and are usually a result of high hydrostatic pressures. It is seen in patients with MI or ischemia, cardiomyopathies, valvular heart disease, and hypertensive emergencies. *Nitroglycerin* acts to decrease the preload of the heart by venous dilation. This lowers the work of the heart so that it can function more effectively. A *loop diuretic* is used to induce diuresis and also is thought to act as a venous dilator. In conjunction, these medications act to improve the overall functional capacity of the heart. If medical interventions are not stabilizing, preparation should be made for endotracheal intubation. Positive air pressure devices (e.g., BiPAP) may also be used as a temporizing measure for oxygen delivery.

(a) Morphine sulfate is thought to act as a venous dilator. However it is a respiratory depressant and should only be given in small quantities for patients with pulmonary edema. Aspirin (d) should be administered if there is suspicion for cardiac ischemia.

61. The answer is e. *(Rosen, pp 986–998.) Legionella* is an intracellular organism that lives in aquatic environments. The organism may live in ordinary tap water and has probably been underdiagnosed in a number of community outbreaks. It is typically seen regionally with the elderly and immune-compromised as the most affected. Legionnaire's disease is more common in the summer, especially in August. Patients often experience a prodrome of 1–2 days of mild headache and myalgias, followed by high fever, chills, and multiple rigors. Cough is present in 90% of cases. Other *pulmonary manifestations* include dyspnea, pleuritic chest pain, and hemoptysis. *GI symptoms* include nausea, vomiting, diarrhea, and anorexia. *Neurologic symptoms* include headache, altered mental status, and rarely, focal symptoms. *Urine antigen testing* is highly specific and sensitive and, if available, very rapid in making the diagnosis.

Streptococcus *pneumoniae* (a) is the most common etiology of community-acquired pneumonia among adults. It is found in the nasopharynx of almost half of the population and may manifest itself as a lobar pneumonia. *Haemophilus influenzae* (b) is common among patients with COPD, alcoholism, malnutrition, or malignancy. *Mycoplasma pneumoniae* (c) is another common cause of community-acquired pneumonia in patients under the age of 40. It presents as a mild nonproductive cough and low-grade temperature with the typical chest x-ray appearing much worse than expected with diffuse infiltrates. Bullous myringitis may also be an associated symptom. *Chlamydia pneumoniae* (d) is an intracellular parasite that is transmitted between humans by respiratory secretions or aerosols. It remains a relatively uncommon cause of pneumonia in the community.

62. The answer is a. *(Rosen, pp 1826–1827.) Respiratory syncytial virus (RSV)* is a common cause of respiratory distress in infants under 6 months of age and usually results in *bronchiolitis* and *pneumonia,* as seen in this clinical scenario. Diagnosis is made by detecting RSV antigens from respiratory secretions, nasal washes, or swabs. The syndromes associated with RSV infections overlap with those of other respiratory tract pathogens including Rhinovirus, Parainfluenza virus, Coronavirus, Echovirus, and Coxsackie virus. Management is largely supportive. Aerosolized ribavirin has been shown to shorten the clinical course. Corticosteroids have not been shown to be beneficial. Respiratory precautions are necessary to limit transmission.

(**b**) COPD is typically a disease of older individuals often secondary to a history of tobacco use. (**c**) It is believed that bronchiolitis is a precursor to asthma and that infants who get bronchiolitis are more likely to develop asthma as they get older. (**d**) Rotavirus is a cause of diarrhea. (**e**) Parvovirus B19 is the etiologic agent of fifth disease. Fifth disease is a mild rash illness that occurs most commonly in children. The child typically has a "slapped-cheek" rash on the face and a lacy red rash on the trunk and limbs.

63. The answer is c. *(Rosen, pp 1210–1223.)* This patient has many risk factors for a PE. These include venous stasis due to recent travel, procoagulant medication such as oral contraceptives and tobacco. Despite her usually healthy state, this etiology is high on the differential diagnosis and should be excluded with either a helical CT scan with contrast of the chest or a V-Q scan. An ECG may show signs of right heart strain. However, sinus tachycardia is the most common rhythm. A chest radiograph may show cardiac enlargement, pleural effusion, elevated hemidiaphragm, atelectasis, and pulmonary infiltrates. A *Hampton's hump* is described as a visible pulmonary infarction and a *Westermark's sign* is the paucity of pulmonary vessels. A D-dimer blood test may be obtained in patients at low-risk for a PE. In high-risk patients, imaging should be obtained. It is important to note that each of these diagnostic tools is not exclusive in and of themselves. Pulmonary emboli may still be present despite negative tests and should remain on the differential if the clinical suspicion is high. Despite many advances in this area of medicine, PE continues to be a difficult condition to diagnose.

A pneumothorax (**a**) or tension pneumothorax (**b**) typically involves loss of breath sounds, which is not seen in this patient. Asthma (**d**) manifests with wheezing on exam with a decreased peak expiratory flow. In severe cases of asthma, wheezing may not be heard due to impending respiratory collapse. A pleural effusion (**e**) should manifest itself on chest radiograph.

64. The answer is e. *(Rosen, pp 1110–1130.)* This patient is showing signs and symptoms of CHF, which is classified as right or left sided. Right-sided heart failure manifests as jugular venous distention, ascites, and peripheral edema. Left-sided heart failure manifests as pulmonary edema or shock. This patient has both as left-sided failure often leads to right-sided failure. Outpatient management for CHF includes a β-blocker to decrease cardiac stress and improve contractility, a loop diuretic to aid in diuresis of excess fluid, and an ACE-inhibitor for both blood pressure management and renal-protective effects. Patients should also take a daily aspirin for cardiac protection. Calcium-channel blockers (c) are not specifically indicated for CHF.

65. The answer is b. *(Rosen, pp 1794–1797.)* Botulism is a rare, life-threatening paralytic illness caused by neurotoxins produced by *Clostridium botulinum.* The illness occurs in four forms: infant, wound, food-borne, and weaponized. *Infant botulism* is the most common form, replacing food-borne as the canning industry is more sophisticated than in the past. Infant botulism occurs in infants *younger than 1 year of age,* with a peak incidence at 2–4 months. Infection mainly occurs because of a weaker immune system. Due to cases of infant botulism linked with honey and corn syrup, it is now recommended to avoid feeding these products to any child less than 12 months of age. After the toxin enters the body, it must be transported from the GI system or wound to the neuron where the toxin binds to the presynaptic membrane and becomes internalized within the neuron. Finally, it blocks the release of acetylcholine, resulting in neuromuscular blockade. Paralysis and respiratory symptoms ensue. This is mainly a clinical diagnosis. Confirmation of the diagnosis is made by detecting botulinum toxin in the blood. Other neurological conditions such as Guillain-Barré, congenital muscular dystrophy, and poliomyelitis should also be considered. The principle of treatment is generally supportive and treatment with antitoxin. Antibiotics are generally not recommended as they may increase cell lysis and promote further toxin release.

Dehydration (a) may mimic signs and symptoms of botulism; however it is not indicated in the infant's history in this clinical scenario. Pneumonia (c), RSV (d), and epiglottitis (e) are also unlikely given the clinical scenario.

66. The answer is c. *(Rosen, pp 986–998.)* PCP is a commonly seen opportunistic infection in the HIV-acquired immunodeficiency syndrome (AIDS) population. It typically presents with mild subjective symptoms of cough and general malaise. Objectively, patients are hypoxic and have a chest radiograph with a bilateral interstitial process. Risk factors include a *CD4 count < 200.* Serum lactate dehydrogenase (LDH) is also considerably higher in AIDS patients with PCP than those without. Other pulmonary infections, such as tuberculosis, Kaposi's sarcoma, cytomegalovirus, and fungal infections, should be considered.

Staphylococcus aureus (a) typically may cause a pulmonary abscess that can be seen on chest x-ray, but may also present as a lobar pneumonia.

Mycoplasma pneumoniae (**c**) is a common cause of community-acquired pneumonia in patients under the age of 40. Legionella (**d**) is an intracellular organism that lives in aquatic environments and is not transmitted person-to-person. *H. influenzae* (**e**) is common among patients with COPD, alcoholism, malnutrition, or malignancy.

67. The answer is b. (*Rosen, pp 1011–1052.*) The ECG is important in delineating this patient's respiratory symptoms and serves as a reminder that not all causes of respiratory distress are necessarily pulmonary in origin. It is important to maintain a broad differential diagnosis in patients that present to the ED.

The ECG is not indicative of an anterolateral infarction (**a**), which presents as ST-segment elevations in leads V2–V6. Pericarditis (**c**) may present with diffuse ST-segment elevations throughout all leads. Hypokalemia (**e**) may present with interval prolongations, U-waves, and clinically as weakness or periodical paralysis causing respiratory distress. ECG changes are generally not seen with pneumothoraces (**d**) unless cardiovascular collapse occurs.

68. The answer is c. (*Rosen, pp 1620–1633.*) The patient is having an *anaphylactic reaction* probably to the shrimp she ate. Anaphylaxis refers to a severe systemic allergic reaction with variable features such as respiratory difficulty, cardiovascular collapse, pruritic skin rash, and abdominal cramping. Anaphylaxis is a hypersensitivity reaction caused by an *IgE-mediated* reaction. Foods are the major cause in cases of anaphylaxis in which a source can be determined. Common foods that cause anaphylaxis include *nuts, shellfish, and eggs.* In the ED, attention is focused on reversing cardiovascular and respiratory disturbances. Epinephrine is the first drug of choice for patients with anaphylaxis. The route of administration is chosen by the severity of the patient's presentation. A patient with upper airway obstruction or hypotension, intravenous epinephrine should be administered. Patients with stable vital signs can receive subcutaneous epinephrine. Epinephrine should be used with caution in the elderly or any patient with coronary artery disease or dysrhythmias. Antihistamines, such as *diphenhydramine* and ranitidine, should be used in all cases. These drugs block the action of circulating histamines at target tissue receptors. Corticosteroids, such as *methylprednisolone,* have an onset of action approximately 4–6 hours after administration and therefore are of limited value in the acute setting. However, giving them early may blunt the biphasic reaction of anaphylaxis and therefore, it is advised to administer in patients in anaphylaxis.

(**d**) and (**e**) are appropriate to give in the setting of anaphylaxis, however, they are adjunctive therapy and should never be given alone to treat anaphylaxis.

69. The answer is c. (*Rosen, pp 481, 1212.*) *Fat embolism* refers to the presence of fat globules within the lung parenchyma and peripheral circulation after a *long bone fracture* or *major trauma*. Symptoms usually appear 1–2 days after the event or intramedullary nailing. Unlike thromboemboli, fat emboli may pass through the pulmonary vasculature into the systemic arterial circulation where any organ may be affected. Respiratory distress is a common initial system with subsequent neurologic manifestations given that the cerebral circulation is at particular risk. Treatment is primarily supportive in an intensive care setting.

This patient is of particularly lower risk of PE (**a**) given that she has been properly anticoagulated. (**b**) Her ECG does not indicate an acute MI. A pneumothorax (**d**) is less likely given her clinical exam, which would involve decreased breath sounds given the severity of her symptoms. There is no history of new trauma to indicate a rib fracture (**e**) in this patient.

70. The answer is d. (*Rosen, pp 757–762, 2255–2256.*) The most likely etiology of this patient's symptoms is a *foreign body aspiration*, given his age and presentation. Patients may present with *cough, wheezing, dyspnea, and stridor.* Depending on the location and degree of impaction, patients may be asymptomatic or present in respiratory arrest. In the stable patient, plain radiography of the neck and chest remains the diagnostic test of choice. It is important to note that a normal radiograph can never rule out an aspirated foreign body in a patient with a suggestive history. Radiographs may show air trapping or atelectasis, narrowing of the subglottic space, or direct foreign body visualization. Classically, coins are commonly aspirated objects. It is said that if the coin is seen head-on on a radiograph, it is in the esophagus and if it is seen in the sagittal plain it is thought to be in the trachea. The Emergency physician may accomplish removal in some patients with more proximal obstructions. With distal obstructions, consultation with a specialist in bronchoscopy is indicated for removal. In critical cases the foreign body may be forced out with expulsion maneuvers. Ultimately, controlling the patient's airway must be obtained.

The patient is outside the age limits for croup (**a**), and does not present with the typical barking cough. A pneumothorax (**b**) should be part of the differential diagnosis, but is unlikely given the clinical presentation. The patient is afebrile and therefore infectious causes such as bacterial tracheitis (**b**) and pneumonia (**e**) are unlikely given the usual gradual progression of these entities.

71. The answer is c. (*Rosen, pp 956–969.*) This clinical scenario paints a typical picture of *emphysema:* a patient in respiratory distress with low oxygen saturation and breathing with *pursed lips.* These patients are often classified as "pink puffers" and use their pursed lips to push air that remains trapped in alveoli due to a prolonged expiratory phase. Corticosteroids, anticholinergic inhalers, and intermittent β_2-agonists act to decrease inflammation, decrease mucous production and relax smooth muscle in an effort to open up the distal airways. Exacerbations should be treated with these agents. Patients with COPD are at higher risk for developing bacterial bronchitis and pneumonia. COPD is generally caused by smoking but may also result from air pollution, occupational exposure, and genetic factors such as α-1 antitrypsin deficiency. Patients may require supplemental outpatient oxygen to function and perform activities of daily living.

Patients with chronic bronchitis (**a**) are considered "blue bloaters" given their mucous overproduction that causes hypoventilation. These patients generally have lowered oxygen saturation levels at baseline. Asthma (**b**) is not classified as COPD due to its reversible natures and lack of structural lung damage. This patient's signs and symptoms are not typical of CHF (**d**) or pneumothorax (**e**).

72. The answer is d. (*Rosen, pp 381–383.*) Given the history of trauma, a *rib fracture* is the most probable etiology in this clinical scenario. Rib fractures usually occur at the *point of impact* or at the *posterior angle,* which is the weakest part of the rib. It is important to note that the true danger of rib fractures involves not the rib itself, but the risk of penetrating injury to underlying structures. A *rib series* is the most effective way to visualize these fractures. Treatment of patients with simple acute rib fractures include pain relief so that respiratory splinting does not occur, which increases the rate of atelectasis and pneumonia. Chest binders should not be used as they promote hypoventilation. For multiple rib fractures, intercostal nerve blocks may be a more effective means of analgesia. Most rib fractures heal uneventfully within 3–6 weeks. The patient should be encouraged to take deep breaths to avoid developing pneumonia.

A chest radiograph (**a**) is valuable for investigating other associated injuries, but often obscures the ribs and fractures may remain hidden.

A chest CT scan (**b**) is not indicated at this time and is only warranted with worsening symptoms or negative radiographs with a high clinical suspicion. An ECG (**c**) may be obtained to evaluate the general health of this patient but is not helpful in diagnosing a rib fracture. A thoracentesis (**e**), whether diagnostic or therapeutic, is indicated only in patients with pleural effusions.

73. The answer is d. (*Rosen, pp 1557–1564.*) The patient has normal vitals, a normal chest x-ray and is stable. In fact, her symptoms self-resolve with time and without intervention. Only with this information can one be comfortable with making the diagnosis of an *anxiety attack* as the precipitant to the patient's symptoms. A history of a stressor may be helpful, but it is important to note that these symptoms are not under the voluntary control of the patient and often patients may not even be able to identify a specific stressor. Her extremity symptoms are typical of *carpal-pedal spasm* seen with tetany, a result of a transient decrease in calcium serum levels secondary to a respiratory alkalosis.

(**a**) A pneumothorax and hemopneumothorax (**b**) are generally seen with trauma and typically present with decreased breath sounds and abnormal oxygen saturation. A pleural effusion (**c**) has many etiologies and usually presents with decreased breath sounds at the point of effusion. Asthma (**e**) generally manifests itself with wheezing on examination.

74. The answer is c. (*Rosen, pp 938–956.*) *Corticosteroids* have been shown to improve asthma symptoms in subsequent days after an exacerbation and prevent acute recurrences in patients who are deemed suitable to be discharged from the ED. An acceptable dosage is 40–60 mg prednisone daily for 3–10 days after the initial event. Inhaled steroids may also be an alternative to prevent relapses in more intractable cases, and should be used daily with the guidance of the patient's primary care provider. Spacers are available to ensure adequate delivery of the medications deep into the alveoli.

There is no indication for β-blockers (**d**) or calcium-channel blockers (**e**) in this clinical scenario. Also, adequate amounts of magnesium (**a**) should be obtained in the patient's diet. Epi-Pens (**b**) are only indicated for those patients who suffer severe allergic reactions that require epinephrine in the hospital and are not given on an outpatient basis in patients with asthma.

75. The answer is e. (*Rosen, pp 2560–2568.*) Attention to airway and breathing is of particular importance in *opioid intoxication*, as indicated by the patient's pinpoint pupils, because respiratory and central nervous system (CNS) depression are the most common life-threatening complications. *Naloxone* is a μ-opioid receptor competitive antagonist and its rapid blockade of those receptors reverses the depressive affects of opioids.

Oxygen (**a**) and respiratory treatments (**c and d**) can aid in bringing saturations up, but will not treat the underlying cause. Flumazenil (**b**) is a benzodiazepine antagonist that works as a competitive inhibitor of the GABA receptor.

76. The answer is d. *(Rosen, pp 1210–1223.)* An ECG may show signs of *right heart strain* in the setting of a *PE*. Classically, although not commonly seen, is the $S_1Q_3T_3$ *pattern* in which there is an S-wave in lead I, a Q-wave in lead III, and an inverted T-wave in lead III. Sinus tachycardia is the most common rhythm. Risk factors for PE include older age, obesity, hypertension, hormone replacement therapy, neoplasm, immobilization, pregnancy and postpartum period, surgery, trauma, collagen vascular disorders, and a hypercoagulable state. Signs may include tachycardia, tachypnea, hypoxia, rales, diaphoresis, lower extremity pain and swelling, jugular venous distention, or an audible heart murmur. Patients may complain of pleuritic chest pain, dyspnea, cough, hemoptysis, or back pain.

(**a**) Patients with pneumonia may be tachycardic due to fever or dehydration. (**b**) There is no specific ECG finding for a tension pneumothorax, although tachycardia is typically observed. (**c**) Diffuse ST elevations may be seen with pericarditis. (**e**) A pleural effusion may also cause tachycardia.

77. The answer is a. *(Rosen, pp 986–998.)* *Aspiration pneumonia* occurs secondary to the inhalation of either oropharyngeal or gastric contents into the lower airways. Aspiration of gastric juices may cause a pulmonary inflammatory response. This type of mechanism of acquiring pneumonia is commonly seen in those with *swallowing difficulties* or a *relaxed cardiac sphincter* due to *alcohol*. Given these factors, this patient is in a high-risk category for aspiration pneumonia. The small degree of angulation of the right mainstem bronchus makes the right lung at higher risk. Most particles easily travel down this route ending up in the *right middle lobe* of the lung. *Antibiotic coverage* should be *broad*, covering for both *gram-positive and negative organisms including anaerobes* which are commonly present in the mouth. Given the severity, these patients may go on to develop acute respiratory distress syndrome, an inflammatory response to infection, and subsequent respiratory failure.

Antiviral therapy (b) does not commonly exist for pneumonia. (c) Immunocompromised patients are at risk for fungal pneumonias; however, treatment should not be initiated unless there is high clinical suspicion. PCP prophylaxis (d), without a known CD4 count, is not indicated. (e) Gram-negative bacteria and gram-positive bacteria should be covered.

78. The answer is c. (*Rosen, pp 977–978.*) All of the above should be performed in the care of this patient; however *securing the airway* should be the initial step in managing this patient with *Ludwig's angina*. This is not anginal symptoms as in cardiac disease, but a progressive cellulitis of the connective tissues of the floor of the mouth and neck that begins in the submandibular space. *Dental disease* is the leading cause of this condition, as dentoalveolar abscesses may easily break through the thin cortex of the mandible and infect the space underneath. Swelling and inflammation of the soft tissues may result in *airway obstruction*. Patients need continuous monitoring as airway impairment may occur suddenly. Fiberoptic-guided nasotracheal intubation is the preferred method of airway control as endotracheal intubation may be difficult due to distortion of the upper airway.

79. The answer is e. (*Rosen, pp 2643–2644.*) *Inhalation anthrax* is a rare but life-threatening disease with mortality rates exceeding 90%. It is caused by inhaling *Bacillus anthracis spores* into the lungs. Initially, the patient develops flu-like symptoms. Within 24–48 hours, the clinical course may abruptly deteriorate to septic shock, respiratory failure, and mediastinitis. Chest x-ray may reveal a widened mediastinum. Death usually results within 3 days. There is no evidence for human to human transmission. Anthrax is normally a disease of sheep, cattle, and horses. Disease in humans occurs when spores are inhaled. Working with untreated animal hides increases the risk for anthrax exposure.

(a and d) *Streptococcus pneumoniae and Haemophilus influenzae* can cause respiratory failure however it is unlikely to a healthy 32-year-old man. (b) Diphtheria is a potentially life-threatening disease that is characterized by a gray-green pseudomembrane that covers the tonsils and pharyngeal mucosa. (c) *Coxiella burnetii* is the organism that causes Q fever. It is similar to *Bacillus anthracis* in which cattle, sheep, and goats are the primary reservoirs. However, Q fever usually does not cause such rapid deterioration as compared to anthrax.

80. The answer is d. *(Rosen, pp 388–391, 1000–1005.)* Given the traumatic nature of this patient's presentation, a puncture in the lung or bleeding is the most likely etiology. The *pleural effusion* visualized on the chest x-ray is most likely a *sanguinous,* rather a serous fluid, secondary to a *hemothorax.* This patient will need a thoracostomy tube given that he is symptomatic. This will optimize his respiratory status and prevent further decompensation.

(a) It is difficult to elucidate if a pneumothorax is present because it may be hidden underneath the layering effect of the effusion. Nonetheless, if the patient is symptomatic, insertion of a thoracostomy tube treats both conditions. A ruptured bladder (b) is indicative of severe trauma and often associated with chest trauma, however it does not directly cause pleural effusions. Pelvic fractures (c) may cause fat emboli, which can affect the lungs. However, these effects are not seen until 2–3 days after the event. Pulmonary edema (e) is either due to the loss of cardiovascular function or fluid overload. This is usually a bilateral effect seen in both lungs on chest radiograph.

81. The answer is b. *(Rosen, pp 1005–1009.)* Given this patient's longstanding history of *tobacco* use and having not seen a doctor for annual examinations, it is likely that the pleural effusion is *exudative* due to an underlying *malignancy.* Other causes of exudative effusions include infection, connective tissue diseases, neoplasm, pulmonary emboli, uremia, pancreatitis, esophageal rupture, postsurgical, trauma, or drug-induced. Pleural fluid analysis includes LDH, glucose, protein, amylase, cell count, gram stain, culture, and cytology. Effusions that have a LDH >200 U, fluid-to-blood LDH ratio >0.6 and a fluid-to-blood protein ratio >0.5 are classified as exudative. Levels less than these are classified as transudative.

(a) Causes of transudative effusions include CHF, hypoalbuminemia, cirrhosis, myxedema, nephrotic syndrome, superior vena cava syndrome, and peritoneal dialysis. (c) An effusion cannot be both exudative and transudative.

82. The answer is a. *(Rosen, pp 1147–1148.)* In a patient with untreated *HIV* and *bilateral infiltrates* on chest x-ray, *PCP* must be considered, in addition to community acquired pneumonia (CAP). In the initial treatment of PCP, corticosteroid therapy is shown to reduce mortality when arterial PaO_2 is below 70 mm Hg, presumably due to blunting of the inflammatory reaction caused by lysed dying organisms.

(b) Immediate treatment with intravenous TMP/SMX would be correct if the PaO$_2$ were greater than 70. (c) Delay of antibiotics is never appropriate in an ill patient with suspected pneumonia. Gram stain is unlikely to be useful in acutely identifying the organism in CAP and silver stain is required to see pneumocystis. (d) Nebulizer treatment is ancillary and may provide relief of symptoms in a wheezing patient with pneumonia, but is not appropriate for initial management of this patient. (e) Epinephrine has no role in the acutely ill patient with PCP whose symptoms are less likely related to severe reactive airway disease.

83. The answer is b. (*Rosen, pp 978–980.*) *Retropharyngeal abscesses* present in patients with difficulty breathing, fever, severe throat pain, stridor, drooling, tender cervical lymph nodes, and an overall toxic appearance. Physical examination may include an erythematous oropharynx without the visualization of any tonsillar swellings, given that the abscess lies behind this space. The diagnosis may be made with a radiograph of the soft tissues of the neck showing prevertebral swelling. A contrast CT scan of the neck is more commonly performed to help delineate the extent of the abscess and soft tissue involvement. Treatment involves broad-spectrum antibiotic coverage. Most importantly, the abscess must be drained in the operating room given the high risk of airway compromise. Continuous monitoring and airway vigilance is important in the ED as these patients may decompensate.

Epiglottitis (a) is a life-threatening inflammatory condition of the epiglottis, aryepiglottic and periglottic folds. The diagnosis of a peritonsillar abscess (c) is made upon physical examination where tonsillar swelling or fluctuance is visualized. Patients often present with a muffled voice, sore throat, trismus, uvular deviation, and cervical adenopathy. Ludwig's angina (d) is an infection of the submandibular space. A simple pharyngitis (e) may present with erythema or exudate of the tonsils, dysphagia, fever, and cough but will not present with airway compromise.

84. The answer is a. (*Rosen, pp 938–956.*) This patient is suffering from an *exercise-induced asthma exacerbation*. Various triggers can cause bronchospasm. These include dust, various perfumes, underlying upper respiratory infections, cigarette smoke, menstrual flow, and various medications including aspirin. The medical intervention in this patient should include a β_2-agonist nebulized solution, corticosteroids and oxygen administration. The most useful measure to track the patient's progress with each treatment is a *peak expiratory flow,* and should be a part of the initial assessment and monitoring. The forced expiratory volume in 1 second from a maximal inspiration (FEV$_1$) may be used in the ED setting. More commonly, peak flow meters are used which measure the peak expiratory flow rate in liters per second starting with fully inflated lungs. Both of these measurements require full patient cooperation whose values should be the average of three consecutive forced expirations. Normalized value ranges are determined by patient's age, sex, and height.

A chest radiograph (**b**) is useful if the patient does not improve after standard asthma treatments and there is suspicion of a different etiology for the patient's dyspnea. Brain-naturietic peptide (**c**) is a natural enzyme produced by the atria of the heart and is elevated when there is stretching of these fibers, as occurs in CHF. The peptide then acts as a natural diuretic and vasodilatory agent in lowering stress on the heart. This value is not elevated in asthma. A rectal temperature (**d**) is not a necessary next step, but may be utilized at a later time when evaluating infection as another trigger. An arterial blood gas (ABG) (**e**) is a useful assessment of oxygenation and the degree of airway obstruction initially, however, it is important to note that pretreatment and posttreatment ABGs do not correlate well with the patient's clinical picture and may take longer to normalize.

85. The answer is c. (*Rosen, pp 956–969.*) This patient's history and physical examination indicates that he has *COPD.* COPD refers to the presence of three processes: airway reaction, airway collapse, and airway inflammation. *Emphysema* is generally referred by airway collapse, due to the overexpansion of alveolar destruction. This is typically indicated on chest radiograph by *hyperinflated lung fields with decreased vascular markings and a small heart. Chronic bronchitis* is generally referred by airway inflammation which can be alleviated with corticosteroids. Other radiographic abnormalities include flattened diaphragms, increased retrosternal airspace and bullae.

(**a**) A right middle lobe pneumonia generally presents with opacification of the lung field overlying the right heart boarder. (**b**) A pneumothorax usually presents with decreased lung markings in the periphery of the lung field with visualization of the collapsed pleural edge of the lung. (**d**) Pleural effusion presents as haziness usually in the costophrenic angles. (**e**) Pulmonary edema is characterized by an enlarged cardiac silhouette and cephalization of the pulmonary vasculature.

Abdominal and Pelvic Pain

Questions

86. As you palpate the right upper quadrant (RUQ) of a 38-year-old woman's abdomen, you notice that she stops her inspiration for a brief moment. During the history, the patient states that over the last 2 days she gets pain in her RUQ that radiates to her back shortly after eating. Her vitals are temperature 100.4°F, heart rate (HR) 95, blood pressure (BP) 130/75, respiratory rate (RR) 16. What is the initial diagnostic modality of choice for this disorder?

a. Plain film radiograph
b. Computed tomography (CT) scan
c. Magnetic resonance imaging (MRI)
d. Radioisotope cholescintigraphy (HIDA scan)
e. Ultrasonography

87. A 31-year-old man from Florida presents to the emergency department (ED) complaining of severe pain that starts in his left flank and radiates to his testicle. The pain lasts for about 1 hour and then improves. He had similar pain last week that resolved spontaneously. He noted some blood in his urine this morning. His BP is 145/75 mm Hg, HR is 90 beats per minute, temperature is 98.9°F, and his RR is 24 breaths per minute. His abdomen is soft and nontender. As you examine the patient, he vomits and has trouble lying still in his stretcher. Which of the following is the most appropriate next step in management?

a. Call surgery consult to evaluate the patient for appendicitis
b. Order an abdominal CT
c. Start intravenous (IV) fluids, administer an IV nonsteroidal anti-inflammatory drug (NSAID), and antiemetic
d. Perform an ultrasound to evaluate for an abdominal aortic aneurysm (AAA)
e. Perform an Ultrasound to evaluate for testicular torsion

88. A 67-year-old man is brought to the ED by emergency medical service (EMS). His wife states that the patient was doing his usual chores around the house when all of a sudden he started complaining of severe abdominal pain. He has a past medical history of coronary artery disease and hypertension. His BP is 90/70 mm Hg, HR is 105 beats per minute, temperature is 98.9°F, and his RR is 18 breaths per minute. On physical exam, he is diaphoretic and in obvious pain. Upon palpating his abdomen, you feel a large pulsatile mass. An electrocardiogram (ECG) reveals sinus tachycardia. You place the patient on a monitor, administer oxygen, insert two large-bore IV's, and send his blood to the laboratory. Which of the following is the most appropriate next step in management?

a. Bring the patient to the CT scanner to evaluate his "acute abdomen"
b. Call the angiography suite and have them prepare the room for the patient
c. Order a portable abdominal radiograph
d. Call surgery and have them prepare the operating room (OR) for an exploratory laparotomy
e. Call the cardiac catherization lab to prepare for stent insertion

89. A 57-year-old woman presents to the ED with a basin in her hand and actively vomiting. You insert an intravenous catheter, start intravenous fluids, and administer an antiemetic agent. The patient feels much better but also complains of severe crampy abdominal pain that comes in waves. You examine her abdomen and note that it is distended and there is a small midline scar in the lower abdomen. Upon auscultation, you hear high pitched noises that sound like "tinkles." Palpation elicits pain in all four quadrants but no rebound tenderness. She is guaiac negative. Which of the following is the most common cause of this patient's presentation?

a. Travel to Mexico
b. Ethanol abuse
c. Hysterectomy
d. Hernia
e. Constipation

90. An undomiciled 41-year-old man walks into the ED complaining of abdominal pain, nausea, and vomiting. He tells you that he has been drinking beer continuously over the previous 18 hours. On exam, his vitals are BP 150/75 mm Hg, HR 104 beats per minute, RR 16 breaths per minute, oxygen saturation 97% on room air, temperature of 100.1°F rectally, and finger stick 81 mg/dL. The patient is alert and oriented, his pupils are anicteric. You notice gynecomastia and spider angiomata. His abdomen is soft but tender in the RUQ. Laboratory tests reveal an aspartate transaminase (AST) of 212 U/L, alanine transaminase (ALT) 170 U/L, alkaline phosphatase of 98 U/L, total bilirubin of 2.1 mg/dL, International Normalized Ratio (INR) of 1.3, white blood cell (WBC) 12,000/μL. Urinalysis shows 1+ protein. Chest x-ray is unremarkable. Which of the following is the most appropriate next step in management?

a. Place a nasogastric tube in the patient's stomach and remove any ethanol remaining in the stomach by suction
b. Call the transplant team for possible liver transplant
c. Administer hepatitis B immune globulin
d. Send viral hepatitis titers
e. Supportive care by correcting any fluid and electrolyte imbalances

91. A 48-year-man with a past medical history for hepatitis C and cirrhosis presents to the ED complaining of acute onset abdominal pain and chills. His BP is 118/75 mm Hg, HR 105 beats per minute, RR 16 breaths per minute, temperature 101°F rectally, and oxygen saturation 97% on room air. His abdomen is distended, and diffusely tender. You decide to perform a paracentesis and retrieve 1-liter of cloudy fluid. Laboratory analysis of the fluid shows a neutrophil count of 550 cells/mm^3. Which of the following is the most appropriate choice of treatment?

a. Metronidazole
b. Vancomycin
c. Sulfamethoxazole/trimethoprim (SMX/TMP)
d. Neomycin and lactulose
e. Cefotaxime

92. A 24-year-old man woke up from sleep 1 hour ago with severe pain in his right testicle. He states that he is sexually active with multiple partners but denies having penile discharge or dysuria. On exam, the right scrotum is swollen, tender, and firm. You cannot elicit a cremasteric reflex. Which of the following is the most appropriate next step in management?

a. Administer one dose of ceftriaxone and doxycycline for 10 days and have him follow up with a urologist
b. Swab his urethra, send a culture for gonorrhea and Chlamydia, and treat if positive
c. Send a urinalysis and treat for a urinary tract infection (UTI) if positive
d. Admit the patient to evaluate for testicular tumor
e. Order a statim (STAT) color Doppler ultrasound and attempt manual detorsion

93. A 28-year-old man presents to the ED complaining of constant vague, diffuse epigastric pain. He describes having a poor appetite and feeling nauseated ever since eating sushi last night. His BP is 125/75 mm Hg, HR is 96 beats per minute, temperature is 100.5°F, and his RR is 16 breaths per minute. On exam, his abdomen is soft and moderately tender in the right lower quadrant (RLQ). Lab results reveal a WBC of 12,000/μL. Urinalysis shows 1+ leukocyte esterase. The patient is convinced that this is food poisoning from the sushi and asks for some antacid. Which of the following is the most appropriate next step in management?

a. Order a plain radiograph to look for dilated bowel loops
b. Administer 40 cc of Maalox and observe for 2 hours
c. Send the patient for an abdominal ultrasound
d. Order an abdominal CT scan with IV and oral contrast
e. Discharge the patient home with ciprofloxacin

94. A 41-year-old woman presents to the ED complaining of pain in her RUQ that is steady but gets worse with eating over the past 2 days. The pain also radiates to the right side of her mid-back. She denies vomiting. Her only medication is an oral contraceptive. Her BP is 140/75 mm Hg, HR is 80 beats per minute, temperature is 98.7°F, and RR is 16 breaths per minute. Laboratory tests are within normal limits. An abdominal ultrasound reveals stones in her gallbladder, but no thickened wall or pericholecystic fluid. What is the most likely diagnosis?

a. Cholangitis
b. Urolithiasis
c. Cholecystitis
d. Biliary colic
e. Peptic ulcer disease

95. A 50-year-old man presents to the ED complaining of abrupt onset of epigastric pain that radiates to his back. He describes the pain as constant and associated with nausea and vomiting. The pain improves mildly if he leans forward. He has a 20-pack-year smoking history and consumes a 6-pack of beer daily for more than 5 years. His BP is 150/80 mm Hg, HR is 98 beats per minute, temperature is 100.1°F, and his RR is 18 breaths per minute. He is tender to palpation in the epigastric area. A chest x-ray reveals a small left sided pleural effusion. His WBC count is 12,000/μL, hematocrit 39%, plasma glucose 225 mg/dL, AST and ALT within normal limits, alkaline phosphatase 96 U/L, and lipase 520 U/L. His CT scan is shown on the next page. What is the most likely diagnosis?

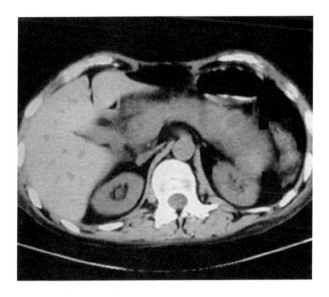

a. Abdominal aortic aneurysm
b. Mesenteric ischemia
c. Pancreatitis
d. Bowel perforation
e. Cholecystitis

96. A 65-year-old woman presents to the ED complaining of abdominal pain. She states that the pain began as a vague aching but has migrated to the left side of her abdomen. She recalls feeling a fever over the past 3 days and just not feeling like herself. She also complains of being more constipated than usual and describes some burning when she urinates. Her BP is 135/70 mm Hg, HR is 90 beats per minute, temperature is 100.9°F, and her RR is 16 breaths per minute. Your abdominal exam reveals normal bowel sounds, mild distension, and tenderness over the left lower quadrant. What is the best test to confirm your diagnosis?

a. Endoscopy
b. Barium enema
c. X-ray
d. CT scan
e. Angiography

97. A 23-year-old woman presents to the ED in moderate pain in her left lower quadrant. She states that the pain began suddenly and is associated with nausea and vomiting. She had a bout of diarrhea yesterday. This is the second time in the month that she experienced pain in this location, however, never with this severity. Her BP is 120/75 mm Hg, HR is 101 beats per minute, temperature is 99.5°F, and RR is 18 breaths per minute. She has a tender left lower quadrant on abdominal exam and a tender adnexa on pelvic exam. Which of the following is the most appropriate diagnostic test for the patient?

a. CT scan
b. MRI
c. X-ray
d. Doppler US
e. Laparoscopy

98. A 35-year-old man presents to the ED complaining of severe left flank pain that began suddenly in the middle of the night. The patient states that the pain begins in his flank region and radiates laterally around his abdomen into his scrotum. He states that the pain occasionally gets better but never completely resolves. His BP is 145/75 mm Hg, HR is 95 beats per minute, temperature is 99.9°F, and his RR is 18 breaths per minute. You observe the patient moving around in the stretcher trying to get comfortable. His abdomen is soft, nontender, and without any masses. The rest of the physical exam is unremarkable. Which of the following tests is most appropriate to confirm the diagnosis?

a. Urinalysis
b. Helical CT scan
c. Intravenous pyelogram
d. Ultrasound
e. Kidney-ureter-bladder (KUB)

99. A 55-year-old man presents to the ED complaining of mild diffuse abdominal pain. He states that he underwent a routine colonoscopy yesterday and was told "everything is fine." The pain began upon waking up and is associated with some nausea. He denies fever, vomiting, diarrhea, and rectal bleeding. His BP is 143/71 mm Hg, HR is 87 beats per minute, temperature is 98.9°F, and RR is 16 breaths per minute. His abdomen is tense but only mildly tender. You order baseline labs. His chest radiograph is seen below. Which of the following is the most likely diagnosis?

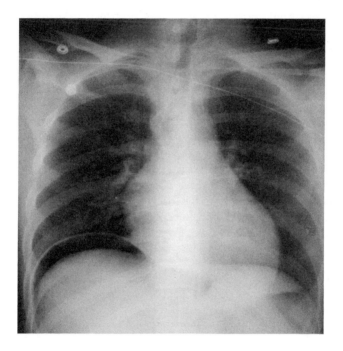

a. Ascending cholangitis
b. Acute pulmonary edema
c. Acute liver failure with ascites
d. Pancreatitis
e. Perforation with pneumoperitoneum

100. A 53-year-old woman presents to the ED with 9 hours of severe left lower quadrant abdominal pain. She describes worsening constipation, tenesmus, and dysuria. Her temperature is 100.9°F, BP is 142/84 mm Hg, HR is 90 beats per minute, RR is 16 breaths per minute, and her oxygen saturation is 98% on room air. Abdominal exam reveals tenderness in the left lower quadrant with focal rebound tenderness and voluntary guarding. WBC is 12,700/μL, urinalysis shows 1+ leukocyte esterase and no bacteria. Abdominal radiographs are nonspecific. Which of the following is the most appropriate next step in management?

a. Immediate transfer to the OR for exploratory laparotomy
b. Consult GI for an emergent colonoscopy
c. Prepare for a barium enema
d. CT scan
e. Admit for intravenous antibiotics and hydration

101. A 33-year-old man presents to the ED complaining of lower abdominal pain. He states that last night he ate pizza with pepperoni for dinner, went to sleep, and awoke several hours later with a vague, periumbilical pain. The pain has been constant since its onset and has migrated to his lower abdomen more on the right than left. Since eating the pizza he has no appetite. He is nauseated and vomited twice in the ED. His BP is 125/70 mm Hg, HR is 88 beats per minute, temperature is 100.4°F, and his RR is 16 breaths per minute. On exam, he is diaphoretic and his RLQ is tender to palpation. Which of the following is most sensitive and specific for appendicitis?

a. Diaphoresis
b. Fever
c. Anorexia
d. Vomiting
e. Nausea

102. A 78-year-old woman is brought to the ED by EMS complaining of vomiting and abdominal pain that began during the night. EMS reports that her BP is 90/50 mm Hg, HR is 110 beats per minute, temperature is 101.2°F, and RR is 18 breaths per minute. After giving her a 500-mL bolus of normal saline, her BP is 115/70 mm Hg. During the exam, you notice that her face and chest appear jaundiced. Her lungs are clear to auscultation and you do not appreciate a murmur on cardiac exam. She winces when you palpate her RUQ. An ultrasound reveals dilation of the common bile duct and stones in the gallbladder. What is the most likely diagnosis?

a. Cholecystitis
b. Acute hepatitis
c. Cholangitis
d. Pancreatic cancer
e. Bowel obstruction

103. A 23-year-old woman presents to the ED complaining of lower abdominal pain and vaginal spotting for 2 days. Her BP is 115/75 mm Hg, HR is 75 beats per minute, temperature is 98.9°F, and RR is 16 breaths per minute. Which of the following tests should be obtained next?

a. Abdominal CT scan
b. β-Human chorionic gonadotropin (β-hCG)
c. Transvaginal ultrasound
d. Abdominal radiograph
e. Chlamydia antigen test

104. A 71-year-old obese man is brought to the ED complaining of constant left middle quadrant abdominal pain with radiation into his back. His past medical history is significant for hypertension, peripheral vascular disease, and kidney stones. He smokes a pack of cigarettes daily. His BP is 145/80 mm Hg, HR is 90 beats per minute, temperature is 98.9°F, and RR is 16 breaths per minute. Abdominal exam is unremarkable. An ECG is read as sinus rhythm with a HR of 88. An abdominal radiograph reveals normal loops of bowel and curvilinear calcification of the aortic wall. Which of the following is the most likely diagnosis?

a. Biliary colic
b. Nephrolithiasis
c. Pancreatitis
d. Small bowel obstruction
e. Abdominal aortic aneurysm

105. A 51-year-old man presents to the ED complaining of epigastric pain that radiates to his back. He states that he drinks a 6-pack of beer daily. You suspect he has pancreatitis. His BP is 135/75 mm Hg, HR is 90 beats per minute, temperature is 100.1°F, and his RR is 17 breaths per minute. Laboratory results reveal WBC 13,000/μL, hematocrit 48%, platelets 110/μL, amylase 1150 U/L, lipase 1450, lactate dehydrogenase (LDH) 150 U/L, sodium 135 mEq/L, potassium 3.5 mEq/L, chloride 105 mEq/L, bicarbonate 23 mEq/L, blood urea nitrogen (BUN) 15 mg/dL, creatinine 1.1 mg/dL, and glucose 125 mg/dL. Which of the following laboratory values are most specific for pancreatitis?

a. Leukocytosis
b. Hyperglycemia
c. Elevated lipase
d. Elevated LDH
e. Elevated amylase

106. A 51-year-old man describes 1 week of gradually worsening scrotal pain and dysuria. He is sexually active with his wife. His temperature is 100.1°F, HR 81 beats per minute, BP 140/75 mm Hg, and oxygen saturation 99% on room air. On physical exam, his scrotal skin is warm and erythematous. A cremasteric reflex is present. The posterior left testicle is swollen and tender to touch. Color Doppler ultrasonography demonstrates increased testicular blood flow. Urinalysis is positive for leukocyte esterase. What is the most likely diagnosis?

a. Epididymitis
b. Testicular torsion
c. UTI
d. Testicular tumor
e. Torsion of testicular appendage

107. A 22-year-old man presents to the ED complaining of dysuria for 3 days. He states that he has never had this feeling before. He is currently sexually active and uses a condom most of the time. He denies hematuria but notes a yellowish discharge from his urethra. His BP is 120/75 mm Hg, HR is 60 beats per minute, and temperature is 98.9°F. You send a clean catch urinalysis to the lab that returns positive for leukocyte esterase and 15 white blood cells per high power field (WBCs/hpf). Which of the following is the most appropriate next step in management?

a. Send a urethral swab for culture and administer 125 mg ceftriaxone intramuscularly and 1 g azithromycin orally
b. Send urine for culture and administer Trimethoprim/Sulfamethoxazole orally
c. Discharge the patient with strict instructions to return if his symptoms worsen
d. Order a CT scan to evaluate for a kidney stone
e. Have him follow up immediately with a urologist to evaluate for testicular cancer

108. A 40-year-old woman presents to the ED complaining of fever and 1 day of increasingly severe pain in her RUQ. She denies nausea or vomiting and has no history of fatty food intolerance. The patient returned from a trip to Mexico 6 months ago. Her BP is 130/80 mm Hg, HR is 107 beats per minute, temperature is 102°F, and RR is 17 breaths per minute. Physical exam reveals decreased breath sounds over the right lung base. Abdominal exam shows tenderness to percussion over the RUQ and normal active bowel sounds. There is no Murphy sign. Her WBC is 20,500/μL with 25% bands, 55% eosinophils, 5% lymphocytes, and 15% monocytes. Chest radiograph reveals a small right pleural effusion. Which of the following is the most likely diagnosis?

a. Amebic abscess
b. Cholecystitis
c. Appendicitis
d. Hepatitis
e. Pyogenic abscess

109. A 44-year-old woman is undergoing a diagnostic evaluation for 3 hours of abdominal pain. She had two similar episodes in the past 2 months. She is tolerating oral intake and is afebrile. As part of this evaluation, a diagnostic ultrasound is performed and is shown below. Which of the following is the most likely diagnosis?

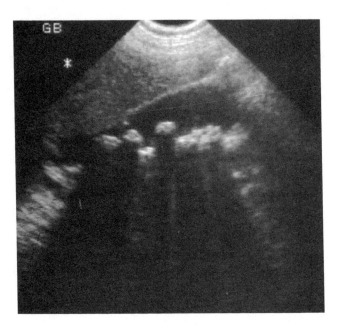

a. Nephrolithiasis
b. Pancreatic pseudocyst
c. Ovarian cysts
d. Cholelithiasis
e. Liver abscess

110. A 53-year-old man with a long history of alcohol abuse presents to the ED with epigastric pain that radiates into his back. He is nauseated and vomiting. You suspect that he has acute pancreatitis so you send off a serum amylase and lipase level. As you suspected, his amylase is 1150 U/L and his lipase is 1275 U/L. What is the most common late complication of pancreatitis?

a. Pseudocyst
b. Abscess
c. Gastric bleed
d. Splenic rupture
e. Splenic vein thrombosis

111. A 59-year-old woman presents to the ED complaining of worsening lower abdominal pain over the previous 3 days. She describes feeling constipated recently and some burning when she urinates. Her BP is 135/75 mm Hg, HR is 89 beats per minute, temperature is 101.2°F, and her RR is 18 breaths per minute. Her abdomen is mildly distended, tender in the left lower quadrant, and positive for rebound tenderness. CT scan is consistent with diverticulitis with a 7 cm abscess. Which of the following is the most appropriate management for this condition?

a. Reserve the OR for emergent laparotomy
b. Start treatment with ciprofloxacin and metronidazole and plan for CT-guided draining of the abscess
c. Give an intravenous dose of ciprofloxacin and have the patient follow up with her primary physician
d. Start treatment with ciprofloxacin and metronidazole and plan for an emergent barium enema
e. Provide pain relief and prep for an emergent colonoscopy

112. A 29-year-old man presents to the ED complaining of RLQ pain for 24 hours. He states that the pain first began as a dull feeling around his umbilicus and slowly migrated to his right side. He has no appetite, is nauseated, and vomited twice. His BP is 130/75 mm Hg, HR is 95 beats per minute, temperature is 100.9°F, and his RR is 16 breaths per minute. His WBC is 14,000/μL. As you palpate the left lower quadrant of the patient's abdomen, he states that his RLQ is painful. What is the name of this sign?

a. Blumberg's sign
b. Psoas sign
c. Obturator sign
d. Raynaud's sign
e. Rovsing's sign

113. A 60-year-old man is brought to the ED complaining of generalized crampy abdominal pain that occurs in waves. He has been vomiting intermittently over the last 6 hours. His BP is 150/75 mm Hg, HR is 90 beats per minute, temperature is 99.8°F, and his RR is 16 breaths per minute. On abdominal exam you notice an old midline scar the length of his abdomen that he states was from surgery after a gunshot wound as a teenager. The abdomen is distended with hyperactive bowel sounds and mild tenderness without rebound. An abdominal plain film confirms your diagnosis. Which of the following is the most appropriate next step in management?

a. Begin fluid resuscitation, bowel decompression with a nasogastric tube, and request a surgical consult
b. Begin fluid resuscitation, administer broad-spectrum antibiotics, and admit the patient to the medical service
c. Begin fluid resuscitation, give the patient stool softener, and administer a rectal enema
d. Begin fluid resuscitation, administer broad-spectrum antibiotics, and observe the patient for 24 hours
e. Order an abdominal ultrasound, administer antiemetics, and provide pain relief

114. A 73-year-old man who is a 1-pack-per-day smoker and a medical history of hypertension and peripheral vascular disease presents to the ED complaining of mid-abdominal and right flank pain. He states that he had this same pain 1 week ago and that it got so bad that he passed out. His BP is 125/75 mm Hg, HR is 85 beats per minute, temperature is 98.7°F, and his RR is 17 breaths per minute. Physical exam reveals a bruit over his abdominal aorta and a pulsatile abdominal mass. Which of the following is the most appropriate initial test to evaluate this patient?

a. Angiography
b. US
c. MRI
d. Plain radiograph
e. D-dimer

115. A 25-year-old G_3P_{1011} presents to the ED with a 6-hour history of worsening lower abdominal pain mostly in the RLQ. She also noticed some vaginal spotting this morning. She is nauseated but did not vomit. Her last menstrual period was 2 months ago but her cycles are irregular. Her BP is 120/75 mm Hg, HR is 95 beats per minute, temperature is 99.2°F, and RR is 16 breaths per minute. Her abdomen is tender in the RLQ. Pelvic exam reveals right adnexal tenderness. Her WBC count is slightly elevated and her β-hCG is positive. After establishing intravenous access, which of the following is the most appropriate next step in management?

a. Call the OR to prepare for laparoscopy
b. Order an emergent CT scan of the abdomen
c. Perform a transvaginal US
d. Order a urinalysis
e. Administer anti-D immune globulin

116. A 59-year-old man presents to the ED complaining of vomiting and sharp abdominal pain in the epigastric area that began abruptly this afternoon. He describes feeling nauseated and has no appetite. Laboratory results reveal WBC 18,000/μL, hematocrit 48%, platelets 110/μL, AST 275 U/L, ALT 125 U/L, alkaline phosphatase 75 U/L, amylase 1150 U/L, lipase 1450, LDH 400 U/L, sodium 135 mEq/L, potassium 3.5 mEq/L, chloride 110 mEq/L, bicarbonate 20 mEq/L, BUN 20 mg/dL, creatinine 1.5 mg/dL, and glucose 250 mg/dL. Which of the following laboratory results correlate with the poorest prognosis?

a. Amylase 950, lipase 1250, LDH 400
b. Lipase 1250, LDH 400, bicarbonate 20
c. Lipase 1250, creatinine 1.5, potassium 3.5
d. WBC 18,000, LDH 400, glucose 250
e. WBC 18,000, amylase 950, lipase 1250

117. A 19-year-old woman presents to the ED with 1 hour of acute onset progressively worsening pain in her RLQ. She developed nausea shortly after the pain and vomited twice over the last hour. She had similar but less severe pain 2 weeks ago that resolved spontaneously. Her BP is 123/78 mm Hg, HR is 99 beats per minute, temperature is 99.1°F, and her RR is 16 breaths per minute. On physical exam, the patient appears uncomfortable, not moving on the gurney. Her abdomen is nondistended, diffusely tender, worst in the RLQ. Pelvic exam reveals a normal sized uterus and moderate right-sided adnexal tenderness. Laboratory results reveal WBC 10,000/μL, hematocrit 38%, a negative urinalysis and β-hCG. Pelvic US reveals an enlarged right ovary with decreased flow. Which of the following is the most appropriate management for this patient?

a. Admit to the gynecology service for observation
b. Administer IV antibiotics and operate once inflammation resolves
c. Discharge and arrange for follow up ultrasound in 2 days
d. Order an abdominal CT
e. Immediate laparoscopic surgery

118. An 18-year-old woman presents to the ED complaining of acute onset of RLQ abdominal pain. She also describes the loss of appetite over the last 12 hours, but denies nausea and vomiting. Her BP is 124/77 mm Hg, HR is 110 beats per minute, temperature is 102.1°F, RR is 16 breaths per minute, and oxygen saturation is 100% on room air. Abdominal exam reveals lower abdominal tenderness bilaterally. On pelvic exam you elicit cervical motion tenderness and note cervical exudates. Her WBC is 20,500/μL and β-hCG is negative. Which of the following is the most appropriate next step in management?

a. Bring her to the OR for an appendectomy
b. Begin antibiotic therapy
c. Perform a culdocentesis
d. Schedule a dilation and curettage
e. Order an abdominal plain film

119. A 73-year-old man is seen in the ED for abdominal pain, nausea, and vomiting. His symptoms have progressively worsened over the past 2–3 days. The pain is diffuse and comes in waves. He denies fever or chills, but has a history of constipation. He reports no flatus for 24 hours. Physical exam is notable for diffuse tenderness and voluntary guarding. There is no rebound tenderness. An abdominal radiograph is seen below. Which of the following is the most likely diagnosis?

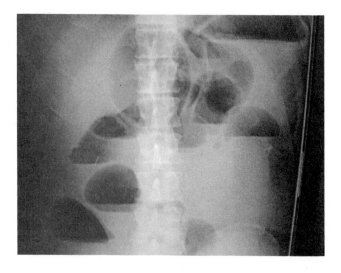

a. Constipation
b. Small bowel obstruction
c. Cholelithiasis
d. Large bowel obstruction
e. Inflammatory bowel disease

120. A 63-year-old woman presents to the ED with pain in her left lower quadrant of her abdomen for the past 3 days. She describes similar episodes on three previous occasions over the past 6 months. Examination shows abdominal tenderness in the left lower quadrant with rebound tenderness. Laboratory results reveal WBC 15,500/μL (82% segmented neutrophils, 18% lymphocytes), hematocrit 41%, platelets 250/μL, AST 51 U/L, ALT 49 U/L, and alkaline phosphatase 75 U/L. Urinalysis shows 5–6 WBC/hpf. Which of the following is the most likely diagnosis?

a. Acute diverticulitis
b. Acute cholecystitis
c. Acute pyelonephritis
d. Appendicitis
e. Spontaneous bacterial peritonitis (*SBP*)

121. A 25-year-old man presents to the ED complaining of dull periumbilical pain that migrated to his RLQ over the last hour. He states that he has no appetite and vomited twice. His BP is 125/75 mm Hg, HR is 87 beats per minute, temperature is 100.6°F, and RR is 16 breaths per minute. Laboratory results reveal WBC 11,000/μL, hematocrit 48%, platelets 170/μL. On physical exam, the patient complains of pain when you flex his knee with internal and external rotation at his hip. What is the name of this sign?

a. Obturator
b. Iliopsoas
c. Rovsing's
d. McBurney
e. Murphy

122. A previously healthy 28-year-old man who returned home 3 days earlier from a vacation in Mexico presents to the ED complaining of frequent, loose stools. His BP is 115/75 mm Hg, HR is 88 beats per minute, temperature is 99.1°F, and his RR is 16 breaths per minute. Stool exam is negative for blood and fecal leukocytes. Laboratory results reveal WBC 9000/μL, hematocrit 45%, platelets 310/μL, AST 42 U/L, ALT 40 U/L, and alkaline phosphatase 75 U/L. Which of the following is the most likely etiology?

a. Campylobacter jejuni
b. Enteroinvasive Escherichia coli
c. Enterotoxigenic E. coli
d. Salmonella
e. Shigella

123. A 27-year-old man is seen in the ED due to leaking around a surgical G-tube that was placed 2 weeks ago and has been used for enteral feeding for 1 week. Inspection reveals the tube is pulled out from the stoma. The abdomen is soft and nondistended and there are no signs of skin infection. Which of the following is the most appropriate next step in management?

a. Insert a Foley catheter into the tract and aspirate. If gastric contents are aspirated the tube can be used for feeding
b. Insert a Foley catheter into the tract, instill water-soluble contrast and obtain an abdominal radiograph prior to using for feeding
c. Remove the tube and admit the patient for observation
d. Remove the tube and immediately obtain a CT scan of the abdomen
e. Return to the OR for closure of gastrotomy and placement of a new tube

124. A 30-year-old man presents to the ED complaining of sudden onset of abdominal bloating and back pain lasting for 2 days. The pain woke him up from sleep 2 nights ago. It radiates from his back to his abdomen and down towards his scrotum. He is in severe pain and is vomiting. His temperature is 101.2°F and HR is 107 beats per minute. A CT scan reveals a 9 mm obstructing stone of the left ureter with hydronephrosis. Urinalysis is positive for 2+ blood, 2+ leukocytes, 2+ nitrites, 40–50 WBCs, and many bacteria. You administer pain medicine, antiemetics, and antibiotics. Which of the following is the most appropriate next step in management?

a. Admit for IV antibiotics and possible surgical removal of stone
b. Observe in ED for another 6 hours to see if stone passes
c. Discharge with antibiotics and pain medicine
d. Discharge patient with instructions to consume large amounts of water
e. Discharge patient with antibiotics, pain medicine, and instructions to drink large amounts of water and cranberry juice

125. For which of the following patients is an abdominal CT scan contraindicated?

a. A 52-year-old man with abdominal pain after blunt trauma, negative focused assessment with sonography for trauma (FAST) exam, BP 125/78 mm Hg, and HR 88 beats per minute
b. A 22-year-old female with RLQ pain, negative β-hCG, temperature 100.6°F
c. A 45-year-old man with abdominal pain, temperature 100.5°F, WBC 11,200/μL, BP 110/70 mm Hg, HR 110, and lipase 250 IU
d. A 70-year-old man with abdominal pain, a 11-cm pulsatile mass in the epigastrium, BP of 70/50 mm Hg, and HR of 110 beats per minute
e. A 65-year-old woman with right flank pain that radiates to her groin, microhematuria, BP 165/85 mm Hg, and HR 105 beats per minute

126. A 71-year-old woman presents to the ED with 12-hours of emesis and abdominal pain. Her temperature is 101.2°F, BP is 100/79 mm Hg, and HR is 104 beats per minute. Physical examination reveals a tender 2 × 2-cm bulge with erythema below the inguinal ligament and abdominal distension. An occasional high-pitched bowel sound is heard. After placing an IV line and nasogastric tube, which of the following is the most appropriate course of management?

a. Administer broad-spectrum antibiotics then obtain a CT scan of abdomen
b. Administer broad-spectrum antibiotics and attempt medical management
c. Administer broad-spectrum antibiotics and prepare the patient for the OR
d. Administer broad-spectrum antibiotics and obtain a plain radiograph
e. Administer broad-spectrum antibiotics

127. You are working in the ED on a Sunday afternoon when four people present with acute onset vomiting and crampy abdominal pain. They were all at the same picnic and ate most of the same foods. The vomiting began approximately 4 hours into the picnic. They deny having any diarrhea. You believe they may have "food poisoning" so you place intravenous lines, administer IV fluids, and observe. Over the next few hours, the patients begin to improve, the vomiting stops and their abdominal pain resolves. Which of the following is the most likely cause of their presentation?

a. Scombroid fish poisoning
b. Staphylococcal food poisoning
c. *Clostridium perfringens* food poisoning
d. Campylobacter
e. Salmonellosis

128. A 63-year-old man is brought to the ED by EMS complaining of severe abdominal pain that began suddenly 6 hours ago. His BP is 145/75 mm Hg, and HR is 105 beats per minute and irregular. On exam, you note mild abdominal distention and diffuse abdominal tenderness without guarding. Stool is heme positive. Laboratory results reveal WBC 12,500/μL, hematocrit 48%, and lactate of 4.2 U/L. ECG shows atrial fibrillation at a rate of 110. A CT scan is shown below. Which of the following is the most likely diagnosis?

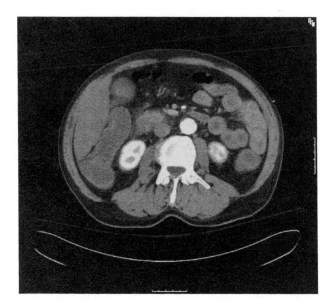

a. Abdominal aortic aneurysm
b. Mesenteric ischemia
c. Diverticulitis
d. Small bowel obstruction
e. Crohn's disease

129. A 19-year-old man from Bangladesh presents to the ED complaining of sudden onset of pain in his scrotum that radiates to his abdomen. He states that the pain began shortly after he finished playing soccer. His abdomen is nontender. There is no penile discharge, lesions, or evidence of a hernia. His right testicle is tender, swollen, and higher than the left testicle.

A Doppler ultrasound reveals decreased flow to the right testicle. Which of the following is associated with an increased likelihood of testicular torsion?

a. Age greater than 50 years
b. Fixed testis
c. Undescended testis
d. Short spermatic cord
e. Epididymitis

130. A 23-year-old woman presents to the ED with RLQ pain for the last 1–2 days. The pain is associated with nausea, vomiting, diarrhea, anorexia, and a fever of 100.9°F. She also reports dysuria. The patient returned 1 month ago from a trip to Mexico. She is sexually active with one partner but does not use contraception. She denies vaginal bleeding or discharge. Her last menstrual period was approximately 1 month ago. She has a history of pyelonephritis. Based on the principles of Emergency Medicine, what are the three priority considerations in the diagnosis of this patient?

a. Perihepatitis, gastroenteritis, cystitis
b. Ectopic pregnancy, appendicitis, pyelonephritis
c. Pelvic inflammatory disease (PID), gastroenteritis, cystitis
d. Ectopic pregnancy, pelvic inflammatory disease, menstrual cramps
e. Gastroenteritis, amebic dysentery, menstrual cramps

131. A 24-year-old woman presents to the ED after being sexually assaulted. She is a college student with no past medical history. Her BP is 130/75 mm Hg, HR is 91 beats per minute, temperature is 98.6°F, and RR is 16 breaths per minute. During the examination, the patient asks which medications she should take to prevent any sexually transmitted diseases. Which of the following medications should be offered to the patient?

a. Ceftriaxone, azithromycin
b. Ceftriaxone, azithromycin, tetanus
c. Ceftriaxone, azithromycin, tetanus, metronidazole
d. Ceftriaxone, azithromycin, tetanus, metronidazole, antiretrovirals
e. Ceftriaxone, azithromycin, tetanus, metronidazole, antiretrovirals, emergency contraception

132. A 71-year-old man presents to the ED with diffuse, crampy abdominal pain that began 1 hour after eating lunch today. The pain is intermittent over the last 8 hours with increasing severity. He also complains of nausea and chills, and vomited once on his way to the ED. He has not had a bowel movement or flatus since the pain began. His past medical history includes prostate cancer, left total hip replacement, appendectomy 25 years ago, right iliac artery aneurysm repair 5 years ago, incisional hernia repair 4 years ago, and irritable bowel syndrome. Which of the following is the most common cause of small bowel obstruction in adults?

a. Bezoar
b. Neoplasm
c. Incarcerated hernia
d. Gallstone ileus
e. Adhesion

133. An 18-year-old man presents to the ED with nausea and vomiting complaining of testicular pain for the past hour that began while playing volleyball. He recalls having similar pain 1 week ago that resolved spontaneously after 10 minutes. He was recently well and reports no fever, diarrhea, urinary frequency, or dysuria. Physical exam reveals vital signs within normal limits. The patient appears in moderate discomfort, holding his scrotum. His abdomen is soft and nontender. His right hemiscrotum is swollen, erythematous, and diffusely tender. It is not possible to palpate the testis separate from the epididymis. The right cremasteric reflex is absent. His left testis has a horizontal lie and is nontender. You suspect testicular torsion. What is the correct way to attempt manual detorsion?

a. Pull down on the painful testis until there is pain relief
b. Rotate the testes in a lateral to medial direction as if you were closing a book
c. Rotate the testes in a medial to lateral direction as if you were opening a book
d. Rotate the testes in an inferior to superior direction
e. Rotate the testes in a superior to inferior direction

134. The following is a radiograph of a 72-year-old man who presented to the ED complaining of gradually worsening back pain that he describes as constant and dull. He denies nausea, vomiting, diarrhea, and hematuria. Which of the following is an important predisposing factor for the development of this condition?

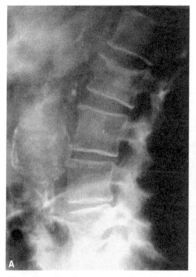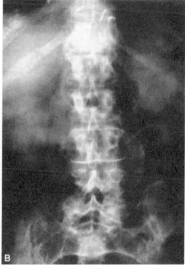

(Reproduced, with permission, from Tintinalli J, Kelen G, and Stapczynski J. Emergency Medicine A Comprehensive Study Guide. *New York, NY: McGraw-Hill, 2004: 407)*

a. Atherosclerosis
b. Hyperparathyroidism
c. Ethanol abuse
d. Prostate cancer
e. Hernia

135. A 22-year-old woman is brought to the ED by ambulance complaining of sudden onset of severe abdominal pain for 1 hour. The pain is in the RLQ and is not associated with nausea, vomiting, fever, or diarrhea. On the pelvic exam you palpate a tender right adnexal mass. The patient's last menstrual period was 6 weeks ago. Her BP is 95/65 mm Hg, HR is 124 beats per minute, temperature is 99.8°F, and RR is 20 breaths per minute. Which of the following are the most appropriate next steps in management?

a. Provide her oxygen via face mask and administer morphine sulfate
b. Administer morphine sulfate, order an abdominal CT with contrast, and call an emergent surgery consult
c. Send the patient's urine for analysis and order an abdominal CT
d. Bolus 2 L normal saline, order a type and crossmatch and β-hCG, and call gynecology for possible surgery
e. Provide oxygen via face mask, give morphine sulfate, and order a transvaginal ultrasound

136. A 33-year-old woman presents to the ED complaining of fever, vomiting, and gradually worsening RUQ pain. She states that her pain radiates to her back. Her BP is 130/75 mm Hg, HR is 90 beats per minute, temperature is 100.9°F, and RR is 17 breaths per minute. While examining her abdomen you palpate her RUQ and notice that she momentarily stops her inspiration. What is the name of this classic sign?

a. Grey-Turner's sign
b. Kernig's sign
c. McMurray's sign
d. Murphy's sign
e. McBurney's sign

137. A 60-year-old woman presents to the ED with progressively worsening left lower quadrant pain over the previous 3 days. Her BP is 130/75 mm Hg, HR is 81 beats per minute, temperature is 99.5°F, and her RR is 16 breaths per minute. An abdominal CT scan reveals pericolonic inflammation consistent with acute diverticulitis. Which of the following symptoms is *least* likely to occur with acute diverticulitis?

a. Urinary symptoms
b. Low-grade fever
c. Gross bleeding
d. Constipation
e. Abdominal pain

138. A 21-year-old girl presents to the ED complaining of diarrhea, abdominal cramps, fever, anorexia, and weight loss for 3 days. Her BP is 127/75 mm Hg, HR is 91 beats per minute, and temperature is 100.8°F. Her abdomen is soft and nontender without rebound or guarding. WBC is 9200/μL, β-hCG negative, urinalysis is unremarkable, and stool is guaiac positive. She tells you that she has had this similar presentation four times over the past 2 months. Which of the following extraintestinal manifestations is associated with Crohn's disease but not ulcerative colitis?

a. Ankylosing spondylitis
b. Erythema nodosum
c. Nephrolithiasis
d. Thromboembolic disease
e. uveitis

139. A 23-year-old woman presents to the ED complaining of pain with urination. She has no other complaints. Her symptoms started 3 weeks ago; she has been to the clinic twice since, and each time urine cultures were negative. Her condition has not improved with antibiotic therapy with sulfonamides or quinolones. Physical examination is normal. Which of the following organisms is most likely responsible for the patient's symptoms?

a. *Staphylococcus aureus*
b. Herpes simplex virus
c. *Trichomonas vaginalis*
d. *E. coli*
e. *Chlamydia trachomatis*

140. A 27-year-old woman presents to the ED with sudden onset severe RLQ pain and pelvic pain that began 4 hours ago. She is nauseated and vomited twice in the ED. She states that her last menstrual period was 3–4 weeks ago. Her BP is 123/78 mm Hg, HR is 94 beats per minute, temperature is 99.1°F, and her RR is 17 breaths per minute. Physical exam is remarkable for right adnexal fullness and tenderness without peritoneal signs. Transvaginal ultrasound reveals a simple 8-cm cyst on the right ovary, without free fluid. Laboratory tests are all within normal limits and her β-hCG is negative. What is the most likely diagnosis?

a. Appendicitis
b. Ectopic pregnancy
c. Tubo-ovarian abscess
d. Mittelschmerz
e. Ovarian torsion

141. A 19-year-old woman presents to the ED complaining of lower abdominal pain over the past 14 hours that is associated with a loss of appetite and mild nausea. She states she is sexually active and is on oral contraceptives. Her last menstrual period was 3 weeks ago. Her temperature is 100.2°F. Her abdomen is tender to palpation in the RLQ of the abdomen and palpation over other areas of the abdomen also results in RLQ pain. Bowel sounds are absent. Pelvic exam reveals scant white discharge from the cervical os. There is no cervical motion tenderness and the adnexae and ovaries appear normal. Which of the following is the most likely diagnosis?

a. Ectopic pregnancy
b. Appendicitis
c. Ovarian cyst
d. Tubo-ovarian abscess
e. Renal calculus

142. A 43-year-old man presents to the ED complaining of progressively worsening abdominal pain over the past 2 days. The pain is constant and radiates to his back. He also describes nausea and vomiting and states he usually drinks a 6-pack of beer daily but has not had a drink for 2 days. His BP is 144/75 mm Hg, HR is 101 beats per minute, temperature is 99.8°F, and RR is 14 breaths per minute. He is lying on his side with his knees flexed. Examination shows voluntary guarding and tenderness to palpation of his epigastrium. Laboratory results reveal WBC 10,500/μL, hematocrit 51%, platelets 225/μL, and lipase 620 IU/L. Which of the following is the most appropriate next step in management?

a. Observe in the ED
b. Send home with analgesic therapy
c. Send home with antibiotic therapy
d. Admit to the hospital for endoscopy
e. Admit to the hospital for medical management and supportive care

Abdominal and Pelvic Pain

Answers

86. The answer is e. (*Rosen, pp 1266–1268.*) The patient's history and physical exam is consistent with *acute cholecystitis*. Because of the poor predictive value of the history, physical and laboratory findings in cholecystitis, the most important test for diagnosis is a strong clinical suspicion and *US imaging*. US may show the presence of gallstones as small as 2 mm, gall bladder wall thickening, distention, and pericholecystic fluid.

(**b**) CT scanning may be useful when there are other intra-abdominal disorders in consideration. However, the sensitivity of a CT is less than that of US when diagnosing acute cholecystitis. (**c**) MRI usually has no role in the diagnosis of acute cholecystitis. (**d**) Radioisotope cholescintigraphy (HIDA scan) has a higher sensitivity and specificity than US; however, it is reserved for cases where US is negative or equivocal. (**e**) Plain film radiographs demonstrate stones in the gall bladder less than 25% of the time.

87. The answer is c. (*Rosen, pp 1414–1422.*) The patient's history of colicky flank pain that radiates to the groin and hematuria is consistent with a *ureteral stone*. Adequate *analgesia* is critical in treating a patient with a ureteral stone. Intravenous *ketorolac*, a NSAID, is frequently administered as a first-line analgesic, but morphine may be necessary for continued pain. In addition to their analgesia, NSAIDs decrease ureterospasm and renal capsular pressure in the obstructed kidney. Antiemetics, such as metoclopramide, help with the nausea and vomiting.

(**a**) Appendicitis is unlikely with a soft, nontender abdomen and no fever. An abdominal CT (**b**) will probably be necessary, but the patient's pain needs to be controlled first. An abdominal aortic aneurysm (**d**) can present with flank pain, however it is very rare in a 31-year-old man. Testicular torsion (**e**) should always be considered in a patient with groin pain. In this case, a stone is more consistent with the history.

88. The answer is d. (*Rosen, pp 1176–1185.*) The *classic triad* of a *ruptured abdominal aortic aneurysm (AAA)* is *pain, hypotension,* and a *pulsatile abdominal* *mass.* Sometimes patients have only one or two of the components and occasionally may have none. Most patients who are diagnosed with AAA are asymptomatic. However, rupture is often the first manifestation of an AAA. Most patients with a ruptured AAA experience pain in the abdomen, back, or flank. It is usually acute in onset and severe. Approximately 20% of the time, patients present to the ED with syncope. Patients with a ruptured AAA are unstable until their aorta is cross clamped in the OR. Therefore, any *hemodynamically unstable* patient with a diagnosed or strongly suspected AAA should be *taken immediately to the OR.*

(**a**) A CT scan is excellent for diagnosing an AAA in stable patients. (**b**) Angiography has no role in the emergent evaluation of a patient suspected of a ruptured AAA. (**c**) An abdominal radiograph can aid in the diagnosis of an AAA. However, when there is high clinical suspicion and the patient is hemodynamically unstable, the patient should be brought to the OR. (**e**) The patient is not complaining of chest pain and his ECG is not consistent with an acute coronary event. Therefore, cardiac catherization is not required.

89. The answer is c. *(Rosen, pp 1283–1287.)* The patient presents with the clinical findings of *small bowel obstruction:* vomiting, intermittent crampy abdominal pain, abdominal distention, hyperactive bowel sounds, and general tenderness. The most common cause of small bowel obstructions in developed countries is *postoperative adhesions,* responsible for more than 50% of all small bowel obstructions. There is a particularly high incidence of small bowel obstruction after *gynecologic surgeries,* such as a *hysterectomy.*

Hernias (**d**) are the second most common cause of obstruction. Traveling to Mexico (**a**) may give you diarrhea and abdominal pain from enteritis. Ethanol abuse (**b**) can lead to abdominal pain due to many causes such as gastritis. Constipation (**e**) will not produce the hyperactive bowel sounds as seen in obstruction.

90. The answer is e. *(Rosen, pp 1256–1258.)* The patient's clinical presentation is consistent with *alcoholic hepatitis,* which is a potentially severe form of alcohol-induced liver disease. Most people remain subclinical, but the presentation ranges from nausea and vomiting to fulminant hepatitis and liver failure. Laboratory tests usually reveal moderate elevations of AST and ALT. Usually in alcoholic hepatitis, the *AST is greater than the ALT* (think Scotch and Tonic for S > L). The patient exhibits stigmata of chronic alcohol disease seen by gynecomastia and spider angiomata. The management is principally *supportive* with correction of any fluid or electrolyte imbalances, paying special attention to blood glucose (ethanol can suppress gluconeogenesis) and magnesium. Thiamine may also be deficient in chronic alcoholics.

Pumping the patient's stomach with a nasogastric tube (**a**) is not indicated and should not be performed. The patient will not require a transplant (**b**) now. His liver, although damaged, is still functioning as demonstrated by the INR of 1.3. Unless this is a known needle stick or mucosal exposure, hepatitis immune globulin (**c**) is not acutely indicated. Viral hepatitis titers (**d**) can be drawn as an outpatient if suspicious for a viral infection.

91. The answer is e. *(Rosen, p 1261.)* Analysis of abdominal fluid and clinical presentation are consistent with *spontaneous bacterial peritonitis (SBP)*. It is recommended to start antibiotic treatment for SBP if the neutrophil count is greater than 250 cell/mm³. Causative organisms include gram negative enterics such as *E. coli, Streptococcus sp.,* Klebsiella, and *S. pneumoniae.* Therefore, the most appropriate antibiotic for treatment is a *third-generation cephalosporin* such as *cefotaxime.*

92. The answer is e. *(Rosen, pp 1422–1423.)* Testicular torsion is a *surgical* emergency. There are two peak periods in which torsion is likely to occur, the first year of life and at puberty. *Manual detorsion* should be attempted in most cases while arranging for definitive care. After appropriate analgesia, the anterior testicle should be twisted laterally, like opening a book. *Color Doppler ultrasound* is the best test of choice in most hospitals. Immediate evaluation and referral to an urologist is essential.

To administer ceftriaxone and doxycycline (**a**) and swab his urethra (**b**) is the correct management for epididymitis. Although epididymitis and torsion have similar presentations, epididymitis usually has more of a gradual onset, reaching a peak over days. A urinalysis (**c**) should be sent on most patients with scrotal pain but in this case the diagnosis of torsion takes precedence. Most testicular tumors (**d**) are painless, although sudden testicular pain can occur with hemorrhage within the tumor.

93. The answer is d. *(Rosen, pp 1293–1297.)* Appendicitis is the most common cause of the acute surgical abdomen. It can occur at any age but is most prevalent in the teens and 20s. It is classically described as starting with the vague onset of dull *periumbilical pain that migrates to the RLQ.* It is associated with anorexia, nausea, and vomiting. A low-grade fever may develop. You should suspect appendicitis in any patient with RLQ pain.

Approximately 90% of patients have a WBC > 10,000 per mm^3. Although, the WBC can be normal in appendicitis. Urinalysis can help differentiate urinary tract disease from acute appendicitis, although a mild pyuria may be seen in appendicitis if the appendix is irritating the ureter. *Abdominal CT with IV and oral or rectal contrast* is reported to have a sensitivity of up to 100% and specificity of 95%. CT findings of appendicitis include an enlarged appendix (>6 mm), pericecal inflammation, and the presence of an appendicolith.

(a) Dilated loops of bowel are suggestive of bowel obstruction. (b) Many patients who ultimately are diagnosed with appendicitis initially believed they had food poisoning. If there is a low clinical suspicion for appendicitis and gastritis is more likely, than administering an antacid and observation is reasonable. However, any change in clinical exam should be attributed to a more significant process. (c) Abdominal ultrasound is commonly used initially in pregnant women with suspected appendicitis. Its sensitivity and specificity approaches 90%, but there may be inadequate studies as a result of body habitus or with a retrocecal appendix. (e) It would be inappropriate to discharge this patient home without first evaluating for appendicitis.

94. The answer is d. *(Rosen, pp 1265–1267.)* The patient's clinical picture is consistent with *biliary colic* due to the passage of small stones from the gallbladder through the cystic duct into the common bile duct. The term colic is a misnomer in that these patients usually have a steady pain rather than an intermittent pain. Pain is present in the RUQ and often is referred to the base of the scapula. Laboratory results are commonly normal. Ultrasound reveals stones in the gallbladder without other pathologies.

Cholangitis (a) usually presents with RUQ pain, jaundice, and fever. Urolithiasis (b) can mimic biliary colic; however the presence of stones in the patient's gallbladder makes biliary colic more likely. Cholecystitis (c) is inflammation of the gallbladder, which can usually be seen on ultrasound as a thickened gallbladder wall, distention, and pericholecystic fluid. Peptic ulcer disease (e) usually presents with burning epigastric pain.

95. The answer is c. *(Rosen, pp 1272–1279.)* The patient's clinical picture is consistent with *acute pancreatitis,* an inflammation and self-destruction of the pancreas by its digestive enzymes. There are many risk factors for pancreatitis, the most common being gallstones and alcohol, which account for more than 80% of cases. Pancreatitis can be divided into mild or severe defined by the presence of organ failure or local complications such as necrosis, pseudocyst, or abscess. It should be suspected in all patients with epigastric pain. Elevation in lipase, a pancreatic enzyme, is used to make the diagnosis of pancreatitis. At five times the upper limit of normal, specificity approaches 100% for pancreatitis.

Abdominal aortic aneurysms (a) may cause epigastric pain with radiation into the back; however lipase elevation is not seen. Mesenteric ischemia (b) can cause pancreatitis by diminished blood flow to the pancreas. Those patients are usually very ill-appearing and complain of abdominal pain that is out of proportion to exam. Bowel perforation (d) usually presents with abrupt generalized abdominal pain associated with a rigid abdomen. Cholecystitis (e) usually presents with RUQ pain due to obstruction of the cystic duct.

96. The answer is d. (*Rosen, pp 1330–1332.*) The patient has *acute diverticulitis*. The clinical presentation reveals a woman in her 60s with abdominal pain localized to the *left lower quadrant,* constipation, and low-grade fever. Urinary symptoms are commonly present secondarily to inflammation near the bladder. The examination of choice is an *abdominal CT scan*. It is also useful in demonstrating or excluding other intra-abdominal pathology. Unlike a barium enema, there is no risk for bowel perforation.

Endoscopy (a) and barium enema (b) are avoided in acute diverticulitis for fear of inducing perforation. An x-ray (c) cannot diagnose diverticulitis but can be used to exclude obstruction and perforation. There is no role for angiography (e) in diagnosing acute diverticulitis.

97. The answer is d. (*Rosen, p 226.*) The patient's clinical picture is consistent with *ovarian torsion*. This phenomenon is most common in women in their mid-20s. It is due to the *ovary twisting on its stalk,* which leads to occlusion of venous draining from the ovary. This leads to ovarian edema, hemorrhage, and necrosis. Most occur in the presence of an enlarged ovary (e.g., cyst, abscess, or tumor). Patients may give a history of similar pain that resolved spontaneously. The first choice to diagnose ovarian torsion is with *Doppler ultrasound* to demonstrate decreased or absent blood flow to the ovary. It can also identify an ovarian mass.

(a) CT scan may be necessary if the Doppler studies are equivocal. (b) MRI and (c) x-ray have no role in the diagnosis of ovarian torsion. If there is high enough clinical suspicion, and diagnostic tests are equivocal, laparoscopy (e) can be used to visualize the ovaries *in vivo.*

98. The answer is b. *(Rosen, pp 1414–1419.) Renal calculi* are common. The prevalence in this country is 7% in men and 3% in women. They primarily occur in people between the ages of 20 and 50 years. The patient in the question presents with typical renal colic. The pain began abruptly in his flank and radiated to his groin. Patients are often in profound pain and may be pale, nauseated, and vomit. Pain control is essential to managing these patients. The best study to make the diagnosis of renal calculi is a *helical noncontrast CT scan,* which has been shown to be 97% sensitive and 96% specific in diagnosing renal stones. It can detect stones as small as 1 mm in diameter and directly visualize complications such as hydronephrosis and hydroureter. CT does not require intravenous contrast and is faster than intravenous pyelogram (IVP). Although CT does not provide information about renal function, this can be obtained from urinalysis and blood BUN and creatinine.

(a) Urinalysis should be obtained in all patients with renal colic. Although it cannot diagnose a renal stone, it provides a considerable amount of information. A urinary pH greater than 7.6 should raise suspicion for the presence of a urea-splitting organism. Red blood cells are found in approximately 20% of patients with renal stones. Pyuria and bacteriuria are important and may suggest a superimposed infection of the stone. **(c)** IVP was used commonly prior to helical CT scanning. It carries some disadvantages, the most important being the use of contrast material which can cause allergy and renal failure. **(d)** US is a fair tool for detecting renal stones, but less reliable at detecting small ureteral and midureteral stones. It has a sensitivity of 65%, although it is very good at detecting hydronephrosis, a complication of renal calculi. **(e)** The KUB has poor sensitivity and specificity for detecting renal stones and is currently not commonly used.

99. The answer is e. *(Tintinalli, p 582.)* Potential complications of colonoscopy include hemorrhage, perforation, retroperitoneal abscess, pneumoscrotum, pneumothorax, volvulus, and infection. *Perforation of the colon with pneumoperitoneum* is usually evident immediately but can take several hours to manifest. Perforation is usually secondary to intrinsic disease of the colon (i.e., diverticulitis) or to vigorous manipulation during the procedure. Most patients require immediate laparotomy. However, some patients with a late presentation (1–2 days later) and without signs of peritonitis, expectant management is appropriate. The radiograph in the figure demonstrates *air under the diaphragm,* which is pathognomonic for pneumoperitoneum.

(a) Ascending cholangitis may occur as a complication from endoscopic retrograde cholangiopancreatography (ERCP). (b) There is no evidence of pulmonary edema in this radiograph. (c) Liver failure with ascites does not cause pneumoperitoneum. (d) Pancreatitis may also occur as a complication from ERCP.

100. The answer is d. *(Rosen, pp 1330–1332.)* The clinical presentation of *acute diverticulitis* depends on the amount of contamination resulting from the perforation and the ability of the host defenses to localize the resulting inflammatory process. When the inflammatory process progresses beyond peridiverticulitis to true abscess formation, the pain and tenderness become more severe and signs of acute peritonitis develop. The peritoneal inflammation remains localized. Abdominal radiographs generally show nonspecific ileus and distention and are commonly performed to exclude obstruction or perforation. The examination of choice to elucidate the extent of acute diverticulitis is an *abdominal CT scan*. It is accurate in demonstrating the presence of abscesses and the extent of pericolonic inflammation, and may demonstrate or exclude other intra-abdominal pathology.

(a) The treatment of generalized peritonitis, perforation, or evidence of gas in the bowel wall is immediate surgical intervention, particularly a bowel resection. The patient in question has focal peritonitis with no signs of sepsis. Although she may be a candidate for bowel resection, it is better to obtain a CT scan to elucidate the extent of her diverticulitis. (b & c) Contrast radiographic studies and colonoscopy are generally avoided in acute diverticulitis for fear of inducing perforation. After resolution of the acute diverticulitis, barium enema examinations are indicated to exclude other colonic pathology and to look for complications of diverticulitis such as fistula formation. (e) Most episodes of diverticulitis are not severe and resolve with medical management including intravenous antibiotics. In a patient with signs of focal peritonitis, it is important to obtain a CT scan to better elucidate the extent of the inflammation from diverticulitis.

101. The answer is c. *(Rosen, pp 1293–1297.)* *Appendicitis* is characterized by abdominal pain, usually beginning as a vague, constant pain in the epigastric or periumbilical region and localizing to the RLQ. The pain is typically associated with anorexia, nausea, vomiting, or low-grade fever. *Anorexia is the most sensitive and specific* of theses symptoms and is usually the first of these to appear. The initial pain of appendicitis is thought to be due to distension of the appendiceal lumen, triggering visceral afferent pain fibers; these fibers enter the spinal cord at the tenth thoracic vertebra, resulting in a patient's perception of vague epigastric or periumbilical pain. As the appendicitis worsens, inflammation of the appendix and surrounding structures triggers somatic pain fibers, resulting in a patient's perception of RLQ pain. Diarrhea is not typically associated with appendicitis, though it is present in some patients.

102. The answer is c. (*Rosen, pp 1268–1269.*) The patient's clinical picture is consistent with *cholangitis*, which is due to an obstruction of the biliary tract leading to bacterial infection. Obstruction is commonly secondary to a stone, but may be due to malignancy or stricture. Cholangitis is a surgical emergency. The classic *triad* of physical findings described by *Charcot* is *RUQ pain, fever, and jaundice*. Sepsis is a common complication. Sonography may demonstrate intrahepatic or ductal dilation. The presence of stones in the gallbladder suggests obstruction as the etiology.

There is overlap in the clinical presentation with cholecystitis (**a**), however the presence of jaundice and evidence of dilated common and intrahepatic ducts is helpful to distinguish it from cholangitis. Acute hepatitis (**b**) will not have the same sonographic findings seen in cholangitis. Pancreatic cancer (**d**) can present with jaundice but it is usually painless. Bowel obstruction (**e**) generally presents with intermittent crampy abdominal pain, vomiting, and distention.

103. The answer is b. (*Rosen, pp 2416–2419.*) β-hCG should be obtained in all women of child-bearing age who present with abdominal pain or vaginal bleeding. A positive pregnancy test in the setting of abdominal pain and vaginal bleeding demands that the physician rule out an ectopic pregnancy.

(**a**) An abdominal CT scan may be indicated later in the workup, but for now there is no urgency for it. (**c**) With a positive pregnancy test, transvaginal ultrasound is the next step in management. This is used to detect an intrauterine pregnancy. If no intrauterine pregnancy is detected, the suspicion for an ectopic pregnancy increases. (**d**) An abdominal radiograph may be obtained later in the workup, but is not currently indicated. (**e**) Women with lower abdominal pain and vaginal discharge may have cervicitis or pelvic inflammatory disease and require a Chlamydia antigen test. However, a pelvic exam should be performed first.

104. The answer is e. (*Rosen, pp 1176–1185.*) The patient presents with multiple risk factors for an *AAA: age > 60, male gender, hypertension, cigarette* *smoking,* and *peripheral artery disease.* Classically, AAA presents with constant abdominal pain, often localizing to the left middle or lower quadrant with radiation to the back. Physical exam may reveal a *pulsatile abdominal mass.* Patients can present unstable if the aneurysm leaks or ruptures requiring emergent management in the OR. Evidence of an AAA is seen on plain radiograph approximately 66–75% of the time. The most common findings are curvilinear calcification of the aortic wall or a paravertebral soft tissue mass. Ultrasound and CT are the best diagnostic tools for the stable patient.

(a) Biliary colic occurs in the RUQ and usually lasts less than 6 hours. (b) The pain of a kidney stone is usually described as colicky in nature. Pain typically begins in the flank and radiates to the groin. (c) Pancreatitis typically presents with mid-epigastric pain that radiates to the back and is associated with nausea and vomiting. (d) Small bowel obstruction is diagnosed by evidence of dilated loops of bowel, air-fluid levels, and thickening of the bowel wall.

105. The answer is c. *(Rosen, p 1276.)* *Lipase* is a *pancreatic enzyme* that hydrolyzes triglycerides. In the presence of pancreatic inflammation it increases within 4–8 hours and peaks at 24 hours. At *five times the upper limits of normal,* lipase is *60% sensitive and 100% specific.* The diagnosis is usually made with a lipase of two times the normal limit, thereby increasing its sensitivity.

(a), (b), and (d) are all laboratory values that are used in the prognosis for pancreatitis, not for its diagnosis. (e) Elevations of amylase are approximately 70% specific for the diagnosis of pancreatitis.

106. The answer is a. *(Rosen, pp 1423–1425.)* The patient has *epididymitis.* It is often difficult to distinguish epididymitis from testicular torsion and the clinician should always rule out torsion first if the diagnosis is in doubt. It is the most common misdiagnosis for testicular torsion. Epididymitis is generally a disease of adult men. The causative organism in men over 35 years old is *E. coli,* while *C. trachomatis* and *N. gonorrhoeae* predominate in men less than 35 years old. The older patient may have a history of gonococcal urethritis (GU) tract manipulation or a history of prostatitis. The onset is usually gradual and urinary tract symptoms may precede the pain.

Testicular torsion (b) should always be on the differential for a patient with scrotal pain. However, it is ruled out in this patient by the presence of blood flow on color Doppler. UTIs in men (c), in the absence of trauma or instrumentation are rare. Scrotal pain is usually not present. Testicular tumors (d) are often mistakenly diagnosed as epididymitis. They usually occur in middle-aged men and have a higher prevalence in patients with cryptorchidism. Color Doppler can often distinguish a tumor from epididymitis. Torsion of a testicular appendage (e) is most commonly seen in males between the ages 3 and 13 years.

107. The answer is a. *(Rosen, pp 1413–1414.)* Dysuria in young men is almost always due to *urethritis*, which is commonly caused by a *sexually transmitted disease*. Urethritis is classically divided into gonococcal (GU) and nongonococcal (NGU) types. Gonococcal urethritis is caused by *Neisseria gonorrhoeae*, while the major pathogen in NGU is *Chlamydia trachomatis*. Nearly all men with GU have purulent urethral discharge. NGU may be asymptomatic or with a yellow, mucopurulent discharge. It was demonstrated in multiple studies that the two pathogens coexist in men with urethritis up to 50% of the time. Therefore, antibiotics should be directed at eliminating both organisms. A third-generation cephalosporin or ciprofloxacin as a one time dose is used to treat GU. Common antibiotics used to treat NGU include azithromycin as a single dose and doxycycline or erythromycin for 7 days.

(b) This choice might be correct if you suspect a patient has a urinary tract infection. However, a young man with dysuria and urethral discharge needs to be treated for a sexually transmitted disease. (c) The patient should not be discharged prior to treatment and culture. In addition, the patient should refer all of their sexual partners for evaluation and treatment. (d and e) There is no clinical suspicion for a kidney stone or testicular cancer.

108. The answer is a. *(Rosen, pp 1263–1264.)* Amebic abscesses are common in countries with tropical and subtropical climates and areas with poor sanitation. *Entamoeba histolytica* causes an intestinal infection, and the liver is seeded via the portal system. The clinical presentation includes abdominal tenderness in the RUQ, leukocytosis, and fever. *Eosinophilia* is often present. Diagnosis is supported by identifying a pathogenic protozoan in the stool. Management consists of supportive care and administering metronidazole. If medical therapy is unsuccessful, percutaneous catheter drainage is required.

(b) Cholecystitis will present with fever, leukocytosis, and pain. However, eosinophilia is not found, and a Murphy's sign is usually present. (c) Appendicitis typically presents with RLQ pain that may start in the periumbilical area. Eosinophilia is not present. (d) Hepatitis usually presents with fever, chills, and pain but not typically associated with eosinophilia. (**e**) Pyogenic abscess is the most common type of liver abscess, however, the history of travel, eosinophilia, and lack of primary source for the pyogenic abscess make it less likely a diagnosis.

109. The answer is d. (*Tintinalli, pp 561–565.*) The ultrasound shows a *gallbladder* with multiple *echogenic gallstones* associated with well-defined *acoustic shadows*. This image is typical for *cholelithiasis*. If the patient was febrile and thought to have cholecystitis, then one may also observe gallbladder distention, wall thickening, and pericholecystic fluid in addition to gallstones. The most common clinical manifestation of cholelithiasis is biliary colic.

(**a**) Renal stones will also appear as echogenic structures casting shadows within a central cavity, but the cavity in the figure does not have the appearance of a renal calyx on ultrasound. In addition, the liver is closely associated with the gallbladder, which is clearly noted in this ultrasound. (**b**) An ultrasound of a pancreatic pseudocyst would show a thick-walled, fluid-filled spherical structure without multiple echogenic structures casting shadows. (**c**) Ovarian cysts would not appear as multiple echogenic structures casting shadows within a central cavity, but rather as spherical, fluid-filled structures. (**e**) A liver abscess can be visualized on ultrasound as a hypoechoic area in one of the lobes of the liver.

110. The answer is a. (*Rosen, p 1275.*) All of the listed answers are late complications (occur after the second week of illness) of pancreatitis. However, the most common is a *pancreatic pseudocyst*, which is an encapsulated fluid collection that develops in 1–8% of patients after 4–6 weeks and is more common in alcoholic pancreatitis. Diagnosis is made with ultrasound or CT scan and treatment is surgical.

111. The answer is b. (*Rosen, pp 1330–1332.*) Management for *complicated acute diverticulitis* involves *admission* and *antibiotic treatment*. Treatment is directed against both anaerobic and gram-negative bacteria. Intra-abdominal *abscess* formation secondary to diverticulitis requires prompt surgical consultation and should be *drained* using CT or ultrasound-guided percutaneous draining. Abscesses less than 5 cm in diameter may be treated with antibiotics alone.

The patient's vital signs are stable and there is no evidence for peritonitis, therefore she does not require an emergent laparotomy (**a**). The patient should not be discharged from the hospital (**c**). Because of the risk for bowel perforation, barium enema and colonoscopy are contraindicated (**d & e**) however, once the diverticulitis is controlled, the patient should undergo one of the procedures to look for other pathology and exclude complications such as fistula formation.

112. The answer is e. *(Rosen, p 1294.)* *Rovsing's sign* is the referred tenderness to the RLQ when the left lower quadrant is palpated. It is seen with *acute appendicitis.*

Blumberg's sign (**a**) is the occurrence of a sharp pain when the examiner presses his or her hand over McBurney's point and then releases the hand pressure suddenly. This sign is indicative of peritoneal inflammation. The Psoas sign (**b**) is the increase of pain when the psoas muscle is stretched as the patient extends his or her hip. The Obturator sign (**c**) is the elicitation of pain as the hip is flexed and internally rotated. Raynaud's sign (**d**) is a condition marked by symmetrical cyanosis of the extremities with persistent, uneven, mottled blue or red discoloration of the skin of the digits, wrists, and ankles and with profuse sweating and coldness of the fingers and toes.

113. The answer is a. *(Rosen, pp 1283–1287.)* The patient's clinical picture is consistent with a *small bowel obstruction. Fluid resuscitation* is important due to the inability of the distended bowel to absorb fluid and electrolytes at a normal rate. Compounded with vomiting, fluid loses can lead to hypovolemia and shock. *Nasogastric suction* provides enteral decompression by removing accumulated gas and fluid proximal to the obstruction. A *surgical consult* is necessary because definitive treatment may require taking the patient to the OR to relieve the obstruction. An old surgical adage states "Never let the sun set or rise on a bowel obstruction." Broad-spectrum antibiotics are appropriate when surgery is planned or when there is suspicion for vascular compromise or bowel perforation.

Stool softener and enemas (**c**) have no role in acute intestinal obstructions due to mechanical causes. Adult small bowel obstructions are diagnosed with an abdominal plain film, or CT scan (**e**).

114. The answer is b. *(Rosen, pp 1176–1185.)* The patient's presentation is worrisome for an *abdominal aortic aneurysm* (AAA). If the patient was hemodynamically unstable, he should be brought immediately to the OR for definitive repair. However, in the *stable* patient, imaging studies can aid in the diagnosis of an AAA. *Ultrasound* (US) is almost 100% *sensitive* in detecting AAA, it is noninvasive, and can be performed rapidly at the patient's bedside. If the entire abdominal aorta is visualized and found to be of normal diameter, it is safe to say that the patient's symptoms are not from an AAA. An alternative to US in the stable patient is a CT scan, which is essentially 100% accurate in determining the presence of an AAA. The CT scan is less subject to technical and interpretation errors than US.

(a) Angiography has no role in the early diagnosis of an AAA. Often the lumen of the aorta is narrowed by mural thrombus and may appear falsely normal. (c) MRI is often used to follow the growth of a known AAA over a period of months or years. (d) An enlarged calcific aorta can sometimes be detected by plain abdominal radiograph; however, the sensitivity is low. (e) D-dimer is not an established marker in the diagnosis of an AAA.

115. The answer is c. *(Rosen, pp 2416–2419.)* Any woman with abdominal pain, vaginal bleeding, and a positive pregnancy test needs to be ruled out for an *ectopic pregnancy*. Her vital signs are stable so that she can undergo a *transvaginal ultrasound*. This is used to document an intrauterine pregnancy and the health of the fetus. If no intrauterine pregnancy is observed, the suspicion for an ectopic pregnancy increases.

(a) Laparoscopy is an accurate diagnostic and therapeutic procedure that can be used in the patient with an unclear ultrasound and peritoneal signs on examination. (b) If an intrauterine pregnancy is documented and there is low suspicion for an ectopic pregnancy, yet the patient complains of severe RLQ pain, then the risks (e.g., radiation exposure to the fetus) and benefits (e.g., diagnosing appendicitis) for performing a CT scan must be discussed. (d) A urinalysis is part of the general workup but is not emergently needed. (e) Anti-D immune globulin should be administered if the patient is Rh-negative (unless the father is known to be Rh-negative). However, this can wait until the patient is diagnosed and further stabilized.

116. The answer is d. *(Rosen, pp 1272–1276.)* The patient's clinical picture is consistent with *acute pancreatitis*. Ranson developed criteria that help *predict mortality rates* in patients with pancreatitis. The presence of more than three criteria equals 1% mortality, while the presence of six or more criteria approaches 100% mortality. *Ranson's Criteria* at admission are age > 55, WBC > 16,000, glucose > 200, LDH > 350, AST > 250. Within 48 hours of admission, hematocrit fall > 10%, BUN rise > 5, serum calcium < 8, arterial PO_2 < 60, base deficit > 4, and fluid sequestration > 6 L. The patient in the case fulfills four of Ranson's criteria and has approximately 15% mortality risk. Note that lipase and amylase are not part of Ranson's criteria despite being relevant in the diagnosis of acute pancreatitis.

117. The answer is e. (*Rosen, p 223.*) The differential diagnosis in a woman with RLQ pain is expansive and includes GI pathology such as appendicitis, inflammatory bowel disease, diverticulitis, and hernia. Gynecologic pathology includes ectopic pregnancy, tubo-ovarian abscess, ruptured corpus luteum cyst, and ovarian torsion. It is often difficult to initially distinguish between GI and gynecological (GYN) pathology and which diagnostic test, abdominal CT, or a pelvic ultrasound, is warranted. Often, the decision is based on the pelvic exam. The patient in the question exhibits *adnexal tenderness* and therefore received a pelvic ultrasound that revealed a *unilateral enlarged ovary with decreased flow,* indicative of *ovarian torsion.* Ovarian torsion is a *gynecologic emergency* and conservative management has no place in the treatment decision of suspected torsion even if pain improves in the ED. Failure to surgically correct this entity may result in ischemia and subsequent necrosis of the involved ovary. Therefore, the mainstay of therapy is *laparoscopy or laparotomy.*

(**a**) Conservative management is not an option in suspected ovarian torsion. (**b**) Antibiotics and delayed surgery may be acceptable for a tubo-ovarian abscess. (**c**) Discharging the patient is unacceptable. (**d**) If pelvic ultrasound was normal and there is suspicion for a GI pathology, then abdominal CT is warranted.

118. The answer is b. (*Tintinalli, pp 697–699.*) *Pelvic inflammatory disease (PID)* comprises a spectrum of infections of the female upper reproductive tract. Although *Neisseria gonorrhoeae* and *Chlamydia trachomatis* are thought to cause the majority of infections, new evidence points to greater rates of polymicrobial infections. Most cases of PID are thought to start with a sexually transmitted disease of the lower genital tract and ascend to the upper tract. Women typically present with lower abdominal pain and may have vaginal discharge, vaginal bleeding, dysuria, and fever. The exam usually reveals *lower abdominal tenderness* and *cervical motion tenderness or adnexal tenderness.* Many patients are treated as outpatients with antibiotics. Considerations for admission include those women who are pregnant, failed outpatient therapy, are toxic appearing, have evidence for a tubo-ovarian abscess, or a surgical emergency cannot be ruled out. Long-term outcomes are improved if antibiotics are begun immediately.

(a) The onset of appendicitis is more insidious than what is presented in this case. The initial symptoms are usually nausea or loss of appetite. Pain typically begins in the periumbilical area and migrates to the RLQ. Fever is usually not significant unless the appendix ruptures. (c) Culdocentesis is used to retrieve fluid in the cul-de-sac. The findings are limited and not specific to PID. (d) A dilation and curettage scrapes the endometrium which may aggravate and perpetuate the pelvic infection. (e) There is no role for a plain film in this patient. It would be useful if you suspected a bowel obstruction or free air.

119. The answer is b. *(Tintinalli, pp 524–526.)* The clinical scenario and radiograph are consistent with *small bowel obstruction (SBO)*. Patients usually present with *diffuse, crampy abdominal pain that* is often episodic in nature. Typically, the patient reports no recent bowel movements or flatus passage. The most common causes of SBO are *adhesions and hernias.* All patients with suspected SBO should have flat and upright abdominal radiographs. Flat-plate abdominal films can show distended loops of small bowel and the upright film can show multiple air-fluid levels in a stepladder appearance.

(a) Constipation is a diagnosis of exclusion, although fecal impaction is a common problem in elderly debilitated patients and may present with symptoms of colonic obstruction. (c) Cholelithiasis typically presents with RUQ pain and fever. Ultrasound is typically used to make the diagnosis of cholecystitis. (d) The most common causes of large bowel obstruction include neoplasm, diverticulitis, and sigmoid volvulus. The large bowel contains folds called haustra that do not cross the entire length of the bowel width. In the above figure, we see *valvulae coniventes,* which are folds of the small bowel that cross the entire width of the bowel. (e) Neither the clinical scenario nor the plain film is consistent with inflammatory bowel disease. Most patients with inflammatory bowel disease are younger.

120. The answer is a. *(Tintinalli, pp 536–537.)* Left lower quadrant tenderness in a *patient older than 60 years* should always suggest the diagnosis of *diverticulitis.* The incidence of diverticulitis increases with age and one-third of the population will have acquired the disease by age 50. *Low-grade fever* and *leukocytosis* are common; rebound tenderness is consistent with peritoneal inflammation. The involved diverticulum may irritate the bladder or ureter, causing the patient to have urinary complaints. CT scan is the diagnostic procedure of choice.

(b) Acute cholecystitis presents with RUQ pain that may radiate to the ipsilateral scapula. (c) Pyelonephritis is in the differential but the localization of this patient's symptoms is far more suggestive of diverticulitis. (d) Appendicitis should always be in the differential of abdominal pain. It usually begins as a dull periumbilical pain that migrates to the RLQ. (e) Spontaneous bacterial peritonitis typically occurs in patients with liver pathology and ascites.

121. The answer is a. (*Rosen, pp 1293–1295.*) The test is the *Obturator sign,* in which the patient is supine with the right thigh flexed; passive internal or external rotation of the hip eliciting pain is a positive test for *appendicitis.* The pain is due to an inflamed appendix that is irritated by stretching the obturator internus muscle.

(b) The iliopsoas sign for appendicitis is tested by having the patient lie on his or her left side; pain caused by passive right thigh extension is a positive result. (c) Rovsing's sign refers to pain in the RLQ elicited by palpation in the LLQ. (d) McBurney's point is the classic location of maximum tenderness to palpation in the RLQ, one-third the distance from the anterior superior iliac crest to the umbilicus. It is common in patients with an anterior appendix. (e) Murphy's sign refers to pain causing cessation of respiration during palpation of the RUQ and is seen in acute cholecystitis.

122. The answer is c. (*Rosen, pp 1301–1307.*) Diarrhea is caused by a variety of organisms including bacteria, viruses, and parasites. *Enterotoxigenic E. coli* (ETEC) is the primary agent identified in *traveler's diarrhea* secondary to the ingestion of *contaminated food or water.* Watery diarrhea typically begins after a few days of travel. Most cases of traveler's diarrhea come from Mexico, South America, or Africa. Fluids and electrolytes, along with antidiarrheal agents, are the mainstay of treatment for traveler's diarrhea.

(a, b, d, e) These organisms invade the intestinal mucosa and cause bloody mucoid stools. The presence of fecal leukocytes and occult blood is a sensitive and specific predictor for an invasive bacterial cause of diarrhea and a likelihood of a positive bacterial stool culture.

123. The answer is b. (*Tintinalli, pp 584–585.*) Although there are no studies stating how long it takes for a tract to mature, tracts that are 7–10 days old probably will remain open long enough to allow replacement. Insertion of a new tube should be performed with water-soluble lubricant. If resistance is met, the attempt should be aborted. After replacing the tube,

20–30 mL bolus of *water soluble contrast* material should be instilled into the tube, and a supine *abdominal radiograph* should demonstrate rugae of the stomach. If there is any question of improper placement, immediate consultation should be obtained.

(a) Aspiration of gastric contents does not confirm proper placement of a G-tube. The intragastric location of a replaced tube should be confirmed by a contrast study before feedings. Many patients have received intraperitoneal feedings in the absence of such a confirmatory test. (c) If the tract is open, a tube should be replaced; otherwise observation would be appropriate until a new tube could be arranged. (d) A CT scan may be helpful to determine if the tube is out, but once it is, clinical signs would be sufficient to evaluate for intraperitoneal soilage. (e) Surgical G-tubes generally involve anchoring the stomach to the anterior abdominal wall. Contamination is unlikely and the tube tract will be patent for a short time. There is no immediate indication for surgery.

124. The answer is a. *(Rosen, pp 11415–11422.)* An *obstructing stone with an overlying infection* is an impending *urologic emergency.* Bacteria in an obstructed collecting system can cause abscess formation, renal destruction, and severe systemic toxicity. The patient requires admission for IV antibiotics and removal and drainage of the stone. In addition to obstruction with infection, other indications for admission include persistent pain, persistent nausea and vomiting, urinary extravasation, and hypercalcemic crisis.

(b) Observation is not recommended. Stones smaller than 4 mm pass 90% of the time, stones 4–6 mm pass 50% of the time, and stones larger than 6 mm pass 10% of the time. The patient requires IV antibiotics and removal of the stone. (c, d, & e) The patient should not be discharged; rather admission is required for an infected obstructing stone. Although it is important to keep the patient well hydrated, no evidence supports the notion that IV hydration increases likelihood of stone passage.

125. The answer is d. *(Tintinalli, pp 1878–1883.)* CT scanning has become an integral part of the ED evaluation of a patient. It is useful to differentiate abdominal pathologies when the history and physical exam are nonspecific or in confirming a diagnosis suspected by the clinical presentation. Contrast materials for CT exams in the ED are usually administered via oral and IV routes, which improves visualization of abdominal organs. *A patient must be relatively stable to undergo a CT scan.* The patient with abdominal pain and a BP of 70/50 mm Hg is not hemodynamically stable. His clinical presentation is consistent with a ruptured abdominal aortic aneurysm. This is a surgical emergency and should be treated in the OR. Obtaining a CT scan first will delay definitive treatment and worsen the patient's hemorrhagic shock and ultimately decrease his chance of survival.

(a) This patient sustained blunt trauma and does not show evidence of an active bleed on the FAST exam. With stable vital signs, a CT scan is safe. (b) This patient may have appendicitis and requires a CT scan. If she was β-hCG positive, you would first perform a pelvic US to evaluate for an ectopic pregnancy. (c) Pancreatitis is high on the differential; a CT scan will help to evaluate his abdominal pain. (e) This patient most likely has a kidney stone, which is seen on abdominal CT scan.

126. The answer is c. *(Rosen, pp 1283–1287.)* The clinical scenario is highly suspicious for a *strangulated loop of bowel* incarcerated in a *femoral hernia.* A closed-loop obstruction implies that a segment of bowel is obstructed at two sequential sites, usually by twisting about a constricting adhesive band or hernia opening. This mechanism of obstruction has a high risk of compromising intestinal blood flow with resulting intestinal ischemia, a condition referred to as *strangulation obstruction.*

(a & d) The physical exam is highly suspicious for the presence of intra-abdominal complications associated with the obstruction; therefore a CT scan or plain film is unlikely to contribute further in the diagnosis. (b) Nonoperative therapy is inappropriate for a patient with suspected complicated bowel strangulation. (e) Antibiotics alone are insufficient, surgery is required.

127. The answer is b. *(Rosen, pp 1301–1313.)* *Staphylococcal-related food poisoning* is caused by an enterotoxin forming strain of *Staphylococcus* organisms in the food before ingestion. Most *protein-rich foods* support the growth of staphylococci, particularly ham, eggs, custard, mayonnaise, and potato salad. The illness has an *abrupt onset,* beginning *1–6 hours* after ingestion of the contaminated food. Cramping and abdominal pain, with *violent and frequent retching and vomiting* are the predominant symptoms. Diarrhea is variable; it is usually mild, and occasionally absent. Although often violent appearing, staphylococcal food poisoning is *short-lived* and usually *subsides in 6–8 hours* and rarely lasts more than 24 hours. The patient is often recovering when first seen by a physician. The *short incubation period* and *multiple cases* in persons eating the same meal are highly suggestive of this disease.

(a) Scombroid fish poisoning results from the ingestion of heat-stable toxins produced by bacterial action on the dark meat of the fish (e.g., tuna and mackerel). The symptoms resemble histamine intoxication, occur abruptly within 20–30 minutes and consist of facial flushing, diarrhea, throbbing headache, palpitations, and abdominal cramps. Antihistamine therapy is usually curative. (c) *Clostridium perfringens* is probably the most common cause of acute food poisoning in the United States. Most cases occur in fairly large outbreaks and are caused by the ingestion of meat and poultry dishes. Symptoms usually appear within 6–12 hours but can occur up to 24 hours after ingestion of the contaminated food. Frequent, watery diarrhea and moderately severe abdominal cramping are the major symptoms. The illness is self-limited and rarely lasts for more than 24 hours. (d) Campylobacter is the most common bacterial cause of diarrhea in patients who seek medical attention. The incubation period is approximately 2–5 days. Onset of symptoms is usually rapid and consists of fever, crampy abdominal pain, and diarrhea. Constitutional symptoms are common. (e) Salmonellosis occurs most during the summer months and is acquired by the ingestion of contaminated food or drink. Poultry products such as turkey, chicken, duck, and eggs constitute the most common sources. Family outbreaks and sporadic cases are more common than large epidemics. The typical patient presents with fever, colicky abdominal pain, and loose, watery diarrhea, occasionally with mucus and blood. Symptoms usually abate within 2–5 days and recovery is uneventful.

128. The answer is b. (*Rosen, pp 1288–1291.*) *Acute mesenteric ischemia* is due to the lack of perfusion to the bowel. It primarily affects patients *over the age of 50 years,* particularly those with significant cardiovascular or systemic disease. Most patients present with abdominal pain that is initially dull and diffuse. In this early state, patients frequently complain of severe pain but have minimal tenderness on exam; the characteristic *"pain out of proportion to exam."* As infarction develops, peritoneal signs develop. Sudden onset of pain suggests arterial vascular occlusion by emboli. This may occur with patients who present in *atrial fibrillation.* Insidious onset suggests venous thrombosis or nonocclusive infarction. Radiographs may reveal dilated loops of bowel, air in the bowel wall, which is known as *pneumatosis intestinalis,* and thickening of the bowel wall, as seen in the CT scan above. Management involves fluid resuscitation, antibiotics, and surgical intervention.

(a) Classically, AAA present with constant abdominal pain, often localizing to the left middle or lower quadrant with radiation to the back. Physical exam may reveal a pulsatile abdominal mass. (c) Diverticulitis usually presents with left lower quadrant abdominal pain and low-grade fever. (d) Patients with a small bowel obstruction present with crampy abdominal pain and distention. Vomiting and obstipation are frequent symptoms. Distended loops of bowel and air-fluid levels are seen on radiographs. (e) Crohn's disease may present with bloody diarrhea, abdominal pain, fevers, anorexia, and weight loss. There is a peak incidence between 15 and 22 years and 55 and 60 years.

129. The answer is c. (*Tintinalli, pp 616–617.*) *Torsion* is twisting of the spermatic cord and testis, occluding the venous system and decreasing arterial flow. It commonly occurs during puberty at an average age of 17 years. Torsion results from maldevelopment of fixation between the enveloping tunica vaginalis and the posterior scrotal wall as seen with an *undescended testicle*. Characteristically, the involved testis is aligned along a horizontal rather than a vertical axis. Frequently there is a history of an athletic event, strenuous physical activity, or trauma just before the onset of scrotal pain. However, it may occur during sleep. The pain usually occurs suddenly, is severe, and is usually felt in the lower abdominal quadrant, the inguinal canal, or the testis.

(a) Peak incidence of torsion occurs at puberty, but may occur at any age. (b & d) Fixed testis or short spermatic cord is not associated with increased likelihood of torsion. (e) Although epididymitis may mimic symptoms of torsion, it does not increase the likelihood for torsion.

130. The answer is b. (*Hamilton, p 6.*) The *emergency physician* (EP) approaches a problem by *considering the most serious disease* consistent with the patient complaint and working to exclude it. Thinking of the *worst* first is a reversal from the sequence in many other specialties. Once the EP rules out the life-threatening processes, are the more benign processes considered. This principle is particularly important when placed in the context of the patient population seen in the ED. Most of the patients are new to the EP; many are intoxicated or are brought to the ED by others. This leads to an array of fragmented histories, masked physical findings, and high emotional levels. In this setting, it is even more important for the EP to maintain a high level of suspicion for serious disease.

All of the conditions listed as answer choices can be responsible for the patient's presentation. As discussed, it is important to first rule out the life-threatening processes. To address these processes, the patient requires a β-hCG to rule out an ectopic pregnancy, either an ultrasound or CT scan to evaluate for appendicitis, and a urinalysis to investigate pyelonephritis.

131. The answer is e. *(Riviello, RJ. Emergency Medicine Reports 26(19) Sept 5 2005.)* When a sexual assault patient is evaluated in the ED, the EP not only has the standard responsibility to care for the patient's physical and psychological health, but also needs to be conscientious that the encounter will have considerable impact once the patient is discharged from the ED. Once life-threatening injuries are addressed, EPs are responsible for collecting physical evidence necessary for prosecuting the assailant by conducting a sexual assault or "rape kit" with the patient's consent.

Most medications provided to sexually assaulted patients are provided as prophylaxis against sexually transmitted infections (STIs), pregnancy, and tetanus. Major STIs of concern are gonorrhea *(ceftriaxone)*, Chlamydia *(azithromycin or doxycycline)*, syphilis, and trichomoniasis *(metronidazole)* because of their relative high incidence. The average risk of HIV transmission per contact of unprotected receptive anal intercourse is approximately 1–5%. For unprotected insertive anal intercourse and receptive vaginal intercourse, the risk is approximately 0.1–1%. The decision to provide *HIV postexposure prophylaxis (PEP)* after sexual assault must take into account the likelihood of exposure to HIV, the interval between exposure and treatment with antiretrovirals, and the risks and benefits of treatment. Some states mandate offering and providing HIV PEP to all sexually assaulted patients. The risk of pregnancy following sexual assault is approximately 5%. *Emergency contraception* is the use of hormone pills to prevent pregnancy. Patients who never received a hepatitis B vaccination, the vaccine should be administered. If vaccination status is unclear, obtain hepatitis serology, and if not immune, proceed with vaccination. For patients that were previously fully vaccinated for hepatitis B, further therapy is not required. Tetanus is administered to patients who sustain tetanus-prone injuries.

132. The answer is e. *(Rosen, pp 1283–1287.)* Overall, adhesions, hernias, and cancer account for more than 90% of cases of small bowel obstruction (SBO). *Postoperative adhesions* are the *most common cause of SBO* (50–55%), followed by incarcerated hernia (25%). Approximately 5% of all postoperative laparotomy patients develop adhesive obstruction, years after surgery. The most common locations of obstruction from a hernia are inguinal followed by femoral. Cancer is the cause 10% of the time. Other less common causes include inflammatory bowel disease, gallstones, volvulus, intussusception, radiation enteritis, abscesses, congenital lesions, and bezoars.

133. The answer is c. (*Rosen, pp 1422–1423.*) *Manual detorsion* is a maneuver used to untwist the spermatic cord to *reestablish blood flow to the testis.* This procedure should be performed in any patient with suspected torsion while the patient is being prepared for the OR. Most testes torse lateral to medial. If you were to stand at the foot of the patient's bed, you would perform detorsion for either testis just as you would *open a book*— rotating each testicle in a *medial to lateral direction.* Successful detorsion results in immediate reduction of pain. In many cases, detorsion is not successful or the testis twists again.

134. The answer is a. (*Rosen, pp 1176–1183.*) The radiograph demonstrates an AAA. Signs of AAA large enough to cause symptoms are seen on plain radiographs approximately 66–75% of the time. The most common findings are *curvilinear calcification of the aortic wall* or a *paravertebral soft tissue mass.* Rarely, with longstanding aneurysms, erosion of one or more vertebral bodies may be seen. *Atherosclerosis,* age > 60, smoking, and family history are all important predisposing factor for the development of AAA.

(**b**) Hyperparathyroidism may be seen in patients with recurring renal calculi. (**c**) Ethanol abuse can cause pancreatitis. (**d**) Prostate cancer can metastasize to the vertebral column causing blastic lesions of the spine. (**e**) Hernias are the second most common cause of bowel obstruction preceded by adhesions.

135. The answer is d. (*Rosen, pp 2416–2418.*) You should be concerned about a *ruptured ectopic pregnancy* in this patient. She *missed her last menstrual period,* has *severe pain in the lower abdomen,* and is *hypotensive.* This is a *life-threatening condition* that needs to be managed aggressively. The patient requires fluid resuscitation with 2 L normal saline. If her BP does not respond to the bolus, then blood should be administered. The patient will most likely be taken to the OR for a salpingectomy/oophorectomy. Risk factors for an ectopic pregnancy include history of pelvic inflammatory disease, prior ectopic pregnancy, pelvic surgery, and intrauterine device (IUD) use.

(**a**) This will treat the pain but not its etiology. The patient is hypotensive and this needs to be addressed. (**b**) This is a plan for acute appendicitis, which is lower on the differential for this presentation than ectopic pregnancy. (c) This is a plan if you are suspecting a renal calculus, which would present with flank pain and microhematuria. (e) If the patient was stable then a pelvic ultrasound might be helpful in diagnosing an ectopic pregnancy.

136. The answer is d. (*Rosen, pp 1266–1268.*) *Murphy's sign* is named after the Chicago surgeon, John B. Murphy. The patient is asked to take a deep breath while the examiner applies pressure over the area of the gallbladder. If the *gallbladder is inflamed,* the descending diaphragm forces it against the examiner's fingertips, causing pain and often a *sudden pause to inspiration.* A sonographic Murphy's sign elicits the same response with an ultrasound probe over the gallbladder.

(a) Grey-Turner's sign is ecchymotic skin in the flank area that indicates retroperitoneal blood. It is commonly associated with hemorrhagic pancreatitis. (b) Kernig's sign may be seen in patients with meningitis; patients cannot extend the leg at the knee when the thigh is flexed because of stiffness in the hamstrings (c) McMurray's sign is present when manipulation of the tibia with the leg flexed produces pain and a pronounced click when the meniscus has been injured. If the click occurs when the foot is rotated inward, the tear is in the lateral meniscus. (d) McBurney's sign represents maximum tenderness and rigidity over McBurney's point, which may be indicative of appendicitis.

137. The answer is c. (*Rosen, pp 1330–1331.*) The clinical signs and symptoms of *acute diverticulitis* vary with the severity of disease. The predominant symptom in patients with sigmoid diverticulitis is persistent *abdominal pain,* which starts as vague and generalized but localizes to the *left lower quadrant. Constipation* and *low-grade fever* are common. *Urinary symptoms* can occur due to intestinal inflammation near the ureter or bladder. Although stool samples may be guaiac positive for occult blood, gross bleeding is unusual. Don't confuse diverticulitis and diverticulosis, the latter is associated with gross bleeding.

138. The answer is c. (*Tintinalli, pp 1547–1551.*) *Crohn's disease* is characterized by *chronic inflammation extending through all layers of the bowel wall.* Onset is generally between the ages of 15 and 40 years. Crohn's disease should be suspected in any patient whose symptoms show a picture consistent with chronic inflammatory colitis. Extraintestinal manifestations are seen in 25–30% of patients. The incidence is similar for Crohn's disease and ulcerative colitis. They include aphthous ulcers, erythema nodosum, iritis or episcleritis, arthritis, and gallstones. *Nephrolithiasis* is seen as a result of hyperoxaluria due to increased oxalate absorption in patients with ileal disease. Because ulcerative colitis affects only the large bowel, this extraintestinal manifestation is seen only in patients with Crohn's disease.

139. The answer is e. (*Tintinalli, pp 606–611.*) *Chlamydia trachomatis urethritis* accounts for 5–20% of cases of dysuria, and its presence may be *suspected when urine cultures are sterile.* If clinical symptoms and urinalysis point to a UTI, urine cultures are sterile, and standard antibiotic regimens effective against most urinary pathogens fail, consider Chlamydia urethritis.

(a) Although group A streptococcus is a possible pathogen, it would be very rare and would be susceptible in most cases to the antibiotics that the patient has taken. **(b)** Initial episodes of herpes simplex virus can result in symptoms that mimic true dysuria secondary to sensitivity of lesions on the external genital surface or near the urethra. Generally, these episodes are accompanied by fever, chills, and systemic symptoms, in addition to extremely painful and tender lesions. Also, urinary frequency would not be common. **(c)** Although *T. vaginalis* would not respond to the previous antibiotic therapy, trichomoniasis presents with a copious frothy vaginal discharge and would have been seen on wet mount preparation of the vaginal secretions. **(d)** *E. coli* accounts for 70–90% of community-acquired UTIs in women. In a woman without recurrent UTIs, the antibiotics taken by this patient would be appropriate. In a patient with recurrent UTIs, it is more likely that the *E. coli* would be resistant to standard antimicrobial regimens. This pathogen should have also been grown on the standard culture medium.

140. The answer is e. (*Rosen, pp 223–224.*) The patient has *ovarian torsion.* Torsion of the ovary around its vascular pedicle almost always occurs in the presence of a pathologically large, *simple cyst that is greater than 6 cm,* or when an ovarian *tumor* is solid or heavily cystic. The onset of pain is classically sudden, sharp, unilateral, and often intermittent. Many patients have a history of a similar pain that resolved spontaneously.

(a) Appendicitis is characterized by abdominal pain, usually beginning as a vague, constant pain in the epigastric or periumbilical region and localizing to the RLQ. **(b)** Ectopic pregnancy is unlikely in a patient with a negative β-hCG. **(c)** Tubo-ovarian abscess develops as a complication of pelvic inflammatory disease and is not sudden in onset. (e) Mittelschmerz is pain secondary to ovulation and should not be the cause in this patient as her last menstruation was 3 weeks ago.

141. The answer is b. *(Tintinalli, pp 520–523.)* This patient presents with a history typical of *appendicitis;* gradual onset of abdominal pain, loss of appetite, and mild nausea. Her physical exam reveals a low-grade fever, RLQ tenderness and a positive Rovsing's sign (pain in the RLQ with palpation in another area). As long as the patient is stable, CT scan is the best test choice as an initial imaging study and appears to change management decisions and decrease unnecessary appendectomies in women.

(a) The patient is using oral contraceptives and her last menstrual period was 3 weeks ago. Ectopic pregnancy is unlikely, however, a β-hCG should be obtained to rule out the possibility of an ectopic pregnancy. (c) Her adnexae and ovaries appear normal on exam so a clinically significant ovarian cyst can be ruled out. (d) A tubo-ovarian abscess (TOA) usually develops from prior PID. Often the infection has gone untreated for a while. A TOA should be suspected if an adnexal mass is palpated or there is tenderness of the adnexae or cervix. (e) 90% of ureteral calculi up to 5 mm in diameter pass spontaneously. Typically, patients present with colicky flank pain that radiates to the groin. They may feel nauseated and are usually in significant pain.

142. The answer is e. *(Tintinalli, pp 573–575.)* Abdominal pain that radiates to the back and is associated with nausea, vomiting, epigastric tenderness, and an elevated lipase in a patient with a history of ethanol abuse all point to a diagnosis of *alcoholic pancreatitis.* Although patients with mild pancreatitis, no evidence of systemic complications, and a low likelihood of biliary tract disease may be managed as outpatients, this patient requires admission for the rapid progression of symptoms, severity of pain, and potential unreliability of the patient. The initial treatment for acute pancreatitis is *supportive: bowel rest, fluid resuscitation, and analgesia.* Ninety percent of patients recover without complications. Surgery is reserved for complications of alcoholic pancreatitis, such as pseudocysts, phlegmons, and abscesses.

(a, b, c) As discussed above, this patient with pancreatitis requires admission to the hospital for medical management. (d) Endoscopy is used for patients with ulcerative disease. ERCP is used in patients in whom the etiology of pancreatitis remains unclear after initial assessment.

Gastrointestinal Bleeding

Questions

143. A 51-year-old man is brought to the emergency department (ED) by emergency medical service (EMS) with a blood pressure (BP) of 90/60 mm Hg, heart rate (HR) 110 beats per minute, respiratory rate (RR) 18 breaths per minute, and oxygen saturation of 97% on room air. The patient tells you that he has a history of bleeding ulcers. On exam, his abdomen is tender in the epigastric area. He is guaiac positive with black stool. He has a bout of hematemesis and you notice that his BP is now 80/50 mm Hg, HR is 114 beats per minute, and the patient is starting to drift off. Which of the following is the most appropriate next step in therapy?

a. Assess airway, establish two large-bore IVs, cross-match for two units of blood, administer 1–2 liters of normal saline, and schedule an emergent endoscopy

b. Assess airway, establish two large-bore IVs, crossmatch for two units of blood, and administer a proton pump inhibitor

c. Place two large-bore IVs, crossmatch for two units of blood, administer a 1–2 liters of normal saline, and schedule an emergent endoscopy

d. Intubate the patient, establish two large-bore IVs, cross-match for two units of blood, administer a 1–2 liters of normal saline, and schedule an emergent endoscopy

e. Intubate the patient, establish two large-bore IVs, crossmatch for two units of blood, and administer a proton pump inhibitor

144. A 68-year-old man presents to the ED with abdominal pain, fever, and diarrhea for the past 2 days. His vitals are HR 95 beats per minute, BP 130/85 mm Hg, RR 18 breaths per minute, and temperature 101°F. He has tenderness to palpation in the left lower quadrant, with mild distention and voluntary guarding. His stool is guaiac positive. Which of the following is the most likely diagnosis?

a. Appendicitis
b. Crohn's disease (CD)
c. Diverticulitis
d. Ogilvie's syndrome
e. Diverticulosis

145. A 45-year-old woman presents to the ED with painful rectal bleeding. The bleeding initially was painless but now, she states, the pain has worsened over the past day, especially with defecation. Review of systems is negative for weight loss, abdominal pain, nausea, and vomiting. On physical exam you note an exquisitely tender swelling with engorgement and a bluish discoloration at the anal verge. Her vital signs are HR 98 beats per minute, BP 140/70 mm Hg, RR 18 breaths per minute, and temperature 99°F. Which of the following is the next best step in management?

a. Recommend warm sitz baths, topical analgesics, stool softeners, and a high-fiber diet, and arrange for surgical follow-up
b. Incision and drainage under local anesthesia or procedural sedation followed by packing and surgical follow-up
c. Obtain a complete blood cell (CBC) count, clotting studies, type and cross, and arrange for emergent colonoscopy
d. Excision under local anesthesia followed by sitz baths and analgesics
e. Surgical consult for immediate operative management

146. A 20-year-old man presents to the ED with fever and severe right lower quadrant (RLQ) pain for 1 day. Prior to this episode, he reports 2 months of crampy abdominal pain, generalized malaise, a 10-lb weight loss, and occasional bloody diarrhea. Vitals are HR 115 beats per minute, BP 125/70 mm Hg, RR of 18 breaths per minute, and temperature of 100.8°F. His only significant past medical history is recurrent perirectal abscesses. On physical exam, the patient appears uncomfortable and has a tender mass is in the RLQ, without guarding or rebound. Rectal exam is positive for trace heme-positive stool. An abdominal computed tomography (CT) scan demonstrates a contrast-filled appendix and inflammation of the distal ileum and several areas of the colon without rectal involvement. Which of the following is the most likely diagnosis?

a. CD
b. Ulcerative colitis (UC)
c. Appendicitis
d. Pseudomembranous enterocolitis
e. Diverticulitis

147. A 62-year-old man with a history of hypertension presents to the ED with severe constant mid-epigastric pain for the past hour. Over the last several months, he has had intermittent pain shortly after eating, but never this severe. He states he now has generalized abdominal pain that began suddenly about 15 minutes ago. He has no history of trauma, has never had surgery, and takes no medications. His vitals are HR 115 beats per minute lying supine and increases to 135 when sitting up, BP 170/105 mm Hg supine and falls to 145/85 mm Hg when sitting up. He appears pale. His abdomen is rigid and diffusely tender with guarding and rebound. Bowel sounds are absent and stool hemoccult is positive. The white blood cell (WBC) count is 8,500/μL, hemoglobin 8.5 mg/dL, hematocrit 27%, and platelets 255/μL. Which of the following is the most likely diagnosis?

a. Diverticulosis
b. Perforated gastric ulcer
c. Abdominal aortic aneurysm (AAA)
d. Inflammatory bowel disease (IBD)
e. Splenic laceration

148. A 60-year-old man with a history of alcohol abuse presents to the ED with hematemesis for 1 day. He denies abdominal or chest pain. On physical exam, his eyes appear reddened and he admits to drinking heavily the night before after which he vomited several times. Vital signs are HR 115 beats per minute, BP 130/85 mm Hg, RR 18 breaths per minute, and temperature 99.5°F. Chest radiograph is unremarkable. Lab results reveal a WBC 10,000/μL, hemoglobin 14 mg/dL, hematocrit 40%, and platelets 210/μL. Endoscopy confirms the diagnosis, which is most likely?

a. Esophageal varices
b. Boerhaave's syndrome
c. Curling ulcer
d. Perforated gastric ulcer
e. Mallory-Weiss tear

149. A 50-year-old man is brought to the ED by ambulance with significant hematemesis. In the ambulance, paramedics placed two large-bore IVs and began infusing normal saline. His vital signs are HR 127 beats per minute, BP 79/45 mm Hg, temperature 97.9°F, RR 24 breaths per minute, and SaO$_2$ 96%. On physical exam, his abdomen is nontender, but you note spider angiomata, palmar erythema, and gynecomastia. Laboratory results reveal WBC 9000/μL, hematocrit 28%, platelets 40/μL, aspartate transaminase (AST) 675 U/L, alanine transaminase (ALT) 325 U/L, alkaline phosphatase 95 U/L, total bilirubin 14.4, conjugated bilirubin 12.9, sodium 135 mEq/L, potassium 3.5 mEq/L, chloride 110 mEq/L, bicarbonate 26 mEq/L, blood urea nitrogen (BUN) 20 mg/dL, creatinine 1.1 mg/dL, and glucose 150 mg/dL. Which of the following is the most likely diagnosis?

a. Perforated gastric ulcer
b. Diverticulosis
c. Splenic laceration
d. Esophageal varices
e. Ruptured abdominal aortic aneurysm

150. A 55-year-old man is brought to the ED by his family. They state that he has been vomiting large amounts of bright red blood. The patient in an alcoholic with cirrhotic liver disease; he has a known history of portal hypertension and esophageal varices. His vitals on arrival are HR 110 beats per minute, BP 80/55 mm Hg, RR 22 breaths per minute, and temperature 99°F. The patient appears pale and is in moderate distress. Which of the following would *not* be considered appropriate in the *initial* management of a hypotensive patient with a history of known esophageal varices presenting with hematemesis?

a. Sengstaken-Blakemore tube placement
b. Two large-bore intravenous (IV) lines and volume repletion with crystalloid solutions
c. Nasogastric (NG) lavage
d. Intravenous (IV) octreotide
e. Gastrointestinal (GI) consult

151. A 70-year-old woman presents to the ED with dark stool for 2 weeks. She occasionally notes bright red blood mixed with the stool. Review of systems is positive for 10-lb weight loss over 2 months and light-headedness when she stands. She denies abdominal pain, nausea, vomiting, and fever. Examination reveals a pale female with a supine BP 100/60 mm Hg, HR of

105 beats per minute. Standing BP is 90/50 mm Hg, with a pulse of 130 beats per minute. The most likely diagnosis in this patient is:

a. Hemorrhoids
b. Diverticulitis
c. Mallory-Weiss tear
d. CD
e. Adenocarcinoma

152. A 65-year-old woman with a history of hypertension and diverticular disease presents with 2 days of constant left lower quadrant pain, worsening constipation, and fever. Her vitals are HR of 100 beats per minute, BP 130/85 mm Hg, RR of 20 breaths per minute, and temperature 100.8°F. On physical exam, she is tender in the left lower quadrant without rebound or guarding, and her stool is trace heme-positive. Which of the following is the most appropriate diagnostic test?

a. Abdominal CT
b. Barium enema
c. Colonoscopy
d. Abdominal radiograph
e. Abdominal ultrasound

153. A 76-year-old woman with a history of congestive heart failure, coronary artery disease, and an "irregular heart beat" is brought to the ED by her family. She has been complaining of increasing abdominal pain over the past several days. She denies nausea or vomiting and bowel movements remain unchanged. Vitals are HR of 114 beats per minute, BP 110/75 mm Hg, and temperature 98°F. On cardiac exam, her HR is irregularly irregular and no murmur is detected. The abdomen is soft, nontender, and nondistended. The stool is heme-positive. This patient is at high risk for which of the following conditions?

a. Perforated gastric ulcer
b. Diverticulitis
c. Acute cholecystitis
d. Mesenteric ischemia
e. Sigmoid volvulus

154. A 70-year-old woman with a history of hypertension, congestive heart failure, and atrial fibrillation presents to the ED with several hours of acute onset diffuse abdominal pain. She denies any nausea or vomiting. The pain is constant but she is unable to localize it. She was diagnosed with a renal artery thrombosis several years ago. Vital signs are HR 95 beats per minute, BP 110/70 mm Hg, and temperature 98°F. Her abdomen is soft and mildly tender, despite her reported severe abdominal pain. Her white blood count is 12,000/μL, hematocrit 38%, platelets 250/μL, and lactate 8 mg/dL. The stool is trace heme-positive. You are concerned for acute mesenteric ischemia. What is the best way to diagnose this condition?

a. Angiography
b. Abdominal radiograph (supine and upright)
c. CT
d. Serial serum lactate and creatine phosphokinase (CPK) levels
e. Barium contrast study

155. A 55-year-old man with hypertension and end-stage renal disease requiring hemodialysis presents with 2 days of painless hematochezia. He reports similar episodes of bleeding in the past, which were attributed to angiodysplasia. He denies abdominal pain, nausea, vomiting, diarrhea, and fever. His vitals are HR 90 beats per minute, BP 145/95 mm Hg, RR 18 breaths per minute, and temperature 98°F. His abdomen is soft and non-tender and his stool is grossly positive for blood. Which of the following statements are true regarding angiodysplasia?

a. They are responsible for over 50% of acute lower GI bleeding
b. They are more common in younger patients
c. Angiography is the most sensitive method for identifying angiodysplasias
d. They are less common in patients with end-stage renal disease
e. The majority of angiodysplasias are located on the right side of the colon

156. A 49-year-old man is brought to the ED by EMS stating that he vomited approximately 3 cups of blood over the last 2 hours. He also complains of epigastric pain. While examining the patient, he has another episode of hematemesis. You decide to place a NG tube. You insert the tube, confirm it placement and attach it to suction. You retrieve 200 mL of coffee-ground blood. What is the most common etiology of an upper GI bleed?

a. Varices
b. Peptic ulcer
c. Gastric erosions

d. Mallory-Weiss tear
e. Esophagitis

157. A 68-year-old man presents to the ED 4 hours after an upper endoscopy performed for 5 months of progressive dysphagia. During the procedure, a 1 cm ulcerated lesion was found and a biopsy was taken. Now, the patient complains of severe neck and chest pain. His vitals are BP 135/80 mm Hg, HR 123 beats per minute, RR 26 breaths per minute, and temperature 101°F. On physical exam, he appears diaphoretic and in moderate distress with crepitus in the neck and a crunching sound over the heart. You obtain an electrocardiogram (ECG), which is notable for sinus tachycardia. After obtaining a surgical consult, the next best step in management is?

a. Perform an immediate bronchoscopy
b. Give aspirin 325 mg and obtain a cardiology consult for possible cardiac catheterization
c. Repeat the endoscopy to evaluate the biopsy site
d. Perform an immediate thoracotomy
e. Order an immediate esophagram with water-soluble agent

158. A 65-year-old man with a history of occasional painless rectal bleeding presents with 2–3 days of constant, dull RLQ pain. He also complains of fever, nausea, and decreased appetite. He had a colonoscopy 2 years ago that was significant for sigmoid and cecal diverticula, but was otherwise normal. On physical examination he has RLQ tenderness with rebound and guarding. His vitals are HR of 95 beats per minute, BP 130/85 mm Hg, and temperature 101.3°F. The abdominal CT demonstrates the presence of sigmoid and cecal diverticula, inflammation of pericolic fat, thickening of the bowel wall, and a fluid-filled appendix. Which of the following is the most appropriate next step in management?

a. Discharge the patient with broad-spectrum oral antibiotics and surgical follow-up
b. Begin IV hydration and broad-spectrum antibiotics, keep the patient NPO (nothing per oral), and admit the patient to the hospital
c. Begin IV antibiotics and call a surgical consult for an emergent operative procedure
d. Arrange for an emergent barium enema to confirm the diagnosis
e. Begin sulfasalazine 3–4 g per day along with intravenous steroid therapy

159. At 3 am, a 47-year-old woman presents to the ED complaining of a steady, burning epigastric pain that radiates to her back. She states the pain awoke her from sleep at 2 AM. This is the second similar incident in a week. Over the past month, she describes similar epigastric pain occurring 2–3 hours after a meal and is usually relieved by antacids. Tonight, antacids did not relieve the pain. She never has this pain in the morning. Her vitals are BP 120/75 mm Hg, HR 79 beats per minute, RR 16 breaths per minute, 99% oxygen saturation, and temperature 97.9°F. She has mild epigastric tenderness and her stool is trace guaiac positive. Her urine is β-human chorionic gonadotropin (β-hCG) negative and chest x-ray shows no free air. What is the most common complication associated with this disease process?

a. Pancreatitis
b. Hemorrhage
c. Gastric outlet obstruction
d. Inflammatory bowel disease
e. Gastric cancer

160. A 58-year-old man presents to the ED with acute onset chest pain and hematemesis 8 hours after endoscopy for peptic ulcer disease (PUD). On physical exam, he appears alert, but in obvious discomfort. Crepitus is present on his anterior thorax. Given his history and physical exam, you are concerned about an esophageal perforation. Which of the following is *not* standard practice in a patient with symptoms suggestive of an esophageal perforation?

a. The diagnostic studies of choice are CT scan and emergent endoscopy
b. Emergent gastroenterology and surgical consultation should be obtained in every patient with a suspected esophageal perforation
c. The patient should be observed for 4 hours and, if the pain improves, discharged home
d. Appropriate resuscitation includes large-bore intravenous (IV) access, hemodynamic stabilization, and airway protection
e. Broad spectrum parenteral antibiotics should be started in the Emergency Department

161. A 20-year-old man presents with several weeks of painful rectal bleeding. He denies fever, nausea, or vomiting. He is sexually active with women only and usually uses condoms. He denies any history of CD, UC, or malignancy. He states that the pain is most severe during and immediately after defecating. Bleeding is bright red and only enough to stain the toilet paper. Which of the following is the most common etiology of painful rectal bleeding?

a. Perianal abscess
b. Anal fissure
c. Anorectal tumor
d. Internal hemorrhoid
e. Venereal proctitis

162. An 18-month-old boy is brought to the ED by the boy's father, who states that his son was playing quietly in his playpen when he suddenly stopped playing, began to cry, and rolled around in obvious discomfort. The father states his son then resumed his play and appeared as content as before the painful episode. The father states this happened two to three more times, with less time between episodes which were of increasingly longer duration. The father denies any vomiting, diarrhea, or a history of black stool or bright red blood per rectum. On Physical exam, the boy appears well and without discomfort. A sausage-shaped mass is palpated in the right upper quadrant (RUQ) and the stool guaiac test is positive for occult blood. Based on the history and physical exam, you suspect intussusception. What is the best way to confirm your diagnosis and potentially treat this child?

a. Air enema
b. Gastrografin enema
c. Water enema
d. Barium enema
e. Ultrasonography

163. A 67-year-old woman with a history of hypertension and congestive heart failure presents with "burning" epigastric pain that began 2 hours after eating a meal. She states she has had similar pain over the past several weeks, and has been taking antacids and a medication that her primary care physician had prescribed with moderate relief. The pain has occurred with increasing frequency and now awakens her from sleep. She states she came to the ED today because the pain was not relieved with her usual medications. She denies nausea, vomiting, diarrhea, or fever. She also denies hematemesis, black stool, or bright red blood per rectum. On physical exam, she is tender at the epigastrium, with an otherwise normal abdominal, pulmonary, and heart exam. Stool guaiac tests positive for occult blood. Which of the following is the most common serious complication of PUD?

a. GI hemorrhage
b. GI perforation
c. GI penetration
d. Gastric outlet obstruction
e. Pernicious anemia

164. A 78-year-old man with a history of atherosclerotic heart disease and congestive heart failure presents with increasing abdominal pain. The pain began suddenly 1 day ago and has progressively worsened since then. He denies nausea, vomiting, and diarrhea, but states that he had black tarry stool this morning. He denies any history of prior episodes of similar pain. Vitals are BP 120/65 mm Hg, HR 105 beats per minute, temperature 99°F. The patient is at high risk for which of the following conditions?

a. Cholecystitis
b. Cecal volvulus
c. Mesenteric ischemia
d. Perforated peptic ulcer
e. Small bowel obstruction

Gastrointestinal Bleeding

Answers

143. The answer is a. *(Rosen, p 197.)* Emergency Medicine always starts with an *assessment of the patient's airway*. For patients suspected of having a significant *GI bleed, two large-bore IV lines* need to be established rapidly. Treating an undifferentiated upper GI bleed is like treating a gun shot wound to the abdomen—you should expect the worse. Immediate volume resuscitation should begin with 1–2 liters of normal saline. If there is no improvement in the BP of a hypotensive patient, then blood should be administered. Sending a crossmatch early is advisable since it can take up to an hour to retrieve.

(b) A proton-pump inhibitor may be administered but priority is to the airways, breathing, circulations (ABCs) and this patient is hypotensive. **(c)** You must assess airway first. **(d)** and **(e)** The patient is maintaining his airway and does not need to be intubated emergently.

144. The answer is c. *(Tintinalli, pp 536–538.)* *Diverticulitis* is an acute inflammation of the wall of a diverticulum that occurs in approximately 10–25% of patients with known diverticular disease. Its incidence increases with age and is rare under the age of 40 years. The common presenting symptom is *pain*, which is usually constant and located in *the left lower quadrant*. A *change in bowel habits*, either *diarrhea or constipation*, is common. Nausea and vomiting, secondary to an associated paralytic ileus, may also be present.

(a) Depending on the location of the sigmoid colon, the presentation of diverticulitis may be indistinguishable from acute appendicitis. This occurs when a patient has a redundant sigmoid, lying on the right side of the abdomen or in the rare case when a cecal diverticulum becomes inflamed. **(b)** CD is a chronic inflammatory disease that can affect any part of the GI tract from mouth to anus. Abdominal pain, diarrhea, and anorexia are common symptoms, but the course is generally chronic with symptoms persisting for months to years often before a diagnosis is made. **(d)** Ogilvie's syndrome is caused by colonic pseudo-obstruction due to marked cecal dilatation. Risk factors include chronic use of opiates, tricyclic antidepressants, anticholinergics, and prolonged bed rest. **(e)** Diverticulosis is the presence of diverticula in the colon. It is most commonly associated with painless lower GI bleeding, and can lead to diverticulitis when diverticula become inflamed.

145. The answer is d. (*Rosen, pp 1343–1350.*) Internal hemorrhoids originate above the dentate line, receive their blood supply from the superior hemorrhoidal plexus, and are generally painless. They are classified by severity: first-degree do not prolapse; second-degree prolapse during defecation, but spontaneously reduce; third-degree must be manually reduced; and fourth-degree permanently prolapse and remain irreducible. First- and second-degree internal hemorrhoids are amenable to medical management, but third- and fourth-degree internal hemorrhoids require surgical correction. External hemorrhoids originate below the dentate line, receive their blood supply from the inferior hemorrhoidal plexus, and may be painful. This patient is suffering from an acutely *thrombosed external hemorrhoid.* These may be *excised* in the ED to provide prompt relief. If not excised, symptoms will most often resolve within several days when the hemorrhoid ulcerates and leaks the dark accumulated blood. Residual skin tags may persist. Excision provides both immediate and long-term relief and prevents the formation of skin tags. The *WASH* regimen should be recommended after excision to provide further relief.

(a) The symptoms of nonthrombosed external and nonprolapsing internal hemorrhoids can be improved by the *WASH* regimen. *Warm water,* via sitz baths or by directing a shower stream at the affected area for several minutes, reduces anal pressures; mild oral *analgesics* relieve pain; *stool softeners* ease the passage of stool to avoid straining; and a *high-fiber diet* produces stool that passes more easily. **(b)** *Incision* of a hemorrhoid (as opposed to *excision*) leads to incomplete clot evacuation, subsequent rebleeding, and swelling of lacerated vessels. **(c)** This patient has a thrombosed external hemorrhoid and presents with normal vital signs and a lack of systemic symptoms. The need for further evaluation of the rectal bleeding has not been established. **(e)** Hemorrhoids rarely require immediate operative management, unless there is evidence of thrombus formation with progression to gangrene.

146. The answer is a. (*Tintinalli, pp 547–555.*) *Inflammatory bowel disease (IBD)* is a chronic inflammatory disease of the GI tract. There are two major types: Crohn's disease (CD) and ulcerative colitis (UC). *CD* can involve any part of the GI tract, from mouth to anus, and is characterized by segmental involvement. The distal ileum is involved in the majority of cases; therefore, acute presentations can mimic appendicitis. CD spares the rectum in 50% of cases. There is a bimodal age distribution, with the first peak occurring in patients 15–22 years of age with a second in patients 55–60 years of age. Definitive diagnosis is by upper GI series, air-contrast barium enema, and colonoscopy. Segmental involvement of the colon with rectal sparing is the most characteristic feature. Other findings on colonoscopy include involvement of all bowel wall layers, *skip lesions* (e.g., interspersed normal and diseased bowel), *aphthous ulcers,* and *cobblestone* appearance from submucosal thickening interspersed with mucosal ulceration. Extraintestinal manifestations are seen in 25–30% of patients with CD.

(**b**) UC primarily involves the mucosa only with formation of crypt abscesses, epithelial necrosis, and mucosal ulceration. Rectal pain and bloody diarrhea are more common in UC than in CD. UC begins in the rectum, and fails to progress beyond this point in one-third of patients. Colonoscopy demonstrates inflammation of the mucosa only and continuous lesions of the GI tract. Although blood loss from sustained bleeding may be the most common complication, toxic megacolon must not be missed. (**c**) While appendicitis may be in the differential diagnosis, the acute on chronic nature of this disease and a normal-appearing appendix on abdominal CT rules it out. (**d**) Pseudomembranous enterocolitis is an inflammatory bowel disorder that results from toxin-producing *Clostridium difficile,* a spore-forming obligate anaerobic bacillus. The disease typically begins 7–10 days after the institution of antibiotic therapy, most often in hospitalized patients. However, incidence in the community is rising. (**e**) Diverticulitis is an acute inflammatory disease caused by bacterial proliferation within existing colonic diverticulae. The most common presentation is pain, often in the left lower quadrant. Abdominal CT demonstrates inflammation of pericolic fat, presence of diverticulae, bowel wall thickening, or peridiverticular abscess.

147. The answer is b. (*Rosen, pp 1241–1244.*) This patient had an untreated *gastric ulcer* that just *perforated.* The history of epigastric pain related to eating points to a gastric ulcer, whereas pain 2–3 hours after eating is more likely due to a duodenal ulcer. The sudden onset of generalized abdominal pain associated with a rigid abdomen is concerning for a perforated viscus, in this case, a perforated gastric ulcer. This is a surgical emergency. An abdominal and upright chest radiograph can be performed quickly to look for *free air,* which will be seen *under the diaphragm* on the chest radiograph. This is useful for the majority of perforations, which are anterior, but may miss posterior perforations because the posterior duodenum is retroperitoneal. The treatment includes IV hydration, antibiotics, and immediate surgical correction.

(a) Diverticula are saclike herniations of colonic mucosa that occur at weak points in the bowel wall. They may bleed (diverticulosis) or become filled with fecal matter and lead to inflammation (diverticulitis). Diverticulosis is most commonly associated with substantial painless rectal bleeding, but not with significant abdominal pain. (c) While the history of untreated hypertension is concerning for a ruptured abdominal aortic aneurysm (AAA) the history clearly points to previously undiagnosed PUD. (d) IBD is a chronic condition affecting the GI tract. The abdominal pain is usually crampy, while GI bleeding is generally associated with bloody diarrhea. (e) A splenic laceration in the absence of trauma would be highly unusual.

148. The answer is e. (*Rosen, pp 179, 1243.*) A *Mallory-Weiss tear* usually follows a forceful bout of retching and vomiting and involves a 1–4 cm area of the mucosa or submucosa of the GI tract; 75% of cases occur in the stomach with the remainder near the gastroesophageal (GE) junction. Bleeding is usually mild and self-limited. However, 3% of deaths from upper GI bleeds result from Mallory-Weiss tears.

(a) Esophageal varices are dilated submucosal veins found in 50% of patients with cirrhosis of the liver. They usually develop due to portal hypertension. Up to 30% of patients with esophageal varices develop upper GI bleeds, and the bleeding is usually massive. Patients are often asymptomatic until the varices rupture and bleed. (b) Boerhaave's syndrome involves a spontaneous full thickness perforation of the esophagus—80% involving the posterolateral aspect of the distal esophagus—that usually results from violent retching. Alcohol ingestion is a risk factor. Because the overlying pleura is torn, esophageal contents can spill into the mediastinum and thorax, leading to severe epigastric and retrosternal chest pain, with radiations to the back, neck, or shoulders. Boerhaave's syndrome represents a surgical emergency, with mortality approaching 50% if surgery is not performed within 24 hours. (c) A Curling ulcer is an ulcer or erosion caused by stress gastritis due to patients with severe burn injuries. The most common finding is painless GI bleeding. There is no evidence of severe burn injury in this patient. (d) A perforated gastric ulcer is a complication of chronic gastritis, which is usually associated with severe, acute abdominal pain. Perforations occur when an ulcer erodes through the wall and leaks air and digestive contents into the peritoneal cavity. Often, pain initially begins in the epigastrium but becomes generalized shortly thereafter. Patients usually lie still and avoid movement that might disturb the peritoneal cavity. An upright chest radiograph may demonstrate air under the diaphragm.

149. The answer is d. (*Tintinalli, pp 504–505 & 512–513.*) *Esophageal varices* develop in patients with *chronic liver disease* in response to portal hypertension. Approximately 60% of patients with portal hypertension will develop varices. Of those who develop varices, 25–30% will experience hemorrhage. Patients who develop varices from alcohol abuse have an even higher risk of bleeding, especially with ongoing alcohol consumption. This patient has evidence of chronic liver disease with thrombocytopenia and elevated bilirubin and liver enzymes. In alcoholic hepatitis, the AST is greater than the ALT by a factor of 2. Spider angiomata, palmar erythema, and gynecomastia further suggest underlying liver disease.

(**a**) A perforated gastric ulcer typically presents with severe sudden abdominal pain in a patient with a history of PUD. (**b**) Diverticulosis results from saclike herniations in the colonic mucosa (diverticula) that occur at weak points in the bowel wall, usually where arteries insert. Diverticulosis is most commonly associated with painless rectal bleeding. (**c**) Splenic laceration generally results from trauma. (**e**) The most common symptom with rupture of an AAA is sudden and severe abdominal pain. Back pain, also sudden and severe, is noted by half of patients. Incidence of AAA increases with age in both men and women, and is typically associated with a history of hypertension.

150. The answer is a. (*Current Medical Diagnosis and Treatment, 45/ed*) Acute GI bleeding develops in less than one-third of patients with portal hypertension and varices. With upper GI bleeds, the initial step is assessment of the hemodynamic status. *Hypotension* with or without tachycardia identifies a *high-risk patient* with severe acute bleeding. This patient requires immediate treatment. If initial resuscitative efforts fail or a patient remains hypotensive, more aggressive measures may be required, including consideration of Sengstaken-Blakemore tube placement to physically tamponade the bleeding source, but this is not part of the initial management and has been associated with adverse reactions.

(**b**) In patients with significant bleeding, two 18-gauge or larger IV lines should be started prior to further diagnostic tests. Blood is sent for complete blood count, coagulation studies (PT with INR), serum creatinine, liver enzymes, and cross-matching for 2–4 units or more of packed red blood cells. Patients with hemodynamic compromise should be resuscitated with crystalloid solutions and cross-matched blood. Cardiac monitoring and supplemental oxygen should also be instituted. (c) A NG tube should be placed in all patients with suspected upper GI bleeding. The aspiration of red blood or "coffee grounds" confirms an upper GI bleeding source, although 10% of patients with confirmed upper GI bleeding have non-bloody aspirates, especially when bleeding originates in the duodenum. An aspirate of bright red blood indicates active bleeding and is associated with the highest risk of bleeding and complications. Efforts to control bleeding by gastric lavage with large volumes of fluid are of no benefit and increase the risk of aspiration. (d) Octreotide reduces splanchnic blood flow and portal blood pressures and is effective in the initial control of bleeding related to portal hypertension. It should be administered promptly to all patients with active upper GI bleeding and evidence of liver disease or portal hypertension until the source of bleeding can be clarified by endoscopy. (e) A GI consult should be obtained in all cases of high-risk upper GI bleeds. Most patients with upper GI bleeding should undergo upper endoscopy after the patient is hemodynamically stable. High-risk patients or those with continued active bleeding require more urgent endoscopic evaluation to identify the source of bleeding, determine the risk of rebleeding, and provide hemostasis via sclerotherapy or rubber band ligation.

151. The answer is e. (*Rosen, pp 179, 1330–1331, 1345.*) The combination of significant blood loss—indicated by the pale skin, orthostatic hypotension, and chronic lower GI bleeding—point to carcinoma, most likely *adenocarcinoma of the colon*. The lack of esophageal, abdominal, or rectal pain makes the other choices unlikely, as does the lack of associated symptoms (nausea, vomiting, or fever). Anemia or rectal bleeding in an elderly person should be assumed to be malignancy until proven otherwise.

(a) Bleeding with defecation is the most common complaint with hemorrhoids and unless the hemorrhoids are thrombosed the bleeding is usually painless. Patients usually report bright red blood on the toilet paper or in the toilet bowl. Weight loss would not be expected, and only in rare circumstances is the blood loss substantial. (b) Diverticulitis occurs with inflammation of a diverticulum, and is the most common complication of diverticulosis. Patients typically present with persistent abdominal pain. Initially, the pain may be vague and generalized, but it often becomes localized to the left lower quadrant. Most patients can be managed medically with bowel rest, hydration, analgesics, and antibiotics. (c) A Mallory-Weiss tear is a partial tear of the esophagus that usually results from significant vomiting or retching. (d) CD is one of two entities that comprise IBD and, unlike UC, is characterized by inflammation through all layers of the bowel wall, not only the mucosa and submucosa. Clinical features include chronic diarrhea associated with abdominal cramps, fever, anorexia, and weight loss.

152. The answer is a. (*Tintinalli, pp 536–538.*) The acute complications of diverticular disease can be divided into two main categories: bleeding (diverticulosis) and inflammation (diverticulitis). With suspected diverticulitis, *abdominal CT* is the diagnostic procedure of choice.

(b) A barium contrast study can demonstrate diverticula, but is less sensitive in detecting diverticulitis. Additionally, barium injected under high pressure carries the risk of perforation and is therefore relatively contraindicated with suspected acute diverticulitis. **(c)** Colonoscopy is also relatively contraindicated in acute diverticulitis because of the risk of perforation and should likewise be avoided. **(d)** With acute diverticulitis, an abdominal plain film may be normal or may demonstrate an associated ileus, partial small bowel obstruction, or free air in the presence of peritonitis from a ruptured viscus or ruptured peridiverticular abscess. **(e)** Abdominal ultrasound is quick and inexpensive, but is operator dependent and lacks specificity for diagnosing diverticulitis.

153. The answer is d. (*Rosen, pp 210, 1391–1392, 1420, 1447, 1498.*) Patients with coronary artery disease, valvular heart disease, and arrhythmias, particularly *atrial fibrillation,* are at high risk for *mesenteric ischemia.* In addition, age greater than 50 years, congestive heart failure, recent myocardial infarction, critically ill patients with sepsis or hypotension, use of diuretics or vasoconstrictive medications, and hypercoagulable states place patients at higher risk. The most common cause of acute mesenteric ischemia is *arterial embolus,* which accounts for 50% of cases. The classic finding is "pain out of proportion to exam findings," that is, a patient complains of severe pain but is not particularly tender on exam. A high degree of suspicion in an elderly patient with abdominal pain is warranted.

(a) Perforated gastric ulcer presents with acute onset of severe epigastric pain and bleeding, generally in someone with PUD. **(b)** Diverticulitis presents as left lower quadrant pain that is usually described as dull and constant. **(c)** Acute cholecystitis occurs with an obstruction of the cystic duct with gallstones and is often accompanied by fever, chills, nausea, and a positive Murphy's sign. It is the most common surgical emergency in elderly patients. **(e)** The classic triad for sigmoid volvulus includes abdominal pain, abdominal distention, and constipation. Nausea and vomiting are often present, and diagnosis can be made on plain radiograph in 80% of cases.

154. The answer is a. (*Rosen, pp 1447–1448.*) *Angiography* remains the "gold standard" in the diagnosis of *mesenteric ischemia*. Unlike any other diagnostic tools, it is capable of both *diagnosing and treating* the problem. It is capable of identifying all four types of acute mesenteric ischemia; arterial embolus, arterial or venous thrombosis, and, under most circumstances, nonocclusive mesenteric ischemia.

(**b**) Abdominal radiographs should be performed on any patient with suspected mesenteric ischemia to rule out bowel obstruction or free air. However, in the early stages, plain radiographs are most often normal in patients with mesenteric ischemia and should not be used to rule out this entity. Positive findings include intraluminal gas or gas in the portal venous system, usually coincide with the development of necrotic bowel, and signify a grim prognosis. (**c**) Because of its availability, speed, and improved quality, CT is often used in the ED for assessing abdominal pain of unclear etiology in high-risk patients. CT may identify indirect signs of ischemia—including edema of the bowel wall or mesentery, abnormal gas patterns, intramural gas, and ascites. Occasionally, CT may accurately identify direct evidence of mesenteric venous thrombosis. As with abdominal radiographs, many patients may have normal or nonspecific findings on CT, so it cannot be used to rule out the diagnosis of mesenteric ischemia. While a few studies have found CT to be as sensitive as angiography, it is not currently the study of choice. (**d**) The sensitivity of serum lactate is high, nearly 100%, in the presence of mesenteric ischemia, but the specificity is low, ranging from 42%–87%. Elevated serum lactate may best be used as a predictor of mortality. Some studies suggest that the presence of an unexplained acidosis should prompt a search for reversible causes of mesenteric ischemia. (**e**) Intraluminal barium contrast studies are contraindicated with suspected mesenteric ischemia because residual contrast material can limit visualization of the vasculature during diagnostic angiography.

155. The answer is e. (*Townsend, p 1256.*) *Angiodysplasias*, also known as *arteriovenous malformations*, are small ectatic blood vessels in the submucosa of the GI tract. More than half of angiodysplasias are located on the *right side of the colon*.

(**a**) Angiodysplasias are responsible for 3–20% of acute lower GI bleeds. (**b**) Although angiodysplasia accounts for the most common cause of lower GI bleeding in younger patients, its incidence overall increases with age over 50 years. (**c**) While angiography may identify angiodysplasias, colonoscopy remains the most sensitive diagnostic modality. On colonoscopy, angiodysplasias appear as red, flat lesions, measuring approximately 2–20 mm in diameter. (**d**) Angiodysplasias are associated with many medical problems, including end-stage renal disease, aortic stenosis, and von Willebrand's disease, among others.

156. The answer is b. *(Rosen, pp 1241–1244.)* The most common cause of upper GI bleeds in adults is *PUD* accounting for approximately 45% of the cases. Hematemesis is the presentation in approximately 50% of patients with upper GI bleeds. The appearance of coffee-grounds in the stomach is due to the conversion of hemoglobin to hematin or other pigments by hydrochloric acid in the stomach.

(**a**) Varices account for 10%, (**c**) erosions 23%, (**d**) Mallory-Weiss tear 7% and (**e**) esophagitis 6%.

157. The answer is e. *(Rosen, p 1385.)* The patient most likely has an *esophageal perforation,* a serious, life-threatening *complication of endoscopy* that must be identified and treated quickly. Although sometimes reported as a result of forceful vomiting (Boerhaave's syndrome), the most common cause is iatrogenic. These usually occur as a complication of GI procedures, including upper endoscopy, dilation, sclerotherapy, and even NG tube placement or endotracheal intubation. The signs and symptoms may include chest pain near the rupture site, fever, respiratory distress, hoarseness, or dysphagia. Most patients have *mediastinal or cervical emphysema,* which may be noted by palpation or by a *crunching sound* heard during auscultation (*Hamman's sign*). An immediate esophagram with a water-soluble agent (e.g., Gastrografin) is indicated.

(**a**) Bronchoscopy is used to evaluate a patient with suspected bronchial obstruction or endobronchial disease. It is not indicated in a case of suspected esophageal perforation. (**b**) The likelihood that this patient's chest pain is cardiac in origin is fairly small and the ECG demonstrates no ischemic changes. The diagnosis in a patient presenting with pain or fever following esophageal instrumentation should be considered esophageal perforation until proven otherwise. Also, if perforation is suspected, aspirin should be withheld. (**c**) Repeating the endoscopy may be useful, especially in cases of trauma; however, small perforations may be difficult or impossible to detect. An esophagram is better to evaluate for a suspected perforation. A chest radiograph and an upright abdominal radiograph are usually obtained first, and may detect abnormalities in up to 90% of patients. These findings may include subcutaneous emphysema, pneumomediastinum, mediastinal widening, pleural effusion, or pulmonary infiltrate, but radiographic changes may not be present in the first few hours after the perforation. (**d**) Thoracotomy is the treatment for an esophageal perforation; however, an immediate esophagram with a water-soluble agent should be performed to confirm the diagnosis.

158. The answer is b. (*Tintinalli, pp 536–538.*) The diagnosis of *diverticulitis* is made by abdominal CT, which may demonstrate inflammation of pericolic fat, bowel wall thickening, the presence of diverticula, or peridiverticular abscess. The treatment of diverticulitis includes *IV hydration, bowel rest, and broad-spectrum antibiotics* to cover both aerobic and anaerobic bacteria. These include an aminoglycoside and either clindamycin or metronidazole, or ticarcillin-clavulanic acid or imipenem. Well-appearing patients can be treated as outpatients with oral antibiotics and close follow-up, but patients with fever, signs of localized peritonitis or obstruction, and those who have failed outpatient therapy must be admitted to the hospital.

(**a**) This patient has systemic signs of infection (fever, rebound tenderness, guarding) and should be admitted for IV antibiotics and observation. If the patient manifests signs of bowel obstruction, a NG tube should also be placed. (**c**) The presentation of diverticulitis may be indistinguishable from acute appendicitis. This occurs when a patient has a redundant sigmoid lying on the right side of the abdomen or, as in this case, when a cecal diverticulum becomes inflamed. In this case, the abdominal CT demonstrates a normal fluid-filled appendix, effectively ruling out appendicitis. A prompt surgical consult should be obtained in the presence of intestinal obstruction, free perforation, abscess, or fistula formation. (**d**) The presence of diverticulitis is demonstrated on abdominal CT, which is more sensitive than a barium enema. Furthermore, both barium injected under high pressure and colonoscopy in the presence of acute diverticulitis carry the risk of perforation and are relatively contraindicated. (**e**) An exacerbation of CD, which may also present with RLQ pain and heme-positive stool, may be treated with sulfasalazine and steroid therapy, but neither is appropriate in the treatment of acute diverticulitis.

159. The answer is b. (*Rosen, pp 1214–1244.*) The patient has *PUD*. The most serious complications of PUD include *hemorrhage, perforation, penetration, and gastric outlet obstruction*. The most common complication is *hemorrhage,* occurring in 15% of patients.

Pancreatitis (**a**) may present clinically similar to PUD, but it is not a complication of PUD. Gastric outlet obstruction (**c**) occurs when a healing ulcer scars and blocks the antral or pyloric outlet. Although gastric outlet obstruction is a complication of PUD, it is not the most common.

IBD **(d)** may cause ulcerative lesions in the GI tract, but is not a complication of PUD. Infection with *H. pylori,* a primary risk factor for developing PUD, increases the risk of gastric carcinoma **(e)** and lymphoma. However, hemorrhage is a more common complication.

160. The answer is c. *(Tintinalli, pp 512–513.)* Perforation of the esophagus may result from a number of causes with iatrogenic injury. Pain is classically acute in onset, severe, constant and located in the chest, neck, or abdomen and may radiate to the back or shoulders. Dysphagia, dyspnea, hematemesis, and cyanosis may also be present. Diagnosis is often delayed as esophageal perforation is often ascribed to acute myocardial infarction, pulmonary embolus, PUD, or acute abdomen. Rapid and aggressive management is critical to minimizing associated morbidity and mortality. Patients require hospitalization for continued care and may require emergent surgery for repair.

(a), (b), (d), and **(e)** Esophageal perforation is a medical, and possibly surgical, emergency. Prompt diagnosis and management is essential. This includes resuscitation, broad-spectrum parenteral antibiotics, and emergent surgical consultation. Chest radiograph may be suggestive of esophageal perforation, but additional studies may be required for definitive diagnosis.

161. The answer is b. *(Tintinalli, pp 539–545.)* Pain and bleeding are common complaints associated with anorectal disorders. A good history and a thorough physical exam, including a digital rectal exam and anoscopy should be performed whenever feasible. *Anal fissures (fissures in ano)* result from lineal tears of the anal canal at or just inferior to the dentate line and extend along the anal canal to the anal verge. This area has a rich supply of somatic sensory never fibers. Consequently, anal fissures are exquisitely painful and represent the *most common cause of painful rectal bleeding.* They are most common in *children* and *young adults.*

(a) Most perianal or perirectal abscesses begin with obstruction of an anal gland. If they persist, fistula formation may develop. Of all anorectal abscesses, perirectal abscesses are most common. Pain is usually worse before defecation, decreases with defecation, and persists in between. They are not associated with rectal bleeding. **(c)** Early anorectal malignancies usually present with nonspecific symptoms, such as pruritis, pain, and bleeding mixed with stool, and represent less than 5% of all large bowel malignancies. **(d)** Internal hemorrhoids are detected by direct visualization using anoscopy. Uncomplicated internal hemorrhoids are painless due to lack of sensory innervation. Consequently, they present with *painless,* bright red bleeding with defecation. **(e)** Most venereal diseases involving the anorectal region present with pruritis, discharge, and mild to moderate pain or irritation, and may intermittently bleed.

162. The answer is a. *(Tintinalli, p 818.)* *Intussusception* is the telescoping of one segment of bowel into another, often at the ileocecal segment. It is most common in *children aged 3 months to 6 years* and has a male to female incidence of 4:1. The classic "currant jelly" stool is a late finding, but most patients test positive for occult blood in the stool. *Air contrast enema* is diagnostic and often curative and is the preferred contrast medium when performing diagnostic and reduction enema for intussusception. An abdominal radiograph may demonstrate a mass or filling defect in the RUQ, but is normal in 30% of cases.

(**b**) and (**c**) Gastrografin is a water-soluble substance. Both gastrografin and water are less preferred contrast agents in neonates and infants due to their potential for fluid shifts and resultant electrolyte abnormalities. (**d**) Barium enema offers the advantage of better contrast visualization under fluoroscopy; however it has an increased risk of peritonitis if perforation occurs with resultant spillage into the peritoneum. For this reason, air enema is preferred. (**e**) Ultrasound is the least invasive and most commonly used modality for visualizing intussusceptions, but cannot be used therapeutically.

163. The answer is a. *(Rosen, pp 1241–1243.)* The most serious complications of PUD include hemorrhage, perforation, penetration, and gastric outlet obstruction. *Hemorrhage,* which occurs in 15% of patients, is the *most common complication.*

(**b**) GI perforation occurs when an ulcer erodes through the stomach or bowel wall and leaks air and digestive contents into the peritoneal cavity. It occurs in approximately 7% of patients, and is the second most common serious complication of PUD. (**c**) GI penetration is similar to perforation, except the ulcer erodes into another organ, such as the liver or pancreas. (**d**) Gastric outlet obstruction, which occurs in 2% of patients, occurs as a result of edema and scarring near the gastric outlet. (**e**) Pernicious anemia results from an autoimmune disease in which the body develops antibodies to the acid-secreting cells in the gastric mucosa with ensuing loss of intrinsic factor, vitamin B12 malabsorption, and the development of anemia. It is not a complication of PUD.

164. The answer is c. *(Tintinalli, p 496.)* The complaint of abdominal pain in the elderly patient should prompt the Emergency physician to lower his or her threshold for considering more serious intra-abdominal conditions. Patients with a history of arrhythmias (especially atrial fibrillation), low cardiac output (such as congestive heart failure), or who take particular medications, such as digoxin, are at high risk for the elusive condition of *mesenteric ischemia*. A history of sudden onset abdominal pain with increasing severity, but with a benign physical exam should prompt consideration of this entity. Mesenteric ischemia is associated with a high mortality rate, and initial diagnosis is often incorrect. The diagnostic study of choice is angiography.

(a) Cholecystitis is the most common surgical emergency in elderly patients, but patients often localize pain to the RUQ. Ultrasonography is the initial diagnostic study of choice. **(b)** Sigmoid volvulus is two to three times more common than cecal volvulus among the elderly and presents with gradually increasing abdominal pain, along with nausea and vomiting. **(d)** Perforated peptic ulcer often presents with acute onset epigastric pain followed by peritonitis and GI bleeding, and can be a similarly challenging condition to diagnose in elderly patients, who may lack dramatic pain or impressive peritoneal findings. The diagnostic study of choice is CT scan, although an upright chest or abdominal radiograph, which may show free air under the diaphragm, should be obtained immediately if the diagnosis is suspected. **(e)** Small bowel obstruction may also present with gradually increasing abdominal pain, nausea, and vomiting. It is not associated with the comorbid conditions listed, but rather with adhesions following abdominal surgery, incarcerated groin hernia, polyps, lymphomas, adenocarcinoma, abdominal abscess, and radiation therapy.

Trauma

Questions

165. A 45-year-old man is brought to the emergency department (ED) by paramedics after being involved in a high-speed motor vehicle collision. His blood pressure (BP) is 75/50 mm Hg and heart rate (HR) is 131 beats per minute despite administering 2 L of normal saline. He is awake but slow in responding to questions. A right upper quadrant (RUQ) ultrasound image is seen below. Which of the following is the most appropriate next step in management?

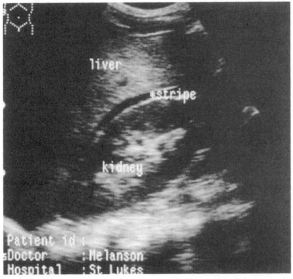

(Reproduced, with permission, from Tintinalli J, Kelen G, and Stapczynski J. Emergency Medicine A Comprehensive Study Guide. New York, NY: McGraw-Hill, 2004: 1875.)

a. Emergent abdominal computed tomography (CT) scan
b. Immediate transfer to the operating room (OR) for laparotomy
c. Perform a diagnostic peritoneal lavage (DPL) to confirm the diagnosis
d. Observe until one more liter of crystalloid fluid is administered
e. Serial abdominal exams

166. A 17-year-old high school football player is brought to the ED by paramedics on a backboard and cervical collar. During a football game, the patient "speared" another player with his helmet and subsequently experienced severe neck pain. He denies paresthesias and is able to move all of his extremities. A cervical spine CT scan reveals multiple fractures of the first cervical vertebra. Which of the following best describes this fracture?

a.   Odontoid fracture
b.   Hangman fracture
c.   Jefferson fracture
d.   Clay-Shoveler's fracture
e.   Teardrop fracture

167. A 20-year-old man presents to the ED with multiple stab wounds to his chest. His BP is 85/50 mm Hg and HR is 123 beats per minute. Two large-bore IVs are established and running wide open. On exam, the patient is mumbling incomprehensibly, has good air entry on lung exam, and you notice jugular venous distension. As you are listening to his heart, the nurse calls out that the patient has lost his pulse and that she cannot get a BP reading. Which of the following is the most appropriate next step in management?

a.   Atropine
b.   Epinephrine
c.   Bilateral chest tubes
d.   ED thoracotomy
e.   Pericardiocentesis

168. A 23-year-old man presents to the ED complaining of finger pain. He states that while playing football, he went to catch a pass and the ball hit the tip of his finger and bent his finger backwards. He thinks his finger is just "jammed". On exam, you notice that the distal phalanx is flexed and there is swelling and tenderness over the distal interphalangeal (DIP) joint as seen on the next page. In addition, he cannot extend his distal finger at the DIP joint. An x-ray does not reveal a fracture. Which of the following is the most appropriate way to manage this injury?

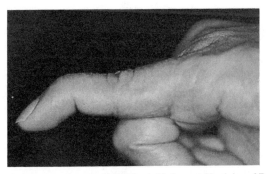

(Reproduced, with permission, from Knoop KJ, Stack LB, Storrow AB. Atlas of Emergency Medicine. New York, NY: McGraw-Hill, 2002: 315.)

a. Place a dorsal splint so that the proximal interphalangeal (PIP) and DIP joints are immobile, remove splint in 1–2 weeks
b. Place a dorsal splint so that the PIP and DIP joints are immobile, remove splint in 1 week
c. Buddy tape the finger
d. Place a dorsal splint to immobilize the interphalangeal (DIP) joint, remove splint in 1–2 weeks
e. Place a dorsal splint to immobilize the DIP joint, remove splint in 6–8 weeks

169. A 38-year-old woman presents to the ED with pain in her right wrist and fingers that is associated with a tingling sensation. The pain is worse after typing on her computer and occasionally awakens her from sleep. The pain improves when the hand is shaken. Her symptoms are reproducible when her wrist is held in flexion for 60 seconds. Which of the following nerves is affected in patients with this syndrome?

a. Ulnar
b. Median
c. Axillary
d. Radial
e. Musculocutaneous

170. A 33-year-old man is brought to the ED by paramedics on a backboard and in a cervical collar after a motor vehicle collision. His BP is 95/60 mm Hg and his HR is 128 beats per minute. You intubate the patient and start two large-bore IVs with fluids running wide open. You reassess the vital signs after 2 L of normal saline and he remains hypotensive. There is no ultrasound available and you believe the patient might be bleeding into his abdomen. You decide to perform a DPL. In the setting of blunt abdominal trauma, which of the following findings is considered a positive DPL?

a. Aspiration of 10 mL of fresh blood
b. Lavage fluid red blood cell (RBC) count of 10,000 cells/mm³
c. Lavage fluid RBC count of 1000 cells/mm³
d. Lavage fluid RBC count of 100 cells/mm³
e. Lavage fluid RBC count of 1 cell/mm³

171. A 23-year-old man presents to the ED complaining of left hand pain. He states that he was mad at a friend and punched the wall in his bedroom. Immediately after he punched the wall, he felt intense pain in his left hand. On physical exam, you note swelling and tenderness over the fifth metacarpal. When you ask him to make a fist, his fifth finger rotates to lie on top of his fourth finger. The radiograph is shown in below. What is the name of this type of fracture?

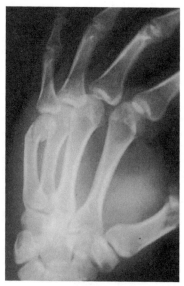

(Reproduced, with permission, from Knoop KJ, Stack LB, Storrow AB. Atlas of Emergency Medicine. New York, NY: McGraw-Hill, 2002: 305.)

a. Colle's fracture
b. Smith's fracture
c. Scaphoid fracture
d. Galeazzi fracture
e. Boxer's fracture

172. A 22-year-old man calls the ED from a local bar stating that he was punched in the face 10 minutes ago and is holding his front incisor tooth in his hand. He wants to know what the best way to preserve the tooth is. Which of the following is the most appropriate advice to give the caller?

a. Place the tooth in a napkin and bring it to the ED
b. Place the tooth in a glass of water and bring it to the ED
c. Place the tooth in a glass of beer and bring it to the ED
d. Pour some water over the tooth and place it immediately back into the socket
e. Place the tooth in a glass of milk and bring it to the ED

173. A 19-year-old man is brought into the trauma room by emergency medical service (EMS) after a head on cycling accident. The patient was not wearing a helmet. Upon presentation his BP is 125/75 mmHg, HR is 105 beats per minute, RR is 19 breaths per minute, and oxygen saturation is 100% on mask. His eyes are closed, but open to command. He can move his arms and legs on command. When you ask him questions, he is disoriented but able to converse. What is this patient's Glasgow Coma Scale (GCS) score?

a. 11
b. 12
c. 13
d. 14
e. 15

174. An 18-year-old man presents to the ED after getting stabbed in his abdomen. His HR is 140 beats per minute and BP is 90/40 mm Hg. He is yelling that he is in pain. Two large-bore IVs are inserted into his antecubital fossa and fluids are running wide open. After 2 L of fluids, his BP does not improve. Which of the following is the most common organ injured in stab wounds?

a. Liver
b. Small bowel
c. Stomach
d. Colon
e. Spleen

175. A 61-year-old man presents to the ED with chest wall pain after a motor vehicle collision. He is speaking full sentences, breath sounds are equal bilaterally, and his extremities are well-perfused. His BP is 150/75 mm Hg, HR is 92 beats per minute, and oxygen saturation is 97% on room air. Chest radiography reveals fractures of the seventh and eight ribs of the right anterolateral chest. He has no other identifiable injuries. Which of the following is the most appropriate treatment for this patient's rib fractures?

a. Apply adhesive tape on the chest wall perpendicular to the rib fractures
b. Insert a chest tube into the right thorax
c. Bring the patient to the OR for surgical fixation
d. Analgesia and incentive spirometry
e. Observation

176. A 27-year-old man arrives to the ED by paramedics after a motor vehicle collision. His RR is 45 breaths per minute, oxygen saturation is 89%, HR is 112 beats per minute, and BP is 115/75 mm Hg. You auscultate his chest and hear decreased breath sounds on the left. Which of the following is the most appropriate next step in management?

a. Perform a tube thoracostomy
b. Perform a pericardiocentesis
c. Perform a DPL
d. Perform an ED thoracotomy
e. Order a chest radiograph

177. A 43-year-old man presents to the ED after falling approximately 6 ft from the roof of his garage. The patient states that he landed on his feet but then fell to the ground. You assess his airway, breathing, and circulation which are all normal. Vital signs are stable. Your secondary survey reveals a swollen and tender right heel. A radiograph reveals a fractured calcaneus. About 6 hours after the initial fall, the patient starts complaining of a constant burning in his right foot. You examine the foot and elicit intense pain with passive movement. There is decreased two-point discrimination. His dorsalis pedis pulse is 2+. Which of the following is the most appropriate next step in management?

a. Place the foot in ice water and administer analgesia
b. Order another radiograph to look for an occult fracture
c. Elevate the leg and place a constrictive bandage around the foot
d. Order a duplex ultrasound for suspicion of a deep vein thrombosis (DVT)
e. Measure the intracompartment pressure of the foot

178. A 41-year-old man is brought into the ED after having a witnessed tonic-clonic seizure. He is alert and oriented and states that he has not taken his seizure medication for the last week. His BP is 140/75 mmHg, HR is 88 beats per minute, temperature is 99.7°F, and his RR is 16 breaths per minute. On exam you notice that his arm is internally rotated and adducted. He cannot externally rotate the arm and any movement of his shoulder elicits pain. Which of the following is the most likely diagnosis?

a. Humerus fracture
b. Clavicular fracture
c. Scapular fracture
d. Posterior shoulder dislocation
e. Anterior shoulder dislocation

179. A 29-year-old man is brought to the ED by EMS after being stabbed in the left side of his back. His BP is 120/80 mm Hg, HR is 105 beats per minute, RR is 16 breaths per minute, and oxygen saturation is 98% on room air. On the secondary survey, you note motor weakness of his left lower extremity and the loss of pain sensation in the right lower extremity. Which of the following is the most likely diagnosis?

a. Spinal shock
b. Central cord syndrome
c. Anterior cord syndrome
d. Brown-Séquard syndrome
e. Cauda equina syndrome

180. A 24-year-old man presents to the ED complaining of right wrist pain that began after he slipped and fell and landed on his outstretched hand. You examine the hand and wrist and note no abnormalities except for snuffbox tenderness. An x-ray does not reveal a fracture. Which of the following is the most appropriate next step in management?

a. Place an elastic wrap around the hand and wrist until the pain resolves
b. Immobilize in a thumb spica splint and have the patient follow up with an orthopedist for repeat radiographs in 10–14 days
c. Continue to ice the wrist for 24–48 hours
d. Immediately order a CT scan to evaluate for an occult fracture
e. Place the wrist and arm in a cast for 6 weeks

181. A 33-year-old man, who was drinking heavily at a bar, presents to the ED after getting into a fight. A bystander tells paramedics that the patient was punched and kicked multiple times and sustained multiple blows to his head with a stool. In the ED, his BP is 150/75 mm Hg, HR is 90 beats per minute, RR is 13 breaths per minute, and oxygen saturation is 100% on nonrebreather. On exam, he opens his eyes to pain and his pupils are equal and reactive. There is a laceration on the right side of his head. He withdraws his arm to pain but otherwise doesn't move. You ask him questions, but he just moans. Which of the following is the most appropriate next step in management?

a. Prepare for intubation
b. Suture repair of head laceration
c. Administer mannitol
d. Bilateral burr holes
e. Neurosurgical intervention

182. A 74-year-old man presents to the ED after being involved in a motor vehicle collision. He states he was wearing his seat belt in the driver's seat when a car hit him from behind. He thinks his chest hit the steering wheel and now complains of pain with breathing. His RR is 20 breaths per minute, oxygen saturation is 98% on room air, BP is 145/75 mm Hg, and HR is 90 beats per minute. On exam, you notice paradoxical respirations. Which of the following best describes a flail chest?

a. One rib with three fracture sites
b. Two adjacent ribs each with two fracture sites
c. Three adjacent ribs each with two fracture sites
d. One fractured right sided rib and one fractured left sided rib
e. Two fractured right sided ribs and two fractured left sided ribs

183. A 29-year-old man presents to the ED after being stabbed in his neck. The patient is speaking in full sentences. His breath sounds are equal bilaterally. His BP is 130/75 mm Hg, HR is 95 beats per minute, RR is 16 breaths per minute, and oxygen saturation is 99% on room air. The stab wound is located between the angle of the mandible and the cricoid cartilage and violates the platysma. There is blood oozing from the site although there is no expanding hematoma. Which of the following is the most appropriate next step in management?

a. Explore the wound and blind clamp any bleeding site
b. Probe the wound looking for injured vessels
c. Apply direct pressure and bring the patient immediately to the OR to explore the zone 1 injury
d. Apply direct pressure and bring the patient immediately to the OR to explore the zone 2 injury
e. Apply direct pressure and bring the patient immediately to the OR to explore the zone 3 injury

184. A 45-year-old man is brought to the ED after a head-on motor vehicle collision. Paramedics at the scene tell you that the front-end of the car is smashed. The patient's BP is 130/80 mm Hg, HR is 100 beats per minute, RR is 15 breaths per minute, and oxygen saturation is 98% on room air. Radiographs of the cervical spine reveal bilateral fractures of the C2 vertebra. The patient's neurologic exam is unremarkable. Which of the following best describes this fracture?

a. Colle's fracture
b. Boxer's fracture
c. Jefferson's fracture
d. Hangman's fracture
e. Clay-Shoveler's fracture

185. A 71-year-old man is found lying on the ground one story below the balcony of his apartment. Paramedics bring the patient into the ED. He is cool to touch with a core body temperature of 96°F. His HR is 119 beats per minute and BP is 90/70 mm Hg. His eyes are closed but they open when you call his name. His limbs move to stimuli and he answers your questions but is confused. On exam, you note clear fluid dripping from his left ear canal and an area of ecchymosis around the mastoid bone. Which of the following is the most likely diagnosis?

a. Lefort fracture
b. Basilar skull fracture
c. Otitis interna
d. Otitis externa
e. Tripod fracture

186. A 34-year-old construction worker is brought to the ED by EMS after falling 30 ft from a scaffold. His vital signs are HR 124 beats per minute, BP 80/40 mm Hg, and oxygen saturation 93% on 100% oxygen. He has obvious head trauma with a scalp laceration overlying a skull fracture on his occiput. He does not speak when asked his name, his respirations are poor and you hear gurgling with each attempted breath. Auscultation of the chest reveals diminished breath sounds on the right. There is no jugular venous distension (JVD) or anterior chest wall crepitus. His pelvis is unstable with movement lateral to medial and you note blood at the urethral meatus. His right leg is grossly deformed at the knee and there is an obvious fracture of his left arm. Which of the following is the most appropriate next step in management?

a. Insert a 32-French chest tube into the right thoracic cavity
b. Perform a DPL to rule out intra-abdominal hemorrhage
c. Create two Burr holes into the cranial vault to treat a potential epidural hematoma
d. Immediately reduce the extremity injuries and place in a splint until the patient is stabilized
e. Plan for endotracheal intubation of the airway with in-line stabilization of the cervical spine

187. A 20-year-old man was found on the ground next to his car after it hit a tree on the side of the road. Bystanders state that the man got out of his car after the collision but collapsed within a few minutes. Paramedics state they found the man unconscious on the side of the road. In the ED, his BP is 175/90 mm Hg, HR is 65 beats per minute, temperature is 99.2°F, RR is 12 breaths per minute, and oxygen saturation is 97% on room air. Physical exam reveals a right-sided fixed and dilated pupil. A head CT is shown on the next page. Which of the following is the most likely diagnosis?

a. Epidural hematoma
b. Subdural hematoma
c. Subarachnoid hemorrhage (SAH)
d. Intracerebral hematoma
e. Cerebral contusion

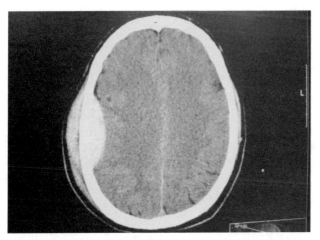

(Reproduced, with permission, from Knoop KJ, Stack LB, Storrow AB. Atlas of Emergency Medicine. New York, NY: McGraw-Hill, 2002: 162.)

188. An 81-year-old woman presents to the ED after tripping over the sidewalk curb and landing on her chin causing a hyperextension of her neck. She was placed in a cervical collar by paramedics. On exam, she has no sensorimotor function of her upper extremities. She cannot wiggle her toes, has 1/5 motor function of her quadriceps, and only patchy sensation. Rectal exam reveals decreased rectal tone. Which of the following is the most likely diagnosis?

a. Central cord syndrome
b. Anterior cord syndrome
c. Brown-Séquard syndrome
d. Transverse myelitis
e. Exacerbation of Parkinson's disease

189. A 29-year-old woman presents to ED complaining of worsening left wrist pain for 1 month. She states that approximately 3 months ago she fell from a ladder and landed on her outstretched hand. She never went to the hospital and just dealt with the pain for a while. On exam, there is no deformity of the wrist, neurovascular status is normal, but there is tenderness when you palpate the snuffbox. What is the most likely reason for this patient's wrist pain?

a. Fracture of the distal ulna
b. Hematoma of the radial artery
c. Avascular necrosis of the scaphoid
d. Transaction of the radial nerve
e. Fracture of the lunate

190. A 22-year-old man presents to the ED after being ejected from his vehicle following a high-speed motor vehicle collision. Upon arrival, his BP is 85/55 mm Hg and HR is 141 beats per minute. Two large-bore IVs are placed in the antecubital veins and lactated ringers solution is being administered. After 3 L of crystalloid fluid, the patient's BP is 83/57 mm Hg. Which of the following statements is most appropriate regarding management of a hypotensive trauma patient who fails to respond to initial volume resuscitation?

a. It is important to wait for fully cross-matched blood prior to transfusion
b. Whole blood should be used rather than packed RBCs
c. Blood transfusion is inappropriate for a trauma patient
d. Only type O blood that is Rh negative should be transfused
e. Unmatched, type-specific blood is preferred to type O blood

191. A 32-year-old male construction worker reports standing on scaffolding when it gave way beneath him. In an attempt to catch his fall, he grabbed on to an overhead beam and now presents with right shoulder pain and decreased range of motion. He denies any loss of consciousness or other sustained trauma. Vital signs are within normal limits, except for the patient's pain scale of 10/10. He is holding his right arm with the contralateral hand. On physical examination, the patient's shoulder appears swollen with no skin breakage. The upper extremity is without obvious deformity. The patient has palpable brachial, radial, and ulnar pulses with good capillary refill. He can wiggle his fingers but cannot internally rotate his shoulder or raise his right arm above his head. Pin-prick testing reveals paresthesias along the lateral deltoid of the affected arm. What is the most likely etiology of this patient's pain and paresthesias?

a. Acromioclavicular joint sprain
b. Posterior shoulder dislocation with axillary nerve impingement
c. Anterior shoulder dislocation with axillary nerve impingement
d. Anterior shoulder dislocation with median nerve impingement
e. Posterior shoulder dislocation with ulnar nerve impingement

192. A 24-year-old man is brought into the ED by paramedics after being run over by a car. His systolic BP is 90 mm Hg by palpation, HR is 121 beats per minute, RR is 28 breaths per minute, and oxygen saturation is 100% on nonrebreather. The airway is patent and breath sounds are equal bilaterally. You establish large-bore access and fluids are running wide open. Secondary survey reveals an unstable pelvis with movement to lateral to medial force.

Bedside focused assessment by sonography for trauma (FAST) is negative for intraperitoneal fluid. Which of the following is the most appropriate immediate next step in management?

a. Bilateral chest tubes
b. Application of external fixator
c. Application of pelvic binding apparatus
d. Venographic embolization
e. Angiographic embolization

193. A 32-year-old man is brought to the ED by paramedics after a diving accident. The lifeguard on duty accompanies the patient and states that he dove head first into the shallow end of the pool and did not resurface. On exam, the patient is speaking but cannot move his arms or legs and cannot feel pain below his clavicle. He is able to feel light touch and position of his four extremities. A cervical spine radiograph does not reveal a fracture. Which of the following is the most likely diagnosis?

a. Brown-Séquard syndrome
b. Central cord syndrome
c. Anterior cord syndrome
d. Cauda equina syndrome
e. Spinal cord injury without radiographic abnormality (SCIWORA)

194. A 22-year-old man is brought to the ED 20 minutes after a head-on motor vehicle collision in which he was the unrestrained driver. On arrival, he is alert and coherent but appears short of breath. His HR is 117 beats per minute, BP is 80/60 mm Hg, and oxygen saturation is 97% on a nonrebreather. Examination reveals bruising over the central portion of his chest. His neck veins are not distended. Breath sounds are present on the left but absent on the right. Following administration of 2 L of lactated ringer solution, his systolic BP remains at 80 mm Hg. Which of the following is the most appropriate next step in management?

a. Sedate, paralyze, and intubate
b. Perform a needle thoracostomy
c. Perform a DPL
d. Perform a FAST examination
e. Perform a pericardiocentesis

195. An 87-year-old man is brought to the ED on a long board and in a cervical collar after falling down a flight of steps. He denies losing consciousness. On arrival, his vital signs are a HR of 99 beats per minute, BP 160/90 mm Hg, and RR of 16 breaths per minute. He is alert and speaking in full sentences. Breath sounds are equal bilaterally. Despite an obvious right arm fracture, his radial pulses are 2+ and symmetric. When examining his cervical spine, he denies tenderness to palpation and you do not feel any bony deformities. Which of the following is a true statement?

a. Epidural hematomas are very common in the elderly age population
b. Cerebral atrophy in the elderly population provides protection against subdural hematomas
c. Increased elasticity of their lungs, allows elderly patients to recover from thoracic trauma more quickly than younger patients
d. The most common cervical spine fracture in this age group is a wedge fracture of the sixth cervical vertebra
e. Despite lack of cervical spine tenderness, imaging of his cervical spine is warranted

196. A 41-year-old man who was a restrained front seat passenger in a high-speed motor vehicle collision is brought to the ED by the paramedics. His vital signs are BP 90/50 mm Hg, HR 125 beats per minute, and RR 20 breaths per minute. On exam, he is alert and answers your questions. His breath sounds are equal bilaterally and chest wall is without contusion or bony crepitus. The abdomen is soft and nondistended. His pelvis is unstable. A FAST exam and DPL are negative for intraperitoneal fluid. Initial radiographs reveal a normal chest film and an open book pelvic fracture. Despite infusion of 2 L of lactated ringer solution, his BP is now 80/40 mm Hg. Which of the following is the most appropriate next step in management?

a. Immediate exploratory laparotomy
b. Pelvic angiography with embolization of the pelvic vessels
c. CT scan
d. Pericardiocentesis
e. Retrograde urethrogram

197. A 45-year-old man is brought into the ED after a head-on motor vehicle collision. His BP is 85/45 mm Hg and HR is 130 beats per minute. He is speaking coherently. His breath sounds are equal bilaterally. After 2 L of fluid resuscitation, his BP is 80/40 mm Hg. A FAST exam reveals fluid in Morison's pouch. Which of the following organs is most likely to be injured in blunt abdominal trauma?

a. Liver
b. Spleen
c. Kidney
d. Small bowel
e. Bladder

198. A 22-year-old college volleyball player presents to the ED complaining of left shoulder pain that began while attempting a serve during a volleyball match. She states this has happened to her before. On exam, the left shoulder looks squared-off. She complains of severe pain when she tries to adduct or internally rotate the shoulder. A radiograph is seen below. What is the most common fracture associated with the patient's diagnosis?

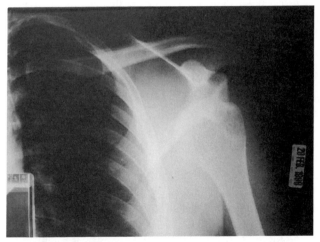

(Reproduced, with permission, from Knoop KJ, Stack LB, Storrow AB. **Atlas of Emergency** **Medicine.** *New York, NY: McGraw-Hill, 2002: 291.)*

a. Bankart fracture
b. Hill-Sachs deformity
c. Clavicular fracture
d. Coranoid fracture
e. Scapular fracture

199. A 47-year-old man is brought into the ED after falling 20 ft from a ladder. His HR is 110 beats per minute, BP is 110/80 mm Hg, RR is 20 breaths per minute, and oxygen saturation is 100% on face mask. He is able to answer your questions without difficulty. His chest is clear with bilateral breath sounds, abdomen is nontender, pelvis is stable, and the FAST exam is negative. You note a large scrotal hematoma and blood at the urethral meatus. Which of the following is the most appropriate next step in management?

a. Scrotal ultrasound
b. Kidney-ureter-bladder (KUB) radiograph
c. Intravenous pyelogram
d. Retrograde cystogram
e. Retrograde urethrogram

200. A 17-year-old man presents to the ED after getting hit in the right eye with a tennis ball during a tennis match. On arrival to the ED, you note periorbital swelling and ecchymosis. The patient's visual acuity is 20/20. When you are testing his extraocular muscles, you note that his right eye cannot look superiorly but his left eye can. He also describes pain in his right eye when attempting to look upward. Which of the following is the most likely diagnosis?

a. Zygomatic arch fracture
b. Orbital floor fracture
c. Retrobulbar hematoma
d. Ruptured globe
e. Mandible fracture

201. A 24-year-old man is brought to the ED after being shot one time in the abdomen. On arrival, his BP is 100/60 mm Hg, HR is 115 beats per minute, and RR is 22 breaths per minute. His airway is patent and you hear breath sounds bilaterally. On abdominal exam, you note a single bullet entry wound approximately 1 cm to the right of the umbilicus. During the log roll, you see a single bullet exit wound approximately 3 cm to the right of the lumbar spine. His GCS score is 15. The patient's BP is now 85/65 mm Hg and HR is 125 beats per minute after 2 L of fluid. Which of the following is the most appropriate next step in management?

a. Probe the entry wound to see if it violates the peritoneum
b. Perform a FAST exam
c. Perform a DPL

d. Take the patient directly to the CT scanner
e. Take the patient directly to the OR

202. A 55-year-old woman presents to the ED stating that her nose has been bleeding profusely for the last 3 hours. After 25 minutes of bilateral pressure on her nasal septum, there is still profuse bleeding. You place anterior nasal packing bilaterally but bleeding still persists. The patient is starting to get anxious. Her BP is 110/70 mm Hg, HR of 80 beats per minute, RR of 18 breaths per minute, and oxygen saturation of 98%. Laboratory results reveal a white blood cell (WBC) count of 9000, hematocrit (HCT) 34%, platelets of 225,000, and International Normalized Ration (INR) 1.1. Under direct visualization, you note the bleeding originating from the posterior aspect of her septum. Which of the following is the most appropriate management?

a. Place posterior nasal packing, start antibiotics, and admit the patient to a monitored hospital bed
b. Place the patient supine and wait for spontaneous resolution of the bleeding
c. Keep pressure on her nasal septum and administer fresh frozen plasma and platelets
d. Place posterior nasal packing, and discharge the patient home with follow-up in 24 hours
e. Apply silver nitrate to the nasal mucosa until the bleeding stops

203. A 44-year-old man is brought to the ED by paramedics. He was found in the middle of the street after being struck by a car. His BP is 70/palp, HR is 125 beats per minute, and oxygen saturation is 89% on room air. The patient's eyes are closed. You ask the patient his name and he doesn't respond. There is no response when you ask him to move his limbs. You notice that his left foot is severely deformed and there is a large laceration to his right arm. Which of the following is the most appropriate next step in management?

a. Prepare for emergent orotracheal intubation
b. Begin fluid resuscitation and administer morphine for pain
c. Apply a tourniquet just above his left foot and begin fluid resuscitation
d. Apply pressure to the laceration, splint the left foot, and order a radiograph
e. Administer two units of packed RBCs and bring him to the CT scanner

204. A 17-year-old boy is found unconscious in a swimming pool. He is brought into the ED by paramedics already intubated. In the ED, the patient is unresponsive with spontaneous abdominal breathing at a rate of 16 breaths per minute, BP of 80/50 mm Hg, and HR of 49 beats per minute. In addition to hypoxemia, what condition must be considered earliest in the management of this patient?

a. Cervical spine injury
b. Electrolyte imbalance
c. Metabolic acidosis
d. Severe atelectasis
e. Toxic ingestion

205. A 26-year-old woman, who was a belted front seat driver in a head-on motor vehicle collision, is brought to the ED. She is speaking but complains of progressively worsening shortness of breath and hemoptysis. Her BP is 135/75 mm Hg, HR is 111 beats per minute, RR is 24 breaths per minute, and oxygen saturation is 96% on nonrebreather. On exam, you note ecchymosis over the right side of her chest. Her breath sounds are equal bilaterally. There is no bony crepitus and the trachea is midline. After placing two large-bore IVs and completing the primary and secondary surveys, you view the chest radiograph seen below. Which of the following is the most likely diagnosis?

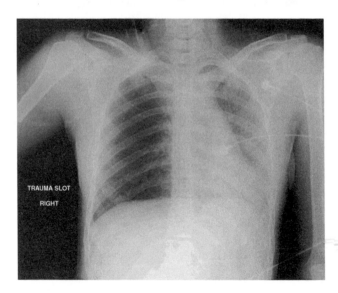

a. Tuberculosis
b. Hemothorax
c. Tension pneumothorax (PTX)
d. Pulmonary contusion
e. Acute respiratory failure syndrome (ARDS)

206. A 22-year-old man is brought to the ED after sustaining a single gun shot wound (GSW) to his right thigh. On arrival, his HR is 105 beats per minute and BP is 115/75 mm Hg. You note a large hematoma of his medial thigh. The patient complains of numbness in his right foot. On extremity exam, the right foot is pale and you cannot palpate a distal pulse but can locate the dorsalis pedis by Doppler. In addition, the patient cannot move the foot. Which of the following is the most appropriate next step in management?

a. Angiography
b. Exploration and repair in the OR
c. Fasciotomy to treat compartment syndrome
d. Wound exploration
e. CT scan of the right extremity

207. A 67-year-old woman is brought to the ED after being struck by a cyclist while crossing the street. On arrival to the ED, her eyes remain closed to stimuli, she makes no verbal sounds, and withdraws only to painful stimuli. You assign her a GCS of 6. Her BP is 175/90 mm Hg and HR is 75 beats per minute. As you open her eye lids, you notice that her right pupil is 8 mm and nonreactive and her left is 4 mm and minimally reactive. Which of the following is the most common manifestation of increasing intracranial pressure (ICP) causing brain herniation?

a. Change in level of consciousness
b. Ipsilateral pupillary dilation
c. Contralateral pupillary dilation
d. Hypertension
e. Hemiparesis

208. A 34-year-old man is brought to the ED after being shot in the right side of his chest. The patient is awake and speaking. Breath sounds are diminished on the right. There is no bony crepitus or tracheal deviation. His BP is 95/65 mm Hg, HR is 121 beats per minute, and RR is 23 breaths per minute. Supine chest radiograph reveals a hazy appearance over the entire right lung field. You place a 36 French chest tube into the right thoracic cavity and note 1200 cc of blood in the Pleur-evac. Which of the following is an indication for thoracotomy?

a. 500 cc of initial chest tube drainage of blood
b. 1200 cc of initial chest tube drainage of blood
c. Persistent bleeding from the chest tube at a rate of 50 cc per hour
d. Chest radiograph with greater than 50% lung field white out
e. Evidence of a PTX

209. A 32-year-old woman is brought to the ED by paramedics after being involved in a motor vehicle collision. The patient was the front seat passenger of the car and was not wearing a seat belt. In the ED, the patient is speaking and complains of abdominal pain. Her breath sounds are equal bilaterally. You note a distended abdomen. A FAST exam is positive for fluid in the left upper quadrant. Her BP is 90/70 mm Hg and HR is 120 beats per minute. You administer 2 L of crystalloid solution. Her repeat BP is 80/60 mm Hg. Which of the following is the most appropriate next step in management?

a. Administer a vasoconstrictor such as epinephrine
b. Administer another 2 L of crystalloid
c. Administer O-negative blood
d. Bring patient to the CT scanner for an emergent scan
e. Perform another FAST exam to see if the fluid is increasing

210. A 27-year-old pregnant woman, in her third trimester, is brought to the ED after being involved in a low-speed motor vehicle collision. The patient was wearing a seat belt in the back seat of a car that was struck in the front by another car. Her BP is 120/70 mm Hg and HR is 107 beats per minute. Her airway is patent, breath sounds equal bilaterally, and skin is warm with 2+ pulses. FAST exam is negative for free fluid. Evaluation of the fetus reveals appropriate fetal HR and fetal movement. Repeat maternal BP is 120/75 mm Hg. Which of the following is the most appropriate next step in management?

a. Perform an immediate cesarean section in the OR
b. Perform an immediate cesarean section in the ED
c. CT scan of the abdomen and pelvis to rule out occult injury
d. Discharge the patient if laboratory testing is normal
e. Monitor the patient and fetus for a minimum of 4 hours

211. A 48-year-old man presents to the ED with low back pain after slipping on an icy sidewalk yesterday. He states the pain started on the left side of his lower back and now involves the right and radiates down both legs. He also noticed difficulty urinating since last night. On neurologic exam, he cannot plantar flex his feet. Rectal exam reveals diminished rectal tone. Which of the following is the best diagnosis?

a. Abdominal aortic aneurysm
b. Disk herniation
c. Spinal stenosis
d. Cauda equina syndrome
e. Osteomyelitis

212. Paramedics bring a 55-year-old woman to the ED after she was struck by a motor vehicle traveling at 30 miles per hour. Her BP is 165/95 mm Hg, HR is 105 beats per minute, and RR is 20 breaths per minute. Upon arrival, she does not open her eyes, is verbal but not making any sense, and withdraws to painful stimuli. You assign her a GCS score of 8. As you prepare to intubate the patient, a colleague notices that her left pupil has become dilated compared to the right. Which of the following has the quickest affect to reduce ICP?

a. Cranial decompression
b. Dexamethasone
c. Furosemide
d. Hyperventilation
e. Mannitol

Trauma

Answers

165. The answer is b. (*Rosen, pp 415–435.*) The image reveals *fluid in Morison's pouch* (the space between the right kidney and liver). Free fluid is seen as an anechoic area (black in color). The *FAST exam* is replacing the DPL in cases of abdominal trauma. It is inexpensive, noninvasive, and confirms the presence of hemoperitoneum in minutes. The minimum amount of intraperitoneal fluid needed for detection by ultrasound is approximately 70 cc. Patients who remain unstable despite volume resuscitation and have intraperitoneal fluid demonstrated by the FAST exam, need to be taken to the OR for a *laparotomy* to identify and treat the source of bleeding.

(a) CT scanning is a very useful diagnostic modality in blunt abdominal trauma allowing for localization of injuries within the abdomen. If the patient's vital signs improved after volume resuscitation or were stable upon presentation, the patient would undergo an abdominal CT scan. (c) If the FAST exam was negative and the patient remained hypotensive despite volume resuscitation, then a DPL should be performed, which may increase the sensitivity of finding an abdominal source of bleeding. (d) With unstable vital signs and a positive FAST exam, the patient requires a laparotomy. Ideally, he will receive another liter of crystalloid fluid or blood on the way to the OR. (e) Serial abdominal exams may be appropriate in certain cases of abdominal trauma with stable vital signs and no obvious internal injuries.

166. The answer is c. (*Rosen, pp 329–342.*) Spearing generates an axial loading force that is transmitted through the occipital condyles to the superior articular surfaces of the lateral masses of the first cervical vertebra (C-1). This fracture is commonly referred to as a *Jefferson fracture.* It is considered an unstable fracture; however, it is not commonly associated with spinal cord injury due to the increased area of the C-1 foramen. It is associated with diving accidents and in this scenario, "spearing" in a football game, which places an increased axial load to the cervical spine. Proper cervical spine precautions should remain in place throughout his management in the ED.

(a) Odontoid fractures occur when there is a fracture through the odontoid process of the C-2 vertebra. (b) A hangman fracture, or traumatic spondylolysis of C-2, occurs when the cervicocranium is thrown into extreme hyperextension secondary to abrupt deceleration. (**d**) Clay-Shoveler's fracture occurs secondary to cervical hyperextension or direct trauma to the posterior neck resulting in an avulsion fracture of the spinous process. (**e**) A teardrop fracture occurs from severe hyperflexion of the cervical spine and is commonly seen after diving accidents. This injury disrupts all of the cervical ligaments, facet joints, and causes a triangular fracture of a portion of the vertebral body. It is associated with anterior cord syndrome.

167. The answer is d. *(Rosen, p 401.)* The vignette describes a traumatic arrest after penetrating chest trauma. The most likely cause is *cardiac tamponade,* which occurs in approximately 2% of anterior penetrating chest trauma. Clinically, patients present with *hypotension, JVD, and muffled heart sounds.* These three signs are called *Beck's triad;* however, it is often difficult to hear heart sounds in the trauma setting. In addition, tachycardia is often present. The most effective method for relieving acute pericardial tamponade in the trauma setting is *thoracotomy* and incision of the pericardium with removal of blood from the pericardial sac. The indications to perform an ED thoracotomy generally include blunt or penetrating trauma patients who lose their vital signs in transport to or in the ED. Patients with penetrating wounds have a significantly better chance of surviving with benefit of thoracotomy and patients with stab wounds are more likely to do better than GSWs.

(**a & b**) The role of advanced cardiac life support (ACLS) drugs in traumatic arrest is unclear. However, patients in traumatic arrest typically require surgical, rather than, medical intervention. (**c**) Chest tube placement will not treat pericardial tamponade. If the patient had evidence of a tension PTX, chest tubes are the treatment of choice. (**e**) Pericardiocentesis may or may not be effective in acute traumatic tamponade because the pericardium is usually distended by clotted blood rather than by free blood. Pericardiocentesis is indicated for patients with suspected cardiac tamponade who have measurable vital signs that are stable.

168. The answer is e. *(Rosen, pp 521–523.)* The patient has a *mallet finger* or a *rupture of the extensor tendon* that inserts into the base of the distal phalanx. This type of injury occurs often from a sudden forceful flexion of an extended finger when an object, such as a football, strikes the tip of the finger. This is the common mechanism among athletes. Clinically, patients present with pain and swelling over the DIP joint, which is held in flexion of up to 40° due to loss of the extensor mechanism. The most important aspect in managing these injuries is to *keep the DIP joint in continuous extension until healing occurs.* Therefore, a splint should be applied so that only the DIP is immobilized in extension for 6–8 weeks. The PIP and metacarpophalangeal (MCP) joints should be mobile. Any disruption of the immobile DIP joint can result in improper healing.

169. The answer is b. *(Rosen, pp 547–549.)* Carpal *tunnel syndrome* is a neuropathy of the *median nerve* that occurs as a result of compression of the nerve within the carpal tunnel of the wrist. Symptoms include *paresthesias and pain* in the distribution of the median nerve; the volar thumb, second, third, and half of the fourth digit. Symptoms are usually worse after strenuous activities and at night. Pain improves with shaking of the hand or holding it in a dependent position. A sensitive test used to diagnose carpal tunnel is *Phalen's test.* Have the patient hold the affected wrist in hyperflexion for 60 seconds. The test is positive if paresthesias or numbness develops in the median nerve distribution.

(a) The ulnar nerve's sensory distribution is over the fourth and fifth digits. (d) The radial nerve's sensory distribution is over the posterior hand. (c) The axillary nerve's sensory distribution is over the proximal arm. (e) The musculocutaneous nerve's sensory distribution is over the lateral forearm.

170. The answer is a. *(Rosen, p 425.)* The patient is hypotensive despite fluid resuscitation in the setting of blunt trauma. The patient most likely has a source of bleeding that is not identified. A common location of bleeding in blunt trauma is the abdomen. In many hospitals, ultrasound is used to detect fluid in the abdomen (e.g., FAST exam). However, in this case, ultrasound is not present so the procedure of choice is a *DPL.* DPL can promptly reveal or exclude the presence of intraperitoneal hemorrhage. A positive aspiration is typically an indication for laparotomy, whereas a negative study allows the clinician to take other steps. In *blunt trauma,* a positive study entails either the *aspiration of 10 cc of fresh blood or a RBC count greater than 100,000/mm³.*

171. The answer is e. *(Simon, pp 123–126.)* A *boxer's fracture* is a fracture of the *neck of the fifth metacarpal.* It is one of the most common fractures of the hand and usually occurs from a direct impact to the hand (e.g., a punch with a closed fist).

(a) Colle's fracture is the most common wrist fracture seen in adults. It is a transverse fracture of the distal radial metaphysis, which is dorsally displaced and angulated. They usually occur from a fall on an outstretched hand. (b) Smith's fracture is a transverse fracture of the metaphysis of the distal radius, with associated volar displacement and angulation (opposite of a Colle's). They typical occur secondary to a direct blow or fall onto the dorsum of the hand. (c) A scaphoid fracture is the most common fracture of the carpal bones. It is typically seen in young adults secondary to a fall on the outstretched hand (FOOSH). (d) A Galeazzi fracture involves a fracture at the junction of the middle and distal thirds of the radius, with an associated dislocation of the distal radial-ulnar joint.

172. The answer is d. *(Rosen, pp 902–904.)* The patient has an *avulsed tooth,* which is a *dental emergency.* When a tooth is missing from a patient, the possibility of aspiration or entrapment in soft tissues should be considered. Avulsed permanent teeth require prompt intervention. The best environment for an avulsed tooth is its socket. *Replantation* is most successful if the tooth is *returned to its socket* within 30 minutes of the avulsion. A 1% chance of successful replantation is lost for every minute that the tooth is outside of its socket. The tooth should only be handled by the crown as not to disrupt the root. If the patient cannot replant the tooth, then they should keep the tooth under his or her tongue or in the buccal pouch so that it is bathed in saliva. If that cannot be achieved, then the tooth can be placed in a cup of milk (e) or in saline. The best transport solution is *Hank's solution.*

(a) The worst situation is to transport the tooth in a dry medium. (b) and (c) water and beer are less than ideal. Saliva, milk, or saline are better solutions.

173. The answer is c. *(Rosen, p 138.)* The GCS score, as seen on the next page, may be used as a tool for classifying head injury and is an objective method for following a patient's neurologic status. The GCS assesses a person's *eye, verbal, and motor responsiveness.* Although the GCS was originally developed to assess head trauma at 6 hours postinjury, it is commonly used in the acute presentation. This patient received a score of 3 for eye opening to verbal command, 4 for disorientation but conversant, and 6 for obeying verbal commands.

A   Glasgow Coma Scale

Eye opening	Spontaneous	4
	To verbal command	3
	To pain	2
	None	1
Verbal responsiveness	Oriented	5
	Confused	4
	Inappropriate words	3
	Incomprehensible sounds	2
	None	1
Motor response	Obeys	6
	Localizes	5
	Withdraws (pain)	4
	Flexion (pain)	3
	Extension (pain)	2
	None	1
	Total:	_____

(Reproduced, with permission, from Stone KC, Humphries RL. Current Emergency Diagnosis & Treatment. New York, NY: McGraw-Hill, 2004: 210.)

174. The answer is a. (Rosen, pp 415–416.) Since most people are right-handed and hold the offending instrument in their right hand, the left upper quadrant is most commonly injured in stab wounds. However, the *liver* occupies the most space in the abdomen and therefore is the most common organ injured.

(b) The small bowel is the second most commonly injured organ in stab wounds and is the most common organ injured in projectile penetrating abdominal trauma. **(c, d, and e)** are less commonly injured than the liver and small bowel in penetrating abdominal trauma.

175. The answer is d. (Rosen, pp 381–382.) *Simple rib fractures* are the most common form of significant chest injury. Ribs usually break at the point of impact or at the posterior angle, which is structurally the weakest area. The fourth through ninth ribs are most commonly involved. Rib fractures occur more commonly in adults than in children due to the relative inelasticity of the adult chest wall compared to the more compliant chest wall of children. The presence of two or more rib fractures at any level is associated with a higher incidence of internal injuries. The treatment of patients with simple acute rib fractures includes *adequate pain relief* and *maintenance of pulmonary function*. Oral pain medications are usually sufficient for young and healthy patients. Older patients may require better analgesia with opioids, trying to avoid oversedation. Continuing daily activities and deep breathing is important to ensure ventilation and prevent atelectasis. If there is a question about the patient's ability to cough, breathe deeply, and maintain activity, particularly if two or more ribs are fractured, it is preferable to admit the patient to the hospital for aggressive pulmonary care.

(a) Attempts to relieve pain by immobilization or splinting should not be used. Although they may decrease pain, they also promote hypoventilation leading to atelectasis and pneumonia. (b) A chest tube is indicated only if a PTX or hemothorax is suspected. (c) Rib fractures heal spontaneously and do not require surgical fixation. (e) The main concern in treating rib fractures is preventing complications such as atelectasis and pneumonia. Therefore, it is important that the patient have adequate analgesia.

176. The answer is a. *(Rosen, pp 388–390.)* A PTX can be divided into three classifications: simple, communicating, and tension. A PTX is considered simple when there is no communication with the atmosphere or any shift of the mediastinum or hemidiaphragm resulting from the accumulation of air within the pleural cavity. A communicating PTX is associated with a defect in the chest wall and is sometimes referred to as a "sucking chest wound." A tension PTX occurs when air enters the pleural cavity on inspiration but cannot exit, which leads to compression of the vena cava and subsequent decreased cardiac output. The progressive accumulation of air under pressure in the pleural cavity may lead to a shift of the mediastinum to the contralateral hemithorax.

Patients with a traumatic PTX typically present with shortness of breath, chest pain, and tachypnea. The physical exam may reveal decreased or absent breath sounds over the involved side as well as subcutaneous emphysema. Any patient with respiratory symptoms in the setting of a PTX should be treated with a *tube thoracostomy (chest tube)*. The preferred site for insertion is the fourth or fifth intercostal space at the anterior or mid-axillary line. The tube should be positioned posteriorly and toward the apex so that it can effectively remove both air and fluid.

(b) A pericardiocentesis is a procedure used to remove fluid from the pericardial sac such as in the case of pericardial tamponade. It is more likely to occur after a penetrating trauma to the chest rather than a blunt trauma. (c) A DPL is used to diagnose fluid in the peritoneum. Although this may be necessary for this patient, it is important to follow the ABC's of resuscitation. In this patient, airway and breathing needs to be addressed first. (d) ED thoracotomy is used in select circumstances such as in blunt or penetrating trauma patients who lose their vital signs in transport to or in the ED. (e) A chest radiograph may be helpful in diagnosing a PTX, however, the patient is unstable in the setting of blunt trauma and intervention should not wait for a chest radiograph. If the patient was stable, then a chest radiograph can be used to confirm the presence of a PTX prior to chest tube insertion.

177. The answer is e. *(Simon, pp 489–491.)* The patient is showing signs and symptoms of *compartment syndrome*. The syndrome occurs due to an increase in pressure within a confined osseofacial space that impedes neurovascular function. The end result is necrosis and damage to tissues. It can occur after crush injuries, circumferential burns, hemorrhage, edema, or any process that increases compartment pressure. Clinically, the patient complains of pain that is out of proportion to the injury. Physical exam may reveal swelling, sensory deficits, and pain with passive motion. The *presence of a pulse does not rule out compartment syndrome*. Late findings include pallor of the skin, diminished or absent pulses, and a cool extremity. The only way to diagnose compartment syndrome is to *measure intracompartmental pressure with a Stryker device*. A pressure *greater than 30 mm Hg* is considered diagnostic and the patient requires a *fasciotomy* to avoid tissue damage.

(a) Ice water may decrease swelling but will not prevent compartment syndrome. (b) There is no reason to suspect that an occult fracture is causing the pain. (c) Elevation to the level of the heart is recommended, however, all constrictive bandages should be removed. (d) A DVT should not cause this pain.

178. The answer is d. *(Rosen, pp 596–597.)* The patient's clinical presentation is consistent with a *posterior shoulder dislocation*. Posterior dislocations are rare and account for only 2% of all glenohumeral dislocations. Posterior dislocations are traditionally associated with *seizure patients* and *lightening injuries*. However, the most common dislocation seen is this population is an anterior dislocation. Classically, the patient holds the dislocated arm across the chest in adduction and internal rotation. Abduction is limited and external rotation is blocked. Radiographs may reveal a "light bulb" sign, which is the light bulb appearance when the humeral head is profiled in internal rotation.

179. The answer is d. *(Rosen, p 349.)* *Brown-Séquard syndrome* or *hemisection* of the spinal cord, typically results from *penetrating trauma* such as a gunshot or knife wound. Patients with this lesion have *ipsilateral motor paralysis* and *contralateral loss of pain and temperature* distal to the level of the injury. This syndrome has the best prognosis for recovery of all of the incomplete spinal cord lesions.

(a) Spinal shock is a clinical syndrome characterized by the loss of neurologic function and autonomic tone below the level of a spinal cord lesion. Patients typically exhibit flaccid paralysis with loss of sensory input, deep tendon reflexes, and urinary bladder tone. Also, they are usually bradycardic, hypotensive, and hypothermic. Spinal shock generally lasts less than 24 hours but may last several days. (b) Central cord syndrome is often seen in patients with degenerative arthritis of the cervical vertebrae, whose necks are subjected to forced hyperextension; typically, a forward fall onto the face in an elderly person. Patients often have greater sensorimotor neurologic deficits in the upper extremities compared to the lower extremities. (c) Anterior cord syndrome results in variable degrees of motor paralysis and absent pain sensation below the level of the lesion. Its hallmark is preservation of vibratory sensation and propioception due to an intact dorsal column. (e) Cauda equina injury causes peripheral nerve injury rather than direct spinal cord damage. Its presentation may include variable motor and sensory loss in the lower extremities, sciatica, bowel and bladder dysfunction, and saddle anesthesia.

180. The answer is b. (*Rosen, pp 538–539.*) The *scaphoid* is the most commonly fractured carpal bone. It is typically seen in patients in their 20s to 30s after a *FOOSH*. Classically, physical exam reveals *tenderness in the anatomic snuffbox,* the space between the extensor pollicis longus and the extensor pollicis brevis. On radiography, however, up to 15% of scaphoid fractures are not detected. As the necrotic bone at the fracture site is resorbed, the fracture line often becomes apparent on radiographs at 10–14 days after injury. Therefore, patients with snuffbox tenderness and an initial radiograph should be splinted in a *thumb spica splint* and return for *repeat radiographs in 10–14 days.*

(a) Placing an elastic wrap will not provide adequate immobilization and will lead to increased complications if a fracture is present. (c) Ice is recommended but immobilization is also required. (d) Even a CT scan will not pick up the fracture immediately after injury. However, if there is snuffbox tenderness after 14 days and the radiograph remains negative, a CT scan is warranted. (e) This is unnecessary because it is not clear if the scaphoid is fractured.

181. The answer is a. (*Tintinalli, pp 1557–1569.*) Head injury severity is assessed on the mechanism of injury and the initial neurologic exam. Although the GCS is currently used in multiple settings, it was initially developed for the clinical evaluation of trauma patients with isolated head trauma, who are hemodynamically stable, and adequately oxygenated.

A score of 14–15 is associated with minor head injury, 9–13 moderate, and *less than 8* is associated with *severe head injury*. His *GCS score is 8* (2 points for eye opening to pain, 2 points for mumbling speech, 4 points for withdrawing from pain). He is classified with a severe head injury. The overall mortality of severe head injury is almost 40%. It is recommended to *intubate* patients with a *GCS score of 8 or less* for airway protection. These patients are at risk for increased ICP and herniation, which can lead to rapid respiratory decline. All patients with severe traumatic brain injury require an emergent CT scan and should be admitted to the intensive care unit in a hospital with neurosurgical capabilities.

(b) Repairing his laceration is not a priority and can take place after diagnosing and stabilizing injuries that are more serious. If there is an active scalp bleed, staples can be rapidly placed to limit bleeding until definitive repair can take place. (c) Mannitol is an osmotic agent that is used to reduce ICP. It is administered if there are signs of impending or actual herniation (i.e., fixed and dilated pupil). (d) Bilateral ED trephination (burr holes) is rarely, if ever, performed and is considered if definitive neurosurgical care is not available. (e) This patient will require neurosurgical intervention if there is any evidence of intracranial hemorrhage or declining neurologic status indicating increased ICP.

182. The answer is c. *(Rosen, p 384.)* *Flail chest* results when *three or more adjacent ribs are fractured at two points,* allowing a freely moving segment of the chest wall to move in a *paradoxical motion*. It is one of the most commonly overlooked injuries resulting from blunt chest trauma. The paradoxical motion of the chest wall is the hallmark of this condition, with the flail segment paradoxically moving inward with inspiration and outward with expiration.

183. The answer is d. *(Rosen, pp 370–374.)* Due to its lack of bony protection, the neck is especially vulnerable to severe, life-threatening injuries. Neck trauma is caused by three major mechanisms penetrating, blunt, and strangulation, which can affect the airway, digestive tract, vascular, and neurologic systems. The neck is divided into three zones as seen in the picture on the next page. Zone 1 extends superiorly from the sternal notch and clavicles to the cricoid cartilage. Injuries to this region can affect both neck and mediastinal structures. Zone 2 is the area between the cricoid cartilage and the angle of the mandible. Zone 3 extends from the angle of the mandible to the base of the skull. Zone 1 and 3 injuries typically pose a greater challenge than zone 2 injuries because zones 1 and 3 and much less exposed than zone 2. *Generally, zone 2 injuries are taken directly to the OR for surgical exploration.* Injuries in zones 1 and 3 may be taken to the OR or managed conservatively using a combination of angiography, bronchoscopy, esophagoscopy, and CT scanning.

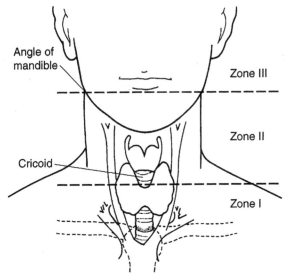

Angle of mandible

Zone III

Cricoid

Zone II

Zone I

(Reproduced, with permission, from Doherty GM, Way LW. Current Surgical Diagnosis & Treatment. New York, NY: McGraw-Hill, 2006: 210.)

Airway management is always given priority in trauma patients, particularly when neck structures are involved due to the potential for rapid airway compromise. Active bleeding sites or wounds with blood clots should not be probed because massive hemorrhage can occur. *Bleeding should be controlled by direct pressure.* Blind clamping should be avoided because of the high concentration of neurovascular structures in the neck.

(**a and b**) Blind clamping and probing the wound are contraindicated. (**c and e**) The injury is in zone 2 of the neck.

184. The answer is d. (*Rosen, pp 337–340.*) *The Hangman's fracture, or traumatic spondylolysis of C2,* occurs when the head is thrown into *extreme hyperextension* as a result of *abrupt deceleration,* resulting in bilateral fractures of the pedicles. The name "hangman's fracture" was derived from judicial hangings, where the knot of the noose was placed under the chin which caused extreme hyperextension of the head on the neck, resulting in a fracture at C2. However, many hangings resulted in death from strangulation rather than spinal cord damage. Today, the most common cause of a Hangman's fracture is the result of *head-on auto-mobile collisions.*

(a) Colle's fracture is the most common wrist fracture seen in adults, It is a transverse fracture of the distal radial metaphysis, which is dorsally displaced and angulated. They usually occur from a fall on an outstretched hand. (b) A boxer's fracture is a fracture of the neck of the fifth metacarpal. It is one of the most common fractures of the hand and usually occurs from a direct impact to the hand (e.g., a punch with a closed fist). (c) A fracture of C1 is called a Jefferson's fracture, which is typically produced by a vertical compression force. (e) Clay-Shoveler's fracture occurs secondary to cervical hyperextension or direct trauma to the posterior neck resulting in an avulsion fracture of the spinous process.

185. The answer is b. *(Tintinalli, pp 1565–1566.)* The skull base comprises the floors of the anterior, middle, and posterior cranial fossae. Fractures in this region typically do not have localized symptoms. However, indirect signs of injury may include visible evidence of bleeding from the fracture into surrounding soft tissue. Ecchymosis around the mastoid bone is often described as *Battle's sign* and periorbital ecchymosis is often described as *"raccoon eyes."* The most common *basilar skull fracture* involves the petrous portion of the temporal bone, the external auditory canal, and the tympanic membrane. It is commonly associated with a torn dura leading to *cerebrospinal fluid (CSF) otorrhea or rhinorrhea.* Other signs and symptoms of a basilar skull fracture include hemotympanum, vertigo, decreased hearing or deafness, and seventh nerve palsy. Periorbital and mastoid ecchymosis develop gradually over hours after an injury and are often absent in the ED. If clear or pink fluid is seen from the nose or ear and a CSF leak is suspected, the fluid can be placed on filter paper and a "halo" or double ring may appear. This is a simple but nonsensitive test to confirm a CSF leak. Evidence of open communication, such as a CSF leak, mandates neurosurgical consultation and admission.

(a) LeFort factures typically result from high-energy facial trauma and are classified according to their location. A LeFort I involves a transverse fracture just above the teeth at the level of the nasal fossa, and allows movement of the alveolar ridge and hard palate. A LeFort II is a pyramidal fracture with its apex just above the bridge of the nose and extending laterally and inferiorly through the infraorbital rims allowing movement of the maxilla, nose, and infraorbital rims. A LeFort III represents complete craniofacial disruption and involves fractures of the zygoma, infraorbital rims, and maxilla. It is rare for these fractures to occur in isolation; they usually occur in combination. (**c and d**) Otitis interna and externa are inflammation of the inner ear and outer ear, respectively, and are not relevant in acute trauma. (**e**) Tripod fractures typically occur from blunt force applied to the lateral face causing fractures of zygomatic arch, the lateral orbital rim, the inferior orbital rim, and the anterior and lateral walls of the maxillary sinus. These fractures present clinically with asymmetrical facial flattening, edema, and ecchymosis.

186. The answer is e. (*Tintinalli, pp 1537–1540.*) Based on the principles of advanced trauma life support (ATLS), injured patients are assessed and treated in a fashion that establishes priorities based on their presenting vital signs, mental status, and injury mechanism. The approach to trauma care consists of a *primary survey,* rapid resuscitation, and a more thorough secondary survey followed by diagnostic testing. The goal of the primary survey is to quickly identify and treat immediately life-threatening injuries. The assessment of the *ABCDEs (airway, breathing, circulation, neurologic disability, exposure)* is a model that should be followed in all patients. Airway patency is first evaluated by listening for vocalizations, asking the patient to speak, and looking in the patient's mouth for signs of obstruction. Breathing is assessed by observing for symmetric rise and fall of the chest and listening for bilateral breath sounds over the anterior chest and axillae. The chest should be palpated for subcutaneous air and bony crepitus. Circulatory function is assessed by noting the patient's mental status, skin color and temperature, and pulses. The patient's neurologic status is assessed by noting level of consciousness and gross motor function. An initial GCS should be calculated in the ED. Lastly, the patient is completely undressed to evaluate for otherwise hidden bruises, lacerations, impaled foreign bodies, and open fractures. Only after the primary survey is complete and life-threatening injuries are addressed, and the patient is resuscitated and stabilized, is the secondary head-to-toe survey undertaken.

(**a**) This patient will require a chest tube for presumed hemo- or pneumothorax demonstrated by decreased breath sounds and oxygen saturation of 93%. However, the airway should first be secured. (**b**) A DPL or FAST exam is used to screen the abdomen for hemoperitoneum. However, airway and breathing take priority in this patient. (**c**) Bilateral ED trephination (burr holes) is rarely, if ever, performed and should only be considered if definitive neurosurgical care is not available. (**d**) Extremity injuries are typically not life-threatening and are assessed after the airway, breathing, and circulation are evaluated.

187. The answer is a. *(Tintinalli, pp 1566–1567.)* *Epidural hematomas* are the result of blood collecting in the potential space between the skull and the dura mater. Most epidural hematomas result from *blunt trauma* to the temporal or temporoparietal area with an associated skull fracture and middle *meningeal artery disruption.* The classic history of an epidural hematoma is a lucent period following immediate loss of consciousness after significant blunt head trauma. However, this clinical pattern occurs in a minority of cases. Most patients either never lose consciousness or never regain consciousness after the injury. On CT scan, epidural hematomas appear *lenticular* or *biconvex (football shaped)*, typically in the temporal region. The high-pressure arterial bleeding of an epidural hematoma can lead to herniation within hours after injury. Therefore, early recognition and evacuation is important to increase survival. Bilateral ED trephination (burr holes) is rarely, if ever, performed and should only be considered if definitive neurosurgical care is not available.

(b) Subdural hematomas appear as hyperdense, crescent-shaped lesions that cross suture lines. They result from a collection of blood below the dura and over the brain. To differentiate the CT finding from an epidural hematoma, think about the high pressure created by the arterial tear of an epidural that causes the hematoma to expand inward. Whereas, the low pressure venous bleed of a subdural hematoma layers along the calvarium. **(c)** Traumatic SAH is probably the most common CT abnormality in patients with moderate to severe traumatic brain injury. **(d and e)** Contusions and intracerebral hematomas occur secondary to traumatic tearing of intracerebral blood vessels. Contusions most commonly occur in the frontal, temporal, and occipital lobes; and may occur at the site of the blunt trauma or the opposite site of the brain, known as a contre-coup injury.

188. The answer is a. *(Rosen, p 349.)* *Central cord syndrome* is often seen in patients with degenerative arthritis of the cervical vertebrae, whose necks are subjected to *forced hyperextension;* typically, a forward fall onto the face in an elderly person. This causes the ligamentum flavum to buckle into the spinal cord, resulting in a contusion to the central portion of the cord. This injury affects the central gray matter and the most central portions of the pyramidal and spinothalamic tracts. Patients often have *greater neurologic deficits in the upper extremities compared to the lower extremities* since nerve fibers that innervate distal structures are located in the periphery of the spinal cord. In severe injuries, patients may appear to be quadriplegic. In addition, patients with central cord syndrome usually have decreased rectal sphincter tone and patchy, unpredictable sensory deficits.

(b) Anterior cord syndrome results in variable degrees of motor paralysis and absent pain sensation below the level of the lesion. Its hallmark is preservation of vibratory sensation and propioception due to an intact dorsal column. (c) Brown-Séquard syndrome results in ipsilateral loss of motor strength, vibratory sensation, and propioception, and contralateral loss of pain and temperature sensation. (d) Transverse myelitis is an inflammatory process that produces complete motor and sensory loss below the level of the lesion. (e) Parkinson's disease develops over years and does not result in paralysis.

189. The answer is c. (*Rosen, pp 538–539.*) *Avascular necrosis* of the *scaphoid* is seen in approximately 3% of scaphoid fractures. The typical presentation of a scaphoid fracture is a FOOSH. On exam patients have *snuffbox tenderness* or tenderness with axial loading of the thumb. Blood supply to the scaphoid is provided by a single artery that flows into the distal portion of the bone leaving the proximal portion vulnerable in the setting of a fracture. This increases the likelihood of complications, particularly avascular necrosis, in the setting of a poorly healed fracture.

(a) A fracture of the distal ulna would heal after 3 months. There is no tenderness over the ulna on exam. (b) A hematoma may have occurred at the time of injury from a venous bleed. However, it would not be present 3 months later. (d) The patient's neurologic exam is normal. (e) Lunate fractures are rare but are also complicated by avascular necrosis. This patient has snuffbox tenderness, which is more likely due to a scaphoid injury.

190. The answer is e. (*American College of Surgeons Committee on Trauma, pp 79–80.*) The decision to begin blood transfusion in a trauma patient is based on the initial response to crystalloid volume resuscitation. *Blood products should be administered if vital signs transiently improve or remain unstable despite resuscitation with 2–3 liters of crystalloid fluid.* The main purpose in transfusing blood is to restore the oxygen-carrying capacity of the intravascular volume. Fully cross-matched blood is preferable (e.g., type B, Rh-negative, antibody negative); however, this process may take more than 1 hour, which is inappropriate for the unstable trauma patient. Type-specific blood (e.g., type A, Rh negative, unknown antibody) can be provided by most blood banks within 10 minutes. This blood is compatible with ABO and Rh blood types, but may be incompatible with other antibodies. If type-specific blood is unavailable, type O packed cells are indicated for patients who are unstable. To reduce sensitization and future complications, type O Rh negative blood is reserved for women of childbearing age.

(a) Fully cross-matched blood may take greater than 1 hour to prepare, which is inappropriate for an unstable patient. (b) Whole blood is rarely used by blood centers and was replaced by blood components such as packed RBCs. (c) Blood transfusion may be life saving and should be administered when appropriate in the setting of trauma. (d) For life-threatening blood loss, type O Rh negative blood is reserved for women of childbearing age. This reduces complications of Rh incompatibility in future pregnancies. Type O Rh positive blood can be administered to women in an emergency.

191. The answer is c. (*Rosen, pp 592–602.*) This patient has an *anterior shoulder dislocation.* The glenohumeral joint is the most commonly dislocated joint in the body, mainly due to the lack of bony stability and its wide range of motion. Anterior dislocations account for 95–97% of cases and are most commonly seen in younger, athletic males and geriatric females. It usually happens by way of an indirect force that involves an abduction/extension/external rotation injury. Directly, it may occur as a result of a posterior blow that forces the humeral head out of the glenoid rim anteriorly. Radiographs obtained must include an axillary view to determine positioning of the humeral head. Patients usually present in severe pain, holding the affected arm with the contralateral hand in slight abduction. The lateral acromial process is prominent giving the shoulder a full or squared-off appearance. Patients typically cannot internally rotate their shoulder. *Axillary nerve injuries* can occur in up to 54% of anterior dislocations; however, these are neuropraxic in nature and tend to resolve on their own. Following the C5/C6 dermatome distribution, patients have a loss of sensation over the lateral aspect of the deltoid with decreased muscle contraction with abduction. After proper muscle relaxation with conscious sedation or intra-articular injection, closed reduction may be attempted using a variety of methods. After reduction, it is imperative to repeat a neurovascular exam and obtain confirmatory radiographs.

AC joint sprains (a) occur primarily in men and account for 25% of all dislocations. However, the mechanism of injury primarily involves a fall or direct blow to the adducted arm causing a downward and medial thrust to the scapula.

Posterior dislocations (b & e) are rare due to the scapular angle on the thoracic ribs. They are seen, however, in convulsive seizures where the large internal rotator muscles overpower the weaker external rotators and cause the dislocation. Median nerve injuries (**d**) mainly involve weakness in the first three finger flexors. Ulnar nerve injuries (**e**) mainly involve weakness in the interossei muscles of the hand and paresthesias along the fifth digit.

192. The answer is c. (*Rosen, pp 625–641.*) This patient is hemodynamically unstable with a pelvic fracture. The retroperitoneum can accommodate up to 4 L of blood after severe pelvic trauma. A few options are useful in managing hemorrhage from an unstable pelvic fracture. However, the initial and simplest modality to use in a patient in shock from a pelvis fracture is placement of a *pelvic-binding garment.* This device can be applied easily and rapidly and is typically effective in tamponading bleeding and stabilizing the pelvis.

(**a**) Bilateral chest tubes would be appropriate if there was evidence for a pneumo- or hemothorax. This patient has bilaterally equal breath sounds. (**b**) Although external fixation is an effective method to stabilize the pelvis, it may delay management of a trauma patient. Because a pelvic binding apparatus is quick and simple, it is preferred. (**d and e**) Angiography is indicated when hypovolemia persists in a patient with a major pelvic fracture, despite control of hemorrhage from other sources. Angiography typically takes place in the angiography suite; therefore, patients should have a pelvic binding device applied then be transferred to angiography. The source of retroperitoneal bleeding with pelvic fractures is typically the venous plexus or smaller veins. However, venography is not useful in managing these patients because even when venous bleeding is localized, embolization is ineffective because of the extensive anastomoses and valveless collateral flow. In contrast, arteriography is a major diagnostic and therapeutic modality for the patient with severe pelvic hemorrhage from arterial sources.

193. The answer is c. (*Rosen, p 349.*) *Anterior cord syndrome* results from *cervical flexion injuries* (diving in shallow water) that cause cord contusion or protrusion of a bony fragment or herniated intervertebral disk into the spinal canal. It may also occur from vascular pathology such as laceration or thrombosis of the anterior spinal artery. The syndrome is characterized by different degrees of paralysis and loss of pain and temperature sensation below the level of injury. Its *hallmark* is the *preservation of the posterior columns, maintaining position, touch, and vibratory sensation.*

(**a**) Brown-Séquard syndrome results in ipsilateral loss of motor strength, vibratory sensation, and propioception, and contralateral loss of pain and temperature sensation. **(b)** Central cord syndrome is often seen in patients with degenerative arthritis of the cervical vertebrae, whose necks are subjected to forced hyperextension; typically, a forward fall onto the face in an elderly person. Patients often have greater sensorimotor neurologic deficits in the upper extremities compared to the lower extremities. **(d)** Cauda equina injury causes peripheral nerve injury rather than direct spinal cord damage. Its presentation may include variable motor and sensory loss in the lower extremities, sciatica, bowel and bladder dysfunction, and saddle anesthesia. **(e)** SCIWORA is reserved for the pediatric population because the spinal cord is less elastic than the bony spine and ligaments. It is associated with parestheisas and generalized weakness.

194. The answer is b. *(Tintinalli, pp 1596–1597.)* The treatment of a *tension PTX* involves immediate reduction in the intrapleural pressure on the affected side of the thoracic cavity. The simplest and quickest way to establish this is by inserting a 14-gauge catheter into the thoracic cavity in the second intercostal space in the midclavicular line. After this procedure, a chest tube should be inserted as definitive management. *Needle thoracostomy* is necessary when a patient's vital signs are unstable; otherwise, direct insertion of a chest tube is adequate for suspicion of a hemo- or pneumothorax. A tension PTX is a life-threatening emergency caused by air entering the pleural space that is not able to escape secondary to the creation of a one-way valve. This increased pressure causes the ipsilateral lung to collapse, shifting the mediastinum away from the injured lung, compromising vena caval blood return to the heart. The severely altered preload results in reduced stroke volume, increased cardiac output, and hypotension.

(a) Airway is the first component addressed in the ABCs; however, the patient is breathing on his own and does not require intubation. **(c and d)** If the BP does not elevate with insertion of a chest tube, then the next area to focus on is an intra-abdominal injury, which can be assessed either by a DPL or FAST exam. **(e)** A pericardiocentesis is indicated in the stable trauma patient when there is suspicion for cardiac tamponade, which may present with tachycardia, hypotension, JVD, and muffled heart sounds.

195. The answer is e. *(Tintinalli, pp 1549–1553.)* The Canadian C-Spine Rule for radiography in alert and stable patients following blunt head or neck trauma identified *age greater than 65 years as a high risk factor for C-spine injury,* even among those with stable vital signs and a GCS score of 15. Therefore, C-spine imaging in all such elderly patients is warranted.

(a) It is thought that elderly patients experience a much lower incidence of epidural hematomas than the general population because of a relatively denser fibrous bond between the dura mater and the inner table of the skull in older individuals. (b) There is, however, a high incidence of subdural hematomas in elderly patients. As the brain mass decreases in size with age, there is greater stretching and tension of the bridging veins that pass from the brain to the dural sinuses. (c) Geriatric patients are more susceptible to the development of hypoxia and respiratory infections following trauma. In the elderly, diminished elasticity of the lungs can lead to a reduction in pulmonary compliance and in the ability to cough effectively resulting in an increased risk for nosocomial gram-negative pneumonia. (d) The most common cervical spine fractures in this age group are upper cervical, particularly fractures of the odontoid, not lower C6 fractures.

196. The answer is b. *(Tintinalli, pp 1715–1716.)* The evaluation of patients with *pelvic fractures* begins with the primary trauma survey (ABCs). Fractured pelvic bones bleed briskly and can lacerate surrounding soft tissues and disrupt their extensive arterial and venous networks. Hemorrhage is a common cause of death in patients with pelvic injuries. Bleeding in the retroperitoneum can accommodate up to 4 L of blood. Most pelvic bleeding is from the fractures and low pressure sacral venous plexus. In the ED, a *stabilizer* can be applied to the pelvis to help control the hemorrhage. Once an abdominal source of bleeding is ruled out as a source of hypotension, the patient should undergo *pelvic angiography with embolization of bleeding vessels.* The patient should also be resuscitated with packed RBCs until the bleeding is controlled.

(a) It is often difficult to discern peritoneal bleeding from pelvic bleeding as a cause of hypotension. A positive FAST exam or DPL in the setting of hypotension requires that the patient undergo exploratory laparotomy to control peritoneal hemorrhage. If a pelvic source of bleeding is also suspected, some facilities are able to perform pelvic angiography in the same OR suite. (c) If the patient was stable, he would undergo a CT scan to better evaluate for internal injuries. However, in the setting of hypotension, the patient requires definitive therapy. (d) A pericardiocentesis is rarely used in the acute trauma setting and is reserved for the treatment of pericardial tamponade. (e) A retrograde urethrogram is performed when there is suspicion for a urethral injury in the stable patient.

197. The answer is b. *(Tintinalli, pp 1613–1614.)* *Blunt trauma* is the most common mechanism of injury seen in the United States. The forces exerted on the abdomen put all of the organs at risk for injury. Motor Vehicle collisions with another vehicle or pedestrian are the major causes of blunt abdominal trauma. The *spleen* is the organ most often injured, and in approximately 66% of these cases, it is the only damaged intraperitoneal organ.

(a) The liver is the second most commonly injured intra-abdominal organ, third is the kidney (c), fourth is the small bowel (d), and fifth is the bladder (e).

198. The answer is b. (*Rosen, pp 593–596.*) The radiograph confirms an *anterior dislocation* of the left shoulder. Patient's typically present in severe pain with the dislocated arm held in slight abduction and external rotation by the opposite extremity. The patient leans away from the injured side and cannot adduct or internally rotate the shoulder without severe pain. Associated fractures may occur in up to 50% of anterior dislocations. The most common of these is a *compression fracture of the humeral head*. This defect is called a *Hill-Sachs deformity*.

a) Fracture of anterior glenoid rim or Bankart's fracture is also associated with anterior dislocations but is present in approximately 5% of cases. Choices c, d, and e are not commonly associated with anterior dislocations.

199. The answer is e. (*Scaletta, pp 229–231.*) *Urethral injuries* make up approximately 10% of genitourinary trauma. Anterior urethral injuries are most often due to falls with straddle injuries or a blunt force to the perineum. Approximately 95% of posterior urethral injuries are secondary to pelvic fractures. Signs and symptoms of urethral injury include perineal pain, inability to void, gross hematuria, blood at the urethral meatus, perineal or scrotal swelling or ecchymosis, and an absent, high-riding, or boggy prostate. A *retrograde urethrogram* is the study of choice when there is suspicion of a urethral injury. This procedure is performed by inserting an 8 Fr urinary catheter 2 cm into the meatus and inflating the catheter balloon with 2 cc saline to create a seal. Then, 30 cc of radiopaque contrast is administered and a radiograph is obtained looking for extravasation of contrast from the urethra.

(a) A scrotal ultrasound may be necessary later on to evaluate for testicular injury, but it is not used to evaluate urethral injury. (b) A KUB is not useful to evaluate the urethra. Prior to CT scanning, it was commonly used to evaluate for kidney stones. (c) An intravenous pyelogram is an alternative to CT scanning for evaluating the kidney and ureter. (d) A retrograde cystogram is a useful study to evaluate the bladder for injury.

200. The answer is b. *(Scaletta, pp 110–111.)* *Orbital floor fractures* typically occur when a blunt object with a radius of curvature less than 5 cm strikes the orbit; often a fist or ball smaller than a softball. The blunt force causes an increase in intraorbital pressure causing a fracture along the weakest part of the orbit, usually the inferior or sometimes medial wall. Patients usually complain of *pain that is greatest with upward eye movement.* They may have *impaired ocular motility* or *diplopia* if the inferior rectus muscle becomes entrapped. They may also present with *infraorbital hypoesthesia* due to compression of the infraorbital nerve. Generally, the patient has normal visual acuity unless there is an associated ocular injury. A classic radiographic finding is the "teardrop sign," which represents herniated orbital fat and muscle in the roof of the maxillary sinus. There may also be an air-fluid level in the maxillary sinus due to bleeding into it. Patients usually do well and recover completely in mild to moderate fractures.

(a) Zygomatic arch fractures usually present with periauricular depression and point tenderness and may be complicated by trismus secondary to impingement of the coronoid process of the mandible on the arch during mouth opening. (c) A retrobulbar hematoma occurs secondary to blunt orbital trauma and typically causes exopthalmos. Patients usually present with periorbital edema, ecchymosis, a decrease in visual acuity, and an afferent papillary defect in the involved eye. (d) Open globe injuries typically result from penetrating trauma to the eye. Patients may present with leakage of aqueous humor, a teardrop-shaped pupil, or prolapse of choroid through the wound. (e) Patients with mandible fractures present with pain and decreased range of motion of the jaw, malocclusion or pain with teeth clenching, and inability to fully open the mouth.

201. The answer is e. *(Tintinalli, p 1617. Scaletta, pp 204–212.)* An important concern with *anterior abdominal GSW* is to determine whether the missile traversed the peritoneal cavity. Patients with transabdominal GSWs nearly all have intra-abdominal injuries requiring surgery. Most of the time, this can be determined by approximating the trajectory. Therefore, a hole in both the anterior and posterior abdomen highly suggests a transabdominal trajectory. If there are a single or odd number of holes, a plain film may help estimate trajectory. In cases of tangential or multiple GSWs, it may be impossible to determine trajectory with any certainty. In a patient with evidence of peritoneal penetration, a missile tract that clearly enters the abdominal cavity, or has a positive diagnostic study (DPL, FAST, CT) in a tangential wound, he or she should undergo exploratory laparotomy. The standard algorithm for *penetrating abdominal trauma* recommends that any patient with *unstable vital signs* be taken directly to the OR to undergo an *exploratory laparotomy.* If their vital signs are stable, they should undergo further diagnostic studies such as a FAST exam, DPL, or CT scan.

(**a**) In general, penetrating abdominal wounds should not be probed. This may worsen the injury and disrupt hemostasis, resulting in uncontrolled hemorrhage. Instead, gently separate the skin edges to see if the base of the wound can be visualized. (**b, c, d**) In the setting of penetrating abdominal trauma, further diagnostic tests should only occur if the patient has stable vital signs. Otherwise, they should go directly to the OR to undergo exploratory laparotomy.

202. The answer is a. *(Rosen, pp 933–935.) Posterior epistaxis* is identified when posterior bleeding occurs with a properly placed anterior nasal packing. Posterior packing is mandated using either a commercially available balloon or a standard Foley catheter inserted into the posterior nares and inflated with water. Patients with posterior nasal packs should be *admitted to a monitored bed.* In addition to cardiac dysrhythmias, myocardial infarctions, cerebrovascular accidents, and aspiration have been reported. *Antibiotics* are often started to prevent sinusitis and toxic shock syndrome from obstruction of the nasal packing.

(**b**) Placing the patient supine increases risk of aspiration and has no benefit to stopping epistaxis. (**c**) If the patient had an elevated INR or was thrombocytopenic, then Fresh Frozen Plasma (FFP) and platelets should be administered. (**d**) Patients with posterior nasal packing require admission. (**e**) Silver nitrate is a therapy for anterior epistaxis. It has no role in posterior epistaxis.

203. The answer is a. *(Hamilton, pp 17–18.)* Patients often present to the ED with life-threatening conditions that require rapid and simultaneous evaluation and treatment. The fundamentals of emergency medicine begin with the *ABCs. Airway assessment and management have priority over all other aspects of resuscitation in the critically ill or injured patient.* Moreover, airway management is not simply the passage of a tube through the trachea. It involves a series of actions ranging from repositioning a patient's head and neck, suctioning secretions in the posterior pharynx to supplying supplemental oxygen or performing an emergent cricothyrotomy. Whatever the intervention, it is important to know how and when to manage an airway. There are many reasons for definitive airway management with an orotracheal tube, the obvious being in patients who are not breathing. However, there are instances that require definitive management even when a patient is spontaneously breathing. Any patient who is at risk of losing the ability to protect their airway should be considered for intubation. This includes intoxicated patients, the poisoned patient, worsening hypoxia, those with evolving laryngeal edema or hematoma near the trachea, and patients with significant head injuries. Once the airway is addressed, it is appropriate to move onto the next critical component of the ABCs.

(**b**) The patient will certainly require volume resuscitation and pain control, but airway management takes priority. (**c and d**) It is important not to get distracted by other injuries in a critical patient who requires definitive airway management. (**e**) Although the patient will require a blood transfusion, the airway must be addressed first.

204. The answer is a. (*Rosen, pp 329–368.*) *Diving injuries* must always be suspected in near-drowning patients. This patient presents with *abdominal breathing* and spontaneous respirations. This pattern provides an important clue to a *cervical spine injury*. The diaphragm is innervated by the phrenic nerve, which originates from the spinal cord at the C3-C4 level, whereas the intercostal muscles of the rib cage are supplied by nerves that originate in the thoracic spine. Therefore, abdominal breathing in the absence of thoracic breathing indicates an injury below C4. His bradycardia in the presence of *hypotension* is suspicious for *neurogenic hypotension,* which is caused by loss of vasomotor tone and *lack of reflex tachycardia* from the disruption of autonomic ganglia. However, this is a diagnosis of exclusion and should only be made once all other forms of shock are ruled out. It is important to maintain **c**-*spine immobilization* to prevent further progression of an injury.

(**b**) Electrolyte abnormalities are typically not a concern in near-drowning injuries. (**c**) Any patient with hypoxia and hypoperfusion generally also has a metabolic acidosis. Treating the underlying pathology will also treat the acidosis.

(**d**) All near-drowning cases (fresh or saltwater) involve the loss of surfactant and subsequent atelectasis with a high potential for hypoxia. (**e**) Although a toxic ingestion should always be considered, there are no specific indications for it in this patient.

205. The answer is d. (*Rosen, pp 387–388.*) *Pulmonary contusions* usually occur after a blunt traumatic force to the chest that causes injury to the lung parenchyma. This is followed by *alveolar edema and hemorrhage.* Pulmonary contusion is reported to be present in 30–75% of patients with significant blunt chest trauma, most often from automobile collisions with *rapid deceleration.* It can also be caused by high-velocity missile wounds and the high-energy shock waves of an explosion in air or water. Pulmonary contusion is the most significant chest injury in children. Clinical manifestations include dyspnea that is usually worsening, tachypnea, cyanosis, tachycardia, hypotension, chest wall bruising, decreasing oxygen saturation, and increasing A-a gradient. Hemoptysis may be present in up to 50% of cases. Typical radiographic findings begin to appear within minutes of injury and range from patchy, irregular, alveolar infiltrate to frank consolidation.

(a) Tuberculosis may present with tachypnea, dyspnea, and hemoptysis. However, in the setting of trauma and the appearance of the chest radiograph, pulmonary contusion is the diagnosis. (b) Hemothorax usually occurs secondary to penetration of pulmonary parenchyma or injury to intercostal or internal mammary vessels that leads to intrathoracic bleeding. Patients may be dyspneic and have pleuritic, chest, shoulder, or back pain. Typically, patients are tachypneic and have absent breath sounds and dullness to percussion of the chest secondary to the accumulation of blood. (c) A tension PTX is a clinical diagnosis in which air can enter the pleural cavity but cannot escape leading to a shift in the mediastinum, which results in impeding venous blood return to the heart. Lung exam generally reveals absent breath sounds on the side of injury. (e) Pulmonary contusion should be differentiated from ARDS with which it is often confused. The contusion usually manifests itself within minutes of the initial injury, is usually localized to a segment or a lobe, is usually apparent on the initial chest radiograph, and tends to last 48–72 hours. ARDS is diffuse, and its development is usually delayed, with onset typically between 24 and 72 hours after injury.

206. The answer is b. (*Scaletta, pp 243–244.*) Clinical manifestations of *penetrating arterial injury of the extremity* are generally divided into "hard signs" and "soft signs". Hard signs include pulsatile bleeding, expanding hematoma, palpable thrill or audible bruit, and evidence of distal ischemia (pain, pallor, pulselessness, paralysis, paresthesia, poikilothermia). Soft signs include diminished ankle-brachial indicies, asymmetrically absent or weak distal pulse, history of moderate hemorrhage or wound close to a major artery, and a peripheral nerve deficit. Emergent surgery is generally necessary when there are *hard signs* of vascular injury. Although the management of penetrating extremity injury is evolving, whenever there is *evidence of distal ischemia*, the patient should be taken to the *OR for exploration and repair.* When severe ischemia is present, the repair must be completed within 6–8 hours to prevent irreversible muscle ischemia and loss of limb function. In the presence of "hard signs" without evidence of ischemia, some surgeons may prefer to first perform angiography to better define the injury.

(a) Angiography is a frequently used modality in penetrating extremity trauma and is the study of choice with some injuries that present with *hard signs*. However, when there is evidence of limb ischemia, the patient should undergo exploration and repair. (c) Fasciotomy is the treatment for compartment syndrome. Although compartment syndrome can occur with blunt and penetrating extremity trauma, it is more common in crush injuries or fractures with marked swelling. It may be required, but should be performed in conjunction with and after the establishment of arterial blood flow. (d) Local wound exploration is not recommended because it may disrupt hemostasis and cause worsening hemorrhage. (e) CT scanning is not appropriate in the setting of limb ischemia.

207. The answer is b. *(Rosen, p 290.)* Cerebral herniation occurs when increased ICP overwhelms the natural compensatory capacities of the central nervous system (CNS). Increased ICP may be the result of posttraumatic brain swelling, edema formation, traumatic mass lesion expansion, or any combination of the three. When increasing ICP cannot be controlled, the intracranial contents will shift and herniate through the cranial foramen. Herniation can occur within minutes or up to days after a traumatic brain injury. Once the signs of herniation are present, mortality approaches 100% without rapid reversal or temporizing measures. *Uncal herniation* is the most common clinically significant form of traumatic herniation and is often associated with traumatic extracranial bleeding. The classic signs and symptoms are caused by compression of the ipsilateral uncus of the temporal lobe. This causes *compression of the third cranial* nerve leading to *aniscoria, ptosis, impaired extraocular movements, and a sluggish pupillary light reflex.* As herniation progresses, compression of the ipsilateral oculomotor nerve eventually causes ipsilateral pupillary dilation and nonreactivity.

(a) An altered level of consciousness is the hallmark of brain insult from any cause and results from an interruption of the reticular-activating-system (RAS) or a global event that affects both cortices. (c) Contralateral dilation is a late manifestation in brain herniation. (d) Progressive hypertension associated with bradycardia and diminished respiratory effort is described as Cushing's reflex and is a late manifestation of herniation. (e) Contralateral hemiparesis develops as herniation progresses.

208. The answer is b. *(Rosen, pp 391–392.)* A *hemothorax* is the accumulation of blood in the pleural space after blunt or penetrating chest trauma.

It can lead to hypovolemic shock and significantly reduce vital capacity if it is not recognized. It is associated with a PTX approximately 25% of the time. Hemorrhage from injured lung parenchyma is the most common cause of hemothorax, but this tends to be self-limiting unless there is a major laceration to the parenchyma. Specific vessels are less often the source of bleeding. A hemothorax is treated with *chest thoracostomy (chest tube)* that is generally placed in the 4th or 5th intercostal space at the anterior or midaxillary line, over the superior portion of the rib. The tube should be directed superior and *posterior* to allow it to drain blood from the dependent portions of the chest. In an isolated PTX, the tube is positioned *anteriorly* to allow it to suction air. Once the tube is inserted, it is important to closely monitor blood output. Indications for thoracotomy include:

- initial chest tube drainage of 1000–1500 cc of blood
- 200 cc per hour of persistent drainage
- Patient remains hypotensive despite adequate blood replacement, and other sites of blood loss have been ruled out
- Patient decompensates after initial response to resuscitation
- Increasing hemothorax seen on chest x-ray studies

209. The answer is c. *(Rosen, pp 248–249.)* This question addresses the "*C*," *circulation,* in the *ABCs.* Initial fluid resuscitation usually begins with crystalloid fluids such as 0.9% normal saline or Ringer's lactate. In general, if the patient remains hemodynamically unstable after 40 cc/kg of crystalloid administration (approximately 2–3 L), then a *blood transfusion* should be started. Fully cross-matched blood is preferable; however, this is generally not available in the early resuscitation period. Therefore, *type-specific blood (O-negative or O-positive)* is a safe alternative and is usually ready within 5–15 minutes. O-negative blood is typically reserved for women in their child-bearing years to prevent Rh sensitization. O-positive blood can be given to all men and women beyond their child-bearing years.

(a) The patient's underlying cause of hypotension is hypovolemia secondary to hemorrhage. Therefore, to treat her hypotension you should treat the underlying cause. She requires fluid resuscitation with blood and eventually may be taken to the OR to stop the bleeding. Epinephrine is used if the patient is in cardiopulmonary arrest and no longer has a pulse. However, the underlying cause, hypovolemia, must be corrected. **(b)** The best resuscitation fluid is blood. ATLS guidelines suggest starting resuscitation with crystalloid solution and adding blood if there is no response after a 40 cc/kg bolus of crystalloid fluid. **(d)** The patient is too unstable to be transferred for a CT scan. If the patient's BP normalizes, then the trauma team may elect for a CT scan. If the patient remains hypotensive despite resuscitation, then definitive measures need to take place, such as an exploratory laparotomy to stop the hemorrhage. **(e)** Once the FAST exam is positive, repeating it will not add valuable information. If the patient remains hypotensive, definitive management is a priority.

210. The answer is e. *(Rosen, pp 256–265.)* Trauma occurs in up to 7% of all pregnancies and is the leading cause of maternal death. It is important to *focus the primary exam on the patient and evaluate the fetus in the secondary exam.* The ABCs are followed in usual fashion. Once the patient is deemed stable, the fetus should be evaluated. Fetal evaluation focuses on the fetal heart rate and fetal movement. Minor trauma to the patient does not rule out injury to the fetus. Therefore, it is important to monitor the fetus. *Cardiotocographic observation of the viable fetus is recommended for a minimum of 4 hours* to detect any intrauterine pathology. The minimum should be extended to 24 hours if, at any time during the first 4 hours, there are more than three uterine contractions per hour, persistent uterine tenderness, a nonreassuring fetal monitor strip, vaginal bleeding, rupture of the membranes, or any serious maternal injury is present.

  (a) Cesarean section in the OR may take place if the patient is stable but the fetus is unstable and greater than 24 weeks gestation. This decision should be made by the obstetrician. **(b)** Cesarean section in the ED, or perimortem cesarean section, is performed if uterine size exceeds the umbilicus, fetal heart tones are present, and maternal decompensation is acute. **(c)** Radiation from CT scanning in the setting of pregnancy is a concern. Shielding of the uterus in head and chest scans allows for an acceptable radiation exposure level. Abdominal and pelvic CT scanning incurs greater radiation exposure and the risks and benefits of these studies should be discussed with the patient. Other diagnostic procedures can be used in the setting of blunt abdominal trauma such as ultrasound, DPL, and MRI. **(d)** Minor trauma does not exempt the fetus from injury and direct impact is not necessary for fetoplacental pathology to occur. The mother with no obvious abdominal injury still requires monitoring.

211. The answer is d. *(Rosen, pp 613–623.)* *Cauda equina syndrome* is an injury to the lumbar, sacral, and coccygeal nerve roots causing peripheral nerve injury that can lead to permanent neurologic defects if not recognized and corrected rapidly. Because of the central location of the disk herniation, symptoms are often bilateral and involve *leg pain, saddle anesthesia,* *and impaired bowel and bladder function (retention or incontinence).* On exam, patients may exhibit *loss of rectal tone* and display other motor and sensory losses in the lower extremities. Patients with suspected cauda equina syndrome require an urgent CT scan or *MRI.*

(a) Abdominal aortic aneurysms (AAA) can present with low back pain and should always be considered in patients over 50 years with low back pain. However, patients should not exhibit new neurologic deficits from an AAA. (b) Disk herniation can result in peripheral nerve root compression and irritation leading to sensory and motor deficits. Patients, however, should not exhibit altered bowel and bladder function, or have decreased rectal tone. If so, there condition is considered cauda equina syndrome and is a neurologic emergency. (c) Spinal stenosis is narrowing of the spinal canal, which may cause spinal cord compression that typically is worse with back extension and relieved with flexion. (e) Osteomyelitis is an infection of the bone that typically presents with fever.

212. The answer is d. *(Rosen, p 295.)* A *unilateral dilated pupil* in the setting of head trauma is an *indicator of increased ICP.* If ICP is not lowered immediately, the patient has little chance of survival. *Hyperventilation* to produce an arterial PCO_2 of 30–35 mm Hg will temporarily reduce ICP by promoting cerebral vasoconstriction and subsequent reduction of cerebral blood flow. The onset of action is within 30 seconds. In most patients, hyperventilation lowers the ICP by 25%. PCO_2 should not fall below 25 mm Hg because this may cause profound vasoconstriction and ischemia in normal and injured areas of the brain. *Hyperventilation is a temporary maneuver* and should only be used for a brief period of time during the acute resuscitation and only in patients demonstrating neurologic deterioration.

(a) ED cranial decompression (Burr Hole) should only be performed under extreme circumstances when all other attempts at reducing ICP have failed. (b) There is no evidence that steroids lower ICP and are not recommended in head trauma. (c) Furosemide has no role in acute traumatic brain injury. (e) Mannitol is the best osmotic agent to reduce ICP. Its onset is within 30 minutes and lasts up to 6–8 hours. Mannitol has the additional benefit of expanding volume, initially reducing hypotension, and improving the blood's oxygen-carrying capacity.

Shock and Resuscitation

Questions

213. A 79-year-old woman with a history of coronary artery disease who underwent a coronary artery bypass graft (CABG) surgery in 2000 is brought to the emergency department (ED) by her family for 2 days of worsening shortness of breath. For the past 2 days, she has not gotten out of bed and is confused. She does not have chest pain, fevers, or cough. Her temperature is 98.1°F, blood pressure (BP) is 85/50 mm Hg, heart rate (HR) is 125 beats per minute, and respiratory rate (RR) is 26 breaths per minute. On exam, she is unable to follow commands and is oriented only to name. The cardiovascular exam reveals tachycardia with no murmurs. Her lungs have rales bilaterally at the bases. The abdomen is soft, nontender, and nondistended. Lower extremities have 2+ edema to the knee bilaterally. Which of the following is the most likely diagnosis?

a. Hypovolemic shock
b. Neurogenic shock
c. Cardiogenic shock
d. Anaphylactic shock
e. Septic shock

214. A 32-year-old man with no past medical problems presents to the ED with palpitations. For the past 2 days he has been feeling weak and over the last 6 hours he has noticed that his heart is racing. He has no chest pain or shortness of breath. He has never felt this way before. His temperature is 98.9°F, BP is 140/82 mm Hg, HR is 180 beats per minute, and RR is 14 breaths per minute. His physical exam is normal. You obtain the following rhythm strip. What is your first-line treatment for this patient?

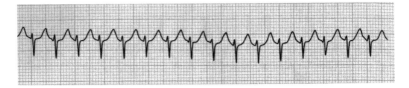

a. Synchronized cardioversion at 100 J
b. Adenosine 6 mg intravenous (IV) push
c. Adenosine 12 mg IV push
d. Valsalva maneuver
e. Verapamil 3 mg IV push

215. You are a passenger aboard an airplane and a 78-year-old woman is complaining of chest pain and difficulty breathing. You are the only medical professional available and volunteer to help. Fortunately, the aircraft is well equipped with basic medical equipment as well as advanced cardiac life support (ACLS) medications and a cardiac monitor. Her BP is 75/40 mm Hg, HR is 180 beats per minute, and RR is 24 breaths per minute. On exam, the patient is in obvious distress, but able to answer basic questions. Her heart is tachycardic, regular, and without murmurs, rubs, or gallops. Physical exam is remarkable for a bounding carotid pulse. You attach the cardiac monitor and see a regular rhythm at 180 beats per minute with wide QRS complexes and no obvious p waves. After asking the pilot to make an emergency landing, what do you do next?

a. Amiodarone IV
b. Synchronized cardioversion
c. Verapamil IV
d. Lidocaine IV
e. Procainamide IV

216. A 41-year-old man is brought into the ED by paramedics in cardiopulmonary arrest. A friend states that the patient is a long-time user of IV heroin. You look at the monitor and see that the patient has pulseless electrical activity (PEA). Cardiopulmonary resuscitation is being performed and the patient is intubated. You decide to administer epinephrine to the patient, but realize that he does not have IV access. Which of the following drugs is *ineffective* when administered through an endotracheal tube (ET)?

a. Atropine
b. Naloxone
c. Lidocaine
d. Epinephrine
e. Sodium bicarbonate

217. A 75-year old man is brought in to the ED by paramedics complaining of chest pain. He is barely able to speak to you because he is short of breath. The nurse immediately attaches him to the monitor, starts an IV, and gives him oxygen. His temperature is 98.9°F, BP is 70/40 mm Hg, HR is 140 beats per minute, RR is 28 breaths per minute, and oxygen saturation is 95% on room air. On exam, he is in mild distress. His heart is irregular and tachycardic. His lungs are clear to auscultation with rales at the bases bilaterally. An ECG is shown below. What is your first-line treatment for this patient?

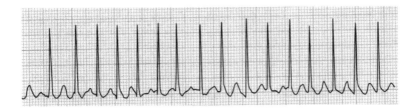

a. Heparin drip
b. Diltiazem 10 mg IV push
c. Metoprolol 5 mg IV push
d. Digoxin 0.5 mg IV
e. Synchronized cardioversion at 100 J

218. A 19-year-old man was struck by a motor vehicle while crossing the street. In the ED, he is awake, alert, and oriented, but complaining of severe right leg pain. His temperature is 98.9°F, BP is 85/50 mm Hg, HR is 125 beats per minute, and RR is 24 breaths per minute. You confirm his airway is patent, breath sounds are equal bilaterally, and his abdomen is soft and nontender. His right leg is shorter than his left leg, slightly angulated, and swollen in his anterior thigh area. There is no open wound. Which of the following is the most likely diagnosis?

a. Hypovolemic shock
b. Neurogenic shock
c. Cardiogenic shock
d. Anaphylactic shock
e. Septic shock

219. You are called to the bedside of a hypotensive patient with altered mental status. The nurse hands you an electrocardiogram (ECG) which shows atrial flutter at 150 beats per minute with 2:1 arteriovenous (AV) block. You feel the patient is unstable and elect to perform emergency cardioversion. You attach the monitor leads to the patient. What is the critical next step in electrical cardioversion?

a. Set the appropriate energy level
b. Position conductor pads or paddles on patient
c. Charge the defibrillator
d. Turn on the synchronization mode
e. Administer 25 μg fentanyl IV

220. Paramedics bring in a 54-year-old man who was found down in his apartment by his wife. He is successfully intubated in the field and paramedics are currently performing cardiopulmonary resuscitation (CPR). He is transferred to an ED gurney and quickly attached to the cardiac monitors. You ask the paramedics to hold CPR and assess the patient and the rhythm strip. The monitor shows sinus bradycardia, but no pulses are palpable. On exam you appreciate bilateral breath sounds with mechanical ventilation, a soft abdomen, no rashes, and a left arm AV graft. In addition to CPR with epinephrine and atropine every 3–5 minutes, which intervention should be performed next?

a. Administer 1 ampule of sodium bicarbonate
b. Administer 1 ampule of calcium gluconate
c. Administer 1 ampule of D50 (dextrose)

d. Place left-sided chest tube
e. Perform pericardiocentesis

221. An 85-year-old man is rambling incoherently and not eating at his nursing home. Records indicate that he has a past medical history of hypertension, diabetes, dementia, and benign prostatic hypertrophy. On arrival to the ED, the patient is combative and oriented only to name. His temperature is 101°F rectally, BP is 85/50 mm Hg, HR is 125 beats per minute, RR is 22 breaths per minute, and blood sugar is 154 mg/dL. He is uncomfortable and cachectic. His lungs are clear to auscultation with scant crackles at the bases and his abdomen is soft, nontender, and nondistended. He has a Foley catheter in place draining cloudy, white urine. He has no peripheral edema. Which of the following is the most likely diagnosis?

a. Hypovolemic shock
b. Neurogenic shock
c. Cardiogenic shock
d. Anaphylactic shock
e. Septic shock

222. A 72-year-old man is in the ED for the evaluation of generalized weakness over the previous 24 hours. He has a past medical history of coronary artery disease with a CABG performed 5 years ago, diabetes mellitus, and arthritis. The nurse places the patient on a cardiac monitor and begins to get his vital signs. While the nurse is obtaining the vital signs, he notices the patient suddenly becomes unresponsive. You arrive at the bedside, look at the monitor, and see the following rhythm. Which of the following is the most appropriate next step in management?

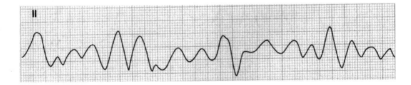

a. Wait 5 minutes to see if he awakens on his own
b. Immediately defibrillate at 200 J
c. Perform synchronized cardioversion at 100 J
d. Immediately intubate the patient
e. Insert an IV line and administer amiodarone

223. As you arrive for your ED shift, you are called to help with a "coding" patient. The senior resident has just intubated the patient and the nurses have established IV access and attached the cardiac monitor. An emergency medical treatment (EMT) student is performing chest compressions. You ask the EMT student to stop compressions. The monitor shows a flat line with no electrical activity. You are unable to detect any pulses. What is your next step in management?

a.   Defibrillate at 360 J
b.   Epinephrine 1 mg IV push
c.   Atropine 1 mg IV push
d.   Ask the nurse to run a rhythm strip in an additional lead
e.   Apply transcutaneous pacers

224. A 34-year-old woman with no known medical problems is having a sushi dinner with her husband. Half-way through dinner, she begins scratching her arms and her husband notices that her face is flushed. The itching intensifies and she begins to feel chest pain, shortness of breath, and dizziness. On arrival to the ED, she can barely talk, her temperature is 100°F, BP is 85/50 mm Hg, HR is 125 beats per minute, and RR is 26 breaths per minute, and O_2 saturation is 91% on room air. Which of the following is the most likely diagnosis?

a.   Hypovolemic shock
b.   Neurogenic shock
c.   Cardiogenic shock
d.   Anaphylactic shock
e.   Septic shock

225. An 82-year-old nursing home patient presents to the ED in septic shock. Her BP is 75/40 mm Hg, HR is 117 beats per minute, temperature is 96.5°F, RR is 29 breaths per minute, and oxygen saturation is 87% on room air. As you perform laryngoscopy to intubate the patient, you easily visualize the vocal cords and subsequently pass the orotracheal tube through the vocal cords. You place the colorimetric end-tidal carbon dioxide device over the tube and get appropriate color change. There are equal, bilateral breath sounds on auscultation and you observe chest wall motion with ventilation. Which of the following is the most reliable method for verifying proper ET placement?

a.   Chest radiograph
b.   Visualization of the ET passing through the vocal cords
c.   Observation of chest wall motion with ventilation

d. Hearing equal, bilateral breath sounds on auscultation
e. End-tidal carbon dioxide color change

226. An 82-year-old man presents to the ED feeling weak and dizzy. He has a past medical history of hypertension and diabetes and both are well controlled on hydrochlorothiazide, benazepril, atenolol, and metformin. On review of systems, he denies chest pain, gastrointestinal bleeding, and syncope, but states he feels short of breath. His temperature is 98.6°F orally, BP is 86/60 mm Hg, HR is 44 beats per minute, RR is 18 breaths per minute, oxygen saturation is 98% on room air, and glucose is 116 mg/dL. He is immediately connected to the cardiac monitor. Which of the following choices best describes the ECG seen below?

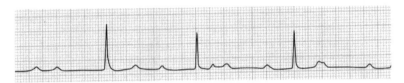

a. Normal sinus rhythm
b. First-degree AV block
c. Second-degree Mobitz I (Wenckebach) AV block
d. Second-degree Mobitz II AV block
e. Third-degree AV block

227. A 25-year-old man fell off his surfboard and landed on rocks. He was pulled from the water by lifeguards and brought to the ED in full cervical and spinal immobilization. He is alert and oriented to person, place, and time. He is complaining of weakness in all his extremities. His temperature is 98.4°F, BP is 85/50 mm Hg, HR is 60 beats per minute, RR is 20 breaths per minute, and O₂ saturation is 98% on room air. On exam, he has no external signs of head injury. His heart is bradycardic without murmurs. The lungs are clear to auscultation and the abdomen is soft and nontender. He has grossly normal peripheral sensation, but no motor strength in all four extremities. Which of the following is the most likely diagnosis?

a. Hypovolemic shock
b. Neurogenic shock
c. Cardiogenic shock
d. Anaphylactic shock
e. Septic shock

228. A 48-year-old man is brought to the ED by paramedics for generalized weakness. His medical history is significant for a CABG last month. He has been unable to get out of bed for the past day because of dizziness when changing position. He denies chest pain, shortness of breath, or syncope. His temperature is 98.9°F, BP is 86/60 mm Hg, HR is 44 beats per minute, RR is 18 breaths per minute, and oxygen saturation is 98% on room air. There is a well-healing midline sternotomy incision. Cardiac exam reveals a III/VI systolic ejection murmur. There are minimal rales at his lung bases. He is immediately attached to the cardiac monitor. His rhythm strip is shown below. What is your initial treatment?

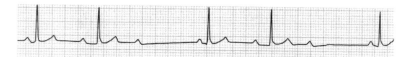

a. Observe on monitor
b. Transcutaneous pacing
c. Transvenous pacing
d. Atropine 0.5 mg IV
e. Epinephrine IV drip at 2 μg/min

229. You are caring for a 54-year-old woman with a history of schizophrenia and coronary artery disease who presents to the ED for chest pain. Her vital signs are within normal limits and her ECG is normal sinus rhythm with nonspecific ST/T wave changes. Her first troponin is sent to the laboratory and you are planning to admit her to the hospital for a complete acute coronary syndrome (ACS) evaluation. She receives aspirin and nitroglycerin and her chest pain resolves. A few minutes later, the nurse alerts you that the patient has become unconscious. You go to the bedside and find the patient awake and alert. You review the rhythm strip below. What is your next step in management?

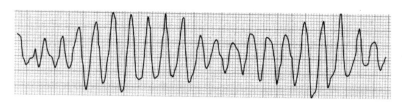

a. Observe patient
b. Magnesium sulfate IV
c. Lidocaine IV
d. Transvenous pacemaker
e. Isoproterenol IV

230. A 101-year-old nursing home resident with a history of dementia and chronic obstructive pulmonary disease (COPD) is brought to the ED by paramedics for difficulty breathing. Workup reveals that the patient is in septic shock secondary to a new right lower lobe pneumonia. He is treated aggressively with rapid sequence intubation, IV fluids, and antibiotics. The chemistry panel returns with a sodium of 136 mEq/L, potassium 4.2 mEq/L, chloride 100 mEq/L, bicarbonate 25 mEq/L, blood urea nitrogen (BUN) 9 mg/dL, creatinine 0.9 mg/dL, and blood sugar 289 mg/dL. Which of the following is the most appropriate management for this patient's hyperglycemia?

a. Continued IV fluids
b. Sliding scale regular insulin
c. Insulin drip
d. Metformin
e. Glipizide

231. A 48-year-old man with a medical history of cirrhosis due to hepatitis C has been vomiting bright red blood for 1 day. On arrival to the ED, the patient is confused and unable to provide more information. His family states that he has been vomiting large amounts of bright red blood every 4 hours and has no prior history of gastrointestinal bleeding. The nurses hook him up to the monitor and start two large-bore IV lines. His BP is 75/43 mm Hg, HR is 130 beats per minute, RR is 24 breaths per minute, and O_2 saturation is 98% on room air. His abdomen is soft with no masses. His rectal exam reveals bright red blood. Which type of fluid is most appropriate to begin his resuscitation?

a. 7% Sodium chloride
b. 0.9% Sodium chloride
c. Type and cross-matched blood
d. Type-specific blood
e. O-positive blood

232. A 19-year-old man is brought into the ED by paramedics with a stab wound to the right lower abdomen. The medics applied a pressure dressing and started an IV line en route to the hospital. On arrival, the patient has no complaints and wants to leave. His temperature is 98.4°F, BP is 130/95 mm Hg, HR is 111 beats per minute, RR is 20 breaths per minute, and O$_2$ saturation 98% on room air. He is alert and oriented to person, place, and time. His abdomen is soft and nontender, with normal bowel sounds. He has a 2 cm stab wound with visible subcutaneous fat in his right lower quadrant (RLQ). You initiate the focused abdominal sonogram for trauma (FAST) exam. Which type of fluid should you start for his initial resuscitation?

a. 7% Sodium chloride
b. 0.9% Sodium chloride
c. 10% Albumin
d. Type and cross-matched blood
e. Type specific blood

233. You are notified that emergency medical service (EMS) is bringing in a patient who collapsed five minutes ago in his house and was intubated at the scene by paramedics. On arrival to the ED, you confirm ET placement and continue CPR. You connect the patient to the cardiac monitor and see the rhythm below. Which of the following is the most appropriate next step in management?

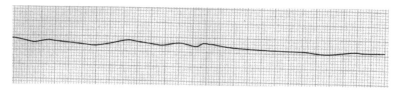

a. Perform synchronized cardioversion at 100 J
b. Immediately defibrillate at 200 J
c. Confirm the rhythm in two leads, begin CPR, defibrillate at 200 J
d. Confirm the rhythm in two leads, begin CPR, administer amiodarone
e. Confirm the rhythm in two leads, begin CPR, administer epinephrine and atropine

234. An 18-year-old college student with no past medical history presents to the ED with a diffuse rash. She also describes having a headache, fever, and arthralgias for 3 days. On exam, her temperature is 101.2°F, BP is 120/63 mm Hg, HR is 110 beats per minute, RR is 24 breaths per minute, and O_2 saturation is 98% on room air. The patient is alert and oriented to person, place, and time. She has nuchal rigidity and photophobia. Her gums are oozing blood. Her abdomen is soft and nontender and her skin has a diffuse, petechial rash. You are concerned about meningococcemia and immediately start ceftriaxone and vancomycin. Her lab results reveal a white blood cell (WBC) count of 13,400/μL, hematocrit 36%, platelets 80/μL, PTT 60 sec, International Normalized Ratio (INR) 1.9, and fibrinogen 250 g/L. Which of the following is the most appropriate next step in management?

a. IV heparin
b. Transfuse cryoprecipitate
c. Transfuse packed red blood cells
d. Transfuse platelets
e. Transfuse fresh frozen plasma (FFP)

235. An 82-year-old man with a history of COPD and hypertension presents with shortness of breath and fever. His medications include albuterol, ipratropium, prednisone, hydrochlorothiazide, and atenolol. His temperature is 102.1°F, BP is 70/40 mm Hg, HR is 110 beats per minute, RR is 24 breaths per minute, and O_2 saturation is 91% on room air. The patient is uncomfortable and mumbling incoherently. On chest exam, you appreciate rales on the left side of his chest. His heart is tachycardic, but regular with no murmurs, rubs, or gallops. His abdomen is soft and nontender. You believe this patient is in septic shock from pneumonia and start IV fluids, broad-spectrum antibiotics, and a dopamine drip. His BP remains at 75/50 mm Hg. Which of the following is the most appropriate next step in management?

a. D5 normal saline IV bolus
b. Phenylephrine IV drip
c. Fludrocortisone IV
d. Hydrocortisone IV
e. Epinephrine IV drip

236. A 64-year-old woman with a history of depression and hypertension was found down by her husband and brought in by paramedics. Her husband says she has recently been depressed and expressed thoughts of suicide. She usually takes fluoxetine for depression and atenolol for hypertension. On arrival, the patient is obtunded, but responds to pain and is maintaining her airway. Her temperature is 98.1°F, BP is 70/40 mm Hg, HR is 42 beats per minute, RR is 12 breaths per minute, and O_2 saturation is 94% on room air. On exam, her pupils are 3 mm and reactive bilaterally. Lungs are clear to auscultation. Heart is bradycardic, but regular, with no murmurs, rubs, or gallops. Extremities have no edema. An electrocardiogram shows first-degree AV block at 42 beats per minute, but no ST or T wave changes. Blood sugar is 112 mg/dL. What is the most specific treatment for this patient's ingestion?

a. Fluid bolus
b. Atropine
c. Glucagon
d. Epinephrine
e. Cardiac pacing

237. A 19-year old man suffers a single gunshot wound to the left chest and is brought in by his friends. He is complaining of chest pain. On exam, his temperature is 99°F, BP is 70/40 mm Hg, HR is 140 beats per minute, RR is 16 breaths per minute, and oxygen saturation is 96% on room air. He has distended neck veins, but his trachea is not deviated. Lungs are clear to auscultation bilaterally. Heart sounds are difficult to appreciate, but you feel a bounding, regular pulse. Abdomen is soft and nontender. Extremity exam is normal. Two large-bore IV lines are placed and the patient is given 2 L of normal saline. Chest radiograph shows a globular cardiac silhouette, but a normal mediastinum and no pneumothorax. What is the definitive management of this patient?

a. Intubation
b. Tube thoracostomy
c. Pericardiocentesis
d. Thoracotomy
e. Blood transfusion

238. An 84-year-old woman with a history of metastatic breast cancer presents to the ED with new-onset dyspnea and exercise intolerance for the past week. She denies fever, chest pain, or cough. On exam, her temperature is 100.3°F, BP is 70/50 mm Hg, HR is 110 beats per minute, RR is 20 breaths per minute, and O_2 saturation is 93% on room air. As your colleague is performing a physical exam, you place the portable ultrasound on the heart and see a thin echo-free area around the heart with right atria and right ventricular collapse. Which of the following is the most likely diagnosis?

a. Pulmonary embolism
b. Congestive heart failure
c. Massive myocardial infarction
d. Cardiac tamponade
e. Dehydration

239. A 50-year-old man with a history of hypertension presents to the ED with severe left-sided chest pain for 1 hour. The pain radiates down his left arm and he feels nauseated. His temperature is 98.3°F, BP is 160/92 mm Hg, HR is 92 beats per minute, RR is 16 breaths per minute, and O_2 saturation is 98% on room air. The physical exam is normal. His electrocardiogram shows ST-segment elevations in leads II, III, and aVF. You administer aspirin, nitroglycerin, and morphine sulfate and wait for his laboratory results. The nurse calls you over 10 minutes later and tells you the patient's BP dropped to 60/30 mm Hg and his HR is 100 beats per minute. Why is this patient hypotensive?

a. Medication-related adverse reaction
b. Cardiogenic shock
c. Papillary muscle rupture
d. Free wall rupture
e. Rupture of the interventricular septum

240. A 25-year-old woman presents to the ED with abdominal pain for 1 day. She is nauseated and reports three episodes of nonbloody, nonbilious vomiting. Her temperature is 99.3°F, HR is 124 beats per minute, BP is 84/44 mm Hg, RR is 18 breaths per minute, and O_2 saturation is 98% on room air. Her abdomen is tender to palpation in the RLQ with rebound and guarding. She has no flank pain. Pelvic exam reveals no vaginal bleeding or cervical motion tenderness, but she does have right adnexal tenderness to palpation. You place two 18-gauge IV lines and fluid resuscitation. She is given IV pain medication and laboratories are sent. Her urine pregnancy test is positive. Using the ultrasound you see no intrauterine pregnancy, but do see fluid in Morrison's pouch. Which of the following is the most appropriate next step in management?

a. Call surgery to bring the patient directly to the operating room (OR)
b. Call obstetrics and gynecology (OB/GYN) to bring the patient directly to the OR
c. Perform a paracentesis and send fluid for analysis
d. Perform a culdocentesis to confirm blood
e. Order a CT scan of the abdomen and pelvis to rule out appendicitis

241. A 35-year-old man was playing soccer when he was stung by a yellow jacket bee. Within minutes, he develops a diffuse pruritic rash and begins to feel his throat closing. He is rushed to the local ED by one of his teammates. Upon arrival, the patient is in moderate respiratory distress. There is scattered wheezing on lung exam with poor air movement. His BP is 100/50 mm Hg, HR 110 beats per minute, RR 22 breaths per minute, and O_2 saturation of 93%. After placing him on a monitor and oxygen by face mask, which of the following is the most appropriate medication to administer first?

a. Diphenhydramine 25 mg intravenously
b. Double the dose of diphenhydramine until the wheezing resolves
c. Methylprednisolone 125 mg IV
d. Dopamine 200 μg/min
e. Epinephrine 0.3 mg 1:100,000 intramuscularly (IM)

242. A car pulls up to your ED and drops off a 19-year-old man who was shot in the chest. He tells you his name and complains of right-sided chest pain and difficulty breathing. On primary survey, his airway is patent and his oropharynx has no blood or displaced teeth. He is breathing at 32 beats per minute with retractions and an oxygen saturation of 88% on 15 L of oxygen. There is a bullet wound to his right mid-chest with another wound in his back. His trachea is deviated to the left. On auscultation, he has diminished breath sounds on the right side. Which of the following is the most appropriate next step in management?

a. Stat portable chest x-ray
b. Intubation
c. Perform ED thoracotomy
d. Call the surgical service
e. Needle decompression

243. An 87-year-woman with a history of dementia, arthritis, and hypertension presents to the ED for abdominal pain. Her caretaker reports that she is having mid-epigastric pain and had one episode of nonbloody, nonbilious vomiting prior to arrival. The patient is oriented to name only. Temperature is 99.8°F, HR is 110 beats per minute, BP is 80/44 mm Hg, RR is 16 breaths per minute, and oxygen saturation is 96% on room air. On exam, the abdomen is soft, nontender, with no masses, rebound or guarding. Stool is brown and guaiac negative. You place two IV lines and begin fluid resuscitation. You send her blood to the lab and order a radiograph of her chest that is shown below. Which of the following is the most appropriate next step in management?

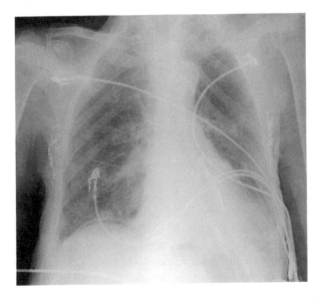

a. Start IV antibiotics
b. Order a CT scan of her abdomen
c. Call the surgery service
d. Place a central venous line
e. Discharge home with Maalox

Shock and Resuscitation

Answers

213. The answer is c. (*Tintinalli, pp 242–247.*) This patient is in *cardiogenic shock* from *decreased cardiac output* producing inadequate tissue perfusion. Support for this diagnosis includes an older patient with a history of coronary artery disease, with new mental status changes coupled with signs of volume overload. Common causes of cardiogenic shock include acute myocardial infarction, pulmonary embolism, COPD exacerbation, and pneumonia. This patient should be stabilized with IV pressors since there is already pulmonary congestion evident on exam. A rapid workup including ECG, chest x-ray (CXR), laboratory tests, echocardiogram, and hemodynamic monitoring should help confirm the etiology and direct specific treatment of the underlying cause.

Hypovolemic shock (**a**) occurs when there is inadequate volume in the circulatory system, resulting in poor oxygen delivery to the tissues. Neurogenic shock (**b**) occurs after an acute spinal cord injury, which disrupts sympathetic innervation resulting in hypotension and bradycardia. Anaphylactic shock (**d**) is a severe systemic hypersensitivity reaction resulting in hypotension and airway compromise. Septic shock (**e**) is a clinical syndrome of hypoperfusion and multiorgan dysfunction caused by infection.

214. The answer is d. (*Tintinalli, pp 185–187.*) This patient has *supraventricular tachycardia (SVT),* a narrow complex, regular tachycardia. It is caused by a re-entry or an ectopic pacemaker in areas of the heart above the bundle of His, usually the atria. Regular p waves will be present, but may be difficult to discern due to the very fast rate. The patient in this case has normal vital signs and exam, and is therefore stable. First line treatment for a patient with stable SVT is *vagal maneuvers to slow conduction and prolong the refractory period in the AV node.* The Valsalva maneuver can be accomplished by asking the patient to bear down as if they are having a bowel movement and hold the strain for at least 10 seconds. Other vagal maneuvers include carotid sinus massage (after auscultating for carotid bruits) and facial immersion in cold water.

If vagal maneuvers fail, the next step is adenosine, a very short-acting AV nodal blocking medication. Initially, adenosine 6 mg (**b**) is rapidly pushed through the IV in an intravenous site as close to the heart as possible. Patients may experience a few seconds of discomfort, including chest pain and facial flushing on receiving the adenosine. If the patient remains in SVT 2 minutes after receiving adenosine, a second dose of adenosine at 12 mg (**C**) is administered. If the second dose of adenosine fails and the patient remains stable, short acting calcium channel blockers (i.e., verapamil), (**e**) β-blockers, or digoxin can be administered. If at any time the patient is considered unstable (hypotension, pulmonary edema, severe chest pain, altered mental status, or other life-threatening concerns), synchronized cardioversion (**a**) should be performed immediately.

215. The answer is b. (*Circulation, IV-67–IV-77, Tintinalli, pp 189–191.*) *Ventricular tachycardia* originates from ectopic ventricular pacemakers and is usually a regular rhythm with rate greater than 100 beats per minute and wide QRS complexes. Treatment of ventricular tachycardia is primarily dependent on whether or not the patient is stable. Evidence of acute altered mental status, hypotension, continued chest pain, or other signs of shock are signs of instability. Unstable patients, such as the passenger on this airplane, should receive immediate *synchronized cardioversion.*

Stable patients can be treated with antidysrhythmics. Amiodarone (**a**) 150 mg IV over 10 minutes is currently first-line treatment as recommended by the American Heart Association (AHA). Lidocaine (**d**) and procainamide (**e**) can also be administered. Verapamil (**c**) should not be used in ventricular tachycardia as it may accelerate the heart rate and cause hypotension.

216. The answer is e. (*Roberts and Hedges, pp 486–493.*) *Endotracheal administration of drugs* is indicated whenever there is a need for emergent pharmacologic intervention in the absence of other access routes, such as IV or intraosseous. There are a limited number of emergency medications that can be administered safely and effectively via the endotracheal route. These include *naloxone, atropine, versed, epinephrine,* and *lidocaine.* This is remembered by the mnemonic *NAVEL.* Specific medications shown to be unsafe include sodium bicarbonate, isoproterenol, and bretylium. The endotracheal dosage of a medication should be at least equivalent to the IV route; and is usually 2–2.5 times the IV dose is administered. The patient in the scenario should receive epinephrine via the ET while IV access is established.

217. The answer is e. (*Tintinalli, pp 184–185.*) This ECG shows *atrial fibrillation with rapid ventricular response (RVR).* Normally, one area of the atria depolarizes and causes uniform contraction of the atria. In atrial fibrillation, multiple areas of the atria continuously depolarize and contract, leading to multiple atrial impulses and an irregular ventricular response. Atrial fibrillation reduces the effectiveness of atrial contractions and may lead to or worsen heart failure in patients with left ventricular failure. Treatment of atrial fibrillation is dependent on whether the patient is stable or not. This patient is clinically *unstable;* the atrial fibrillation with RVR has pushed him into heart failure and he is hypotensive and tachypneic. Unstable patients like this should undergo *synchronized cardioversion.* Synchronized cardioversion is performed at 100 J and then at 200 J if the first attempt fails.

The focus of emergency management in stable patients with atrial fibrillation with RVR is ventricular rate control. Diltiazem (b) or verapamil are excellent choices for rate control. Metoprolol (c) or digoxin (d) may also be used, but may depress BP. Recall that patients in atrial fibrillation for longer than 48 hours are at risk for atrial thrombi. If these patients are cardioverted (electrically or chemically) they have a 1–2% risk of arterial embolism. Since it is often difficult to determine time of onset, ED patients are generally only cardioverted if they are unstable. Stable patients with atrial fibrillation should be anticoagulated with a loading dose of (a) heparin and oral coumadin for at least one month prior to elective cardioversion.

218. The answer is a. (*Tintinalli, pp 1722–1725.*) This patient is in *hypovolemic shock* secondary to blood loss from a *femoral fracture.* Hypovolemic shock occurs when there is inadequate volume in the circulatory system, resulting in poor oxygen delivery to the tissues. Hemorrhage, gastrointestinal losses, burns, and environmental exposures can all be responsible for hypovolemic shock. In trauma, hemorrhage is the most common cause of hypovolemic shock. This patient fractured his femur, disrupting the nearby vascular supply, resulting in significant blood collection in the soft tissue.

This patient's hypovolemic shock can be treated with aggressive fluid and blood product replacement. In the meantime, pain control and x-rays of the hip, femur, and knee should be performed. Once the femur fracture is confirmed, a Sager or Hare traction splint should be applied and orthopedics consulted. Other areas of life-threatening hemorrhage in trauma include the chest, abdomen, retroperitoneum, pelvis, and outside the body.

Neurogenic shock (**b**) occurs after an acute spinal cord injury, which disrupts sympathetic innervation resulting in hypotension and bradycardia. Cardiogenic shock (**c**) is caused by decreased cardiac output producing inadequate tissue perfusion. Anaphylactic shock (**d**) is a severe systemic hypersensitivity reaction resulting in hypotension and airway compromise. Septic shock (**e**) is a clinical syndrome of hypoperfusion and multiorgan dysfunction caused by infection.

219. The answer is d. (*Chauhan V, eMedicine 2006.*) Low-energy cardioversion is very successful in converting atrial flutter to sinus rhythm. Remember, cardioversion is different than defibrillation. Cardioversion is performed on patients with organized cardiac electrical activity with pulses, whereas defibrillation is performed on patients without pulses (ventricular fibrillation and ventricular tachycardia without a pulse). Patients with heart beats who receive electrical energy during their heart's relative refractory period are at risk for ventricular fibrillation. Therefore, cardioversion is a timed shock designed to avoid delivering a shock during the heart's relative refractory period. By activating *synchronization mode,* the machine will identify the patient's R waves and not deliver electrical energy during these times. The key step when cardioverting is to activate the synchronization mode and confirm the presence of sync markers on the R waves prior to delivering electrical energy.

220. The answer is b. (*Circulation, IV-58–IV-66.*) This patient has cardiac electrical activity (sinus bradycardia), but no detectable pulses. He is therefore in *PEA* and management should be directed by the AHA PEA algorithm. Patients in PEA should be treated with CPR, epinephrine every 3–5 minutes, and atropine every 3–5 minutes (if PEA rate is less than 60 per minute), but a search for an underlying etiology with targeted interventions should be performed.

Common etiologies for PEA are shown in the table on the next page along with their specific treatments. Many find the *H's and T's* in the table an easy way to remember the differential. Each etiology should be considered for every patient with PEA and causes that are more likely given a patient's history and physical should be treated first. This patient has an AV graft indicating he has a history of renal disease. Since patient's with end-stage renal disease are at risk for *hyperkalemia* and hyperkalemia can cause PEA, *calcium gluconate* should be given first to stabilize the cardiac membranes.

PEA Etiology and Treatments

H's	Tx	T's	Tx
Hypovolemia	IV fluids	Toxins	Antidotes
Hypoxia	Ventilation	Tamponade (cardiac)	Pericardiocentesis
Hydrogen ion (acidosis)	Sodium bicarbonate	Tension pneumothorax	Tube thoracostomy
Hypokalemia and Hyperkalemia	KCl calcium	Thrombosis (coronary and pulmonary)	Thrombolysis
Hypoglycemia	Dextrose	Trauma (hypovolemia and increased ICP)	IV fluids
Hypothermia	Warming		

If the patient does not improve with calcium, sodium bicarbonate (**a**) could be given to treat for metabolic acidosis and 50% dextrose (**c**) can be given for suspected hypoglycemia. Cardiac tamponade is a possible etiology in a patient with renal disease and pericardiocentesis (**e**) can be attempted if the patient is not improving with the above treatments. A bedside ultrasound may also be helpful to look for right ventricular collapse or other signs of tamponade. Pneumothorax is a less likely etiology in this particular patient. It is treated with a (**d**) chest tube.

221. The answer is e. (*Tintinalli, pp 231–237.*) *Septic shock* is a clinical syndrome of *hypoperfusion, hypotension, and multiorgan dysfunction caused by infection.* This patient is clearly in shock with hypotension, tachycardia, tachypnea, and acute mental status changes. He also has fever and pus in his urine, making a urine infection the likely source of the infection. He requires immediate hydration, broad-spectrum antibiotics, possible intubation, pressors, and admission to the intensive care unit. Remember, elderly patients with comorbid conditions, such as diabetes are more prone to developing sepsis. In addition, patients with indwelling lines, such as Foley catheters, are at an even higher risk of infection.

Hypovolemic shock (**a**) occurs when there is inadequate volume in the circulatory system, resulting in poor oxygen delivery to the tissues. Neurogenic shock (**b**) occurs after an acute spinal cord injury, which disrupts sympathetic innervation resulting in hypotension and bradycardia. Cardiogenic shock (c) is caused by decreased cardiac output producing inadequate tissue perfusion. Anaphylactic shock (d) is a severe systemic hypersensitivity reaction resulting in hypotension and airway compromise.

222. The answer is b. (*Rosen, pp 71–72.*) The rhythm is *ventricular fibrillation (VF)*. Along with pulseless ventricular tachycardia (VT), these are *nonperfusing rhythms* that are treated identically because it is thought to be due to the same mechanisms. A patient who develops VF or pulseless VT while on a cardiac monitor may remain conscious for 15–30 seconds. If a *defibrillator* is not present, the patient should be encouraged to cough vigorously and continuously until one is found. The earlier a "shock" is administered in cardiac arrest, the more likely the patient will return to spontaneous circulation with a perfusing rhythm. If there is a delay to defibrillation (>4 minutes), CPR should be administered for 60–90 seconds before defibrillation. If after defibrillation (200 J biphasic or 360 J monophasic) the patient's rhythm is still VF or pulseless VT, then assisted ventilation and chest compressions should be started. Intubation should be performed and IV access obtained for administration of epinephrine or vasopressin. If the rhythm is unchanged after administration of vasopressor therapy, then another attempt at defibrillation at 360 J (or 200 J biphasic) with subsequent administration of an antidysrhythmic (i.e., amiodarone) is recommended.

(a) There is no role for observation with ventricular fibrillation. Successful return of a perfusing rhythm is most likely to result with immediate defibrillation. (c) Synchronized cardioversion is energy delivered to match the QRS complex. This reduces the chance that a shock will induce VF. Synchronization is used to treat tachydysrhythmias (i.e., rapid atrial fibrillation) in hemodynamically unstable patients. It should not be used in VF or pulseless VT. (d) The most beneficial intervention for this patient is immediate defibrillation. If this fails, the patient's airway management (ABCs) will require him to be intubated. (e) Amiodarone, an antidysrhythmic, is used in patients with VF or pulseless VT after appropriate defibrillation and administration of vasopressor therapy.

223. The answer is d. (*Circulation, IV-58–V-66. Tintinalli, p 62.*) *Asystole* is absent heart rhythm or more colloquially, flat line. A common cause of asystole is a disconnected lead or malfunctioning equipment, so the AHA recommends confirmation of asystole by *switching to another lead*. Confirmation can also be achieved with a 12-lead electrocardiogram if the equipment is readily available.

Defibrillation (a) is never recommended for asystole. Transcutaneous pacing (e) failed to show benefit in several randomized controlled trials and is no longer recommended in the 2005 AHA guidelines for asystole. The appropriate treatment for asystole includes good cardiopulmonary resuscitation (CPR), coupled with epinephrine (b) every 3–5 minutes and atropine (c) every 3–5 minutes. A search and treatment of possible underlying etiologies is recommended.

224. The answer is d. *(Tintinalli, pp 247–250.)* This patient is in *anaphylactic shock* from a food allergy while dining. Anaphylaxis is a severe *systemic hypersensitivity* reaction leading to shock from hypotension and respiratory compromise. The diagnosis is made clinically. This patient's reaction began classically with urticarial symptoms of pruritis and flushing. She then progressed to shock with hypotension and respiratory edema. She should be treated immediately with oxygen, IV epinephrine, corticosteroids, diphenhydramine, and IV fluids. Supplies should also be ready for intubation and surgical cricothyrotomy.

Hypovolemic shock (a) occurs when there is inadequate volume in the circulatory system, resulting in poor oxygen delivery to the tissues. Neurogenic shock (b) occurs after an acute spinal cord injury, which disrupts sympathetic innervation resulting in hypotension and bradycardia. Cardiogenic shock (c) is caused by decreased cardiac output producing inadequate tissue perfusion. Septic shock (e) is a clinical syndrome of hypoperfusion, hypotension, or multiorgan dysfunction caused by infection.

225. The answer is b. *(Roberts and Hedges, pp 78–80.)* The most serious complication of ET intubation is unrecognized intubation with resultant hypoxic brain injury. Esophageal placement is not always obvious. The best assurance that the tube is placed into the trachea is to *see it pass through the vocal cords.*

(a) The chest radiograph can be misleading and is essentially only useful to identify endobronchial intubation (i.e., right main stem bronchus intubation). (c) Although the chest wall should expand with positive pressure and relax with expiration, this may not occur in patients with small tidal volumes or severe bronchospasm. (d) You may hear normal breath sounds if only the midline of the thorax is auscultated. (e) In cardiac arrest situations, low exhaled carbon dioxide levels are seen in both very-low-flow states and in esophageal intubation. In addition, colorimetric changes may be difficult to discern in reduced lighting situations, and secretions can interfere with color change.

226. The answer is e. (*Tintinalli, pp 193–194.*) This ECG shows *third degree, or complete, AV block.* Note that there is *no relationship between the p waves and QRS complexes.* The p waves occur regularly, but since there is no AV conduction, the ventricles do not respond to the p waves. An escape pacemaker at a rate slower than the atrial rate drives the ventricles producing regular QRS complexes independent of the p waves.

In contrast, normal sinus rhythm (**a**) has a rate between 60 and 100 beats per minute with every p wave followed immediately by a QRS complex (1:1 conduction). First degree AV block (**b**) has a PR interval greater than 0.20 seconds. Every p wave is still followed by a QRS complex (1:1 conduction). Second degree Mobitz I (Wenckebach) AV block (**c**) occurs when there is a progressive delay in AV conduction, manifested by a gradually increasing PR interval, followed by a dropped QRS complex. The pattern then spontaneously repeats. Second degree Mobitz II AV block (**d**) occurs when there is a constant delay in AV conduction (prolonged PR interval), followed by a dropped QRS complex. It is important to recognize these distinct dysrhythmias as their etiologies are different and subtle treatment differences exist.

227. The answer is b. (*Tintinalli, pp 252–255.*) This patient is in *neurogenic shock.* He suffered an acute cervical spine injury after his fall onto rocks and has *hypotension* and *bradycardia.* The pathophysiology behind neurogenic shock is still under investigation but it's thought to be partially caused by *disrupted sympathetic outflow tracts* and *unopposed vagal tone.* Note that all other forms of shock attempt to compensate for hypotension with tachycardia. Neurogenic shock lacks sympathetic innervation; therefore, bradycardia results. Given that this is a trauma patient, all other sources for hypotension must be ruled out. He should be treated with cervical spine immobilization and IV fluids. Pressors may be needed if hypotension does not respond to fluids or fluid overload becomes a concern.

Hypovolemic shock (**a**) occurs when there is inadequate volume in the circulatory system, resulting in poor oxygen delivery to the tissues. Cardiogenic shock (**c**) is caused by decreased cardiac output producing inadequate tissue perfusion. Anaphylactic shock (**d**) is a severe systemic hypersensitivity reaction resulting in hypotension and airway compromise. Septic shock (**e**) is a clinical syndrome of hypoperfusion, hypotension, or multiorgan dysfunction caused by infection.

228. The answer is d. (*Tintinalli, p 194.*) *Atropine* is the initial treatment of choice for patients in second-degree, Mobitz I AV block. The majority of patients respond to atropine without further treatment. Mobitz I is commonly seen with acute inferior MI, digoxin toxicity, myocarditis, and after cardiac surgery.

Observation alone (**a**) is appropriate for stable patients. However, this patient is hypotensive and needs more aggressive management. Transcutaneous (**b**) or transvenous pacing (**c**) is an appropriate treatment and should be attempted if atropine is unsuccessful. Finally, if all else fails, epinephrine (**e**) or dopamine drips can be started. These treatments should be applied judiciously as the resulting increased heart rate may worsen patients with active ischemia as the etiology for their bradycardia. Furthermore, patients with acute inferior wall myocardial infarction may have right ventricular failure and may be hypotensive due to decreased preload, not bradycardia. IV fluids would be the therapy of choice in patients with inferior MI.

229. The answer is b. (*Tintinalli, pp 189–191.*) This patient had a run of *Torsades de Pointes,* an atypical ventricular tachycardia where the QRS axis swings from positive to negative within a single ECG lead. This dysrhythmia is frequently seen in patients with significant heart disease who have a prolonged QT interval. There are many possible causes of prolonged QT; however, common etiologies include drugs (e.g., antidysrhythmics, psychotropics), electrolyte abnormalities, and coronary heart disease. This patient was likely on a phenothiazine for her schizophrenia leading to prolonged QT syndrome and an episode of Torsade de Pointes. Administration of *magnesium sulfate* has been shown to decrease runs of Torsades.

Observation alone (**a**), is not adequate. Conventional ventricular tachycardia treatments, such as lidocaine (**c**) are often ineffective. Procainamide can actually further prolong the QT interval. If magnesium is unsuccessful, the next strategy involves increasing the heart rate from 90 to 120 beats per minute and thereby reducing the QT interval and preventing recurrence of Torsade de Pointes. Increased heart rate is best achieved by placing a transvenous pacemaker (**d**); this technique is sometimes called overdrive pacing. During the time it takes for transvenous pacemaker placement, unstable patients can be started on isoproterenol (**e**), a β-adrenergic receptor agonist to medically increase the heart rate.

230. The answer is c. (*van den Berghe G, pp 1359–1367.*) A randomized controlled study of surgical ICU patients on mechanical ventilation found that patients receiving intensive insulin therapy (maintenance of blood glucose at a level between 80 and 110 mg/dL) had decreased mortality compared with those receiving conventional treatment. The best way to achieve intense control of blood sugar levels in a ventilated patient is via an *insulin drip*. It is important to realize that hyperglycemia can be present in septic patients, even without a history of diabetes. The increased levels of catecholamines, cortisol, and glucagons coupled with decreased insulin production, and increased insulin resistance common in shock may contribute to hyperglycemia. However, you should always first address the ABC during the resuscitation.

Sliding scale insulin use (**b**) is more difficult to achieve tight control. Oral agents, such as metformin (**d**) and glipizde (**e**), are not appropriate for an intubated patient and will not permit tight control. Continued IV fluids (**a**) will not correct this patient's hyperglycemia.

231. The answer is e. (*Tintinalli, p 229.*) This patient has significant hypotension and tachycardia with mental status changes and needs *O-positive blood* now. His *hypovolemic shock* is most likely due to a brisk upper GI bleeding, secondary to variceal bleeding. While his blood is being processed in the laboratory, including type and cross, complete blood count, chemistry panel, liver function tests, and coagulation profile, a nasogastric tube should be placed and octreotide should be started. A gastroenterologist and surgeon should also be consulted. O-negative blood is reserved for women in their child-bearing years to prevent potential Rh sensitization.

Isotonic crystalloid (**b**), such as 0.9% normal saline, should run concurrently with the packed red blood cell transfusion, but will not replace the oxygen carrying capacity of lost red blood cells. Hypertonic sodium chloride (**a**) is unlikely to be helpful in an acute GI bleed. There is not enough time to wait for cross-matched (**c**) or type specific blood (**d**).

232. The answer is b. (*Tintinalli, pp 228–231.*) Crystalloids such as *normal saline (0.9% sodium chloride)* or *lactated ringers* are the preferred resuscitation fluid in the United States. The patient is currently stable; however, he is tachycardic and has suffered an injury with the potential for significant injury. The FAST exam will help illustrate the extent of this patient's injury. In the meantime, the patient should be started on isotonic crystalloid solution. There is no convincing evidence that normal saline or Ringers lactate is superior to the other.

Hypertonic saline (**a**) helps prevent the extravascular fluid shift seen with isotonic crystalloids, but is volume limited due to the risk of hypernatremia.

Furthermore, clinical studies have not shown clear evidence of improved outcome using hypertonic saline. Colloid solutions (c), such as albumin, FFP, and dextran solutions have larger protein components and would therefore be expected to remain in the intravascular space. However, this is a theoretical benefit, as numerous studies have not shown improved outcome using colloid solutions. Blood (d and e) is the best resuscitation fluid. Cross-matched blood is preferred over type specific blood, if time is available to perform the cross-match. In this case, the patient has only minimal tachycardia. He can receive crystalloid first with continuous monitoring while the diagnostic workup continues. Blood is indicated after 2–3 L of crystalloid infusion and only minimal improvement in vital signs or when the patient has obviously suffered significant blood loss.

233. The answer is e. (*Rosen, pp 73–74.*) The rhythm is *asystole*. This rhythm represents *complete cessation of myocardial electrical activity*. Although asystole may occur early in cardiac arrest because of progressive bradycardia, it generally represents the end-stage rhythm after prolonged cardiac arrest secondary to VF or PEA. Because the potential exists for an organized rhythm or VF to appear as asystole in a single lead, asystole should always be *confirmed in at least two limb leads*. It may be difficult to distinguish between extremely fine VF and asystole. Treatment includes CPR, intubation, IV access, and the administration of epinephrine or vasopressin and atropine.

(a) Synchronized cardioversion is energy delivered to match the QRS complex. This reduces the chance that a shock will induce VF. Synchronization is used to treat tachydysrhythmias (i.e., rapid atrial fibrillation) in hemodynamically unstable patients. It should not be used in asystole. (b and c) Immediate defibrillation is used in VF and VT. Although some clinicians shock asystole in the event it is actually fine VF, this has not been shown to improve patient outcome. Epinephrine and atropine should be administered first. (d) Amiodarone is an antidysrhythmic that is only effective if there is a rhythm (i.e., ventricular tachycardia); asystole is the lack of a rhythm.

234. The answer is e. (*Tintinalli, pp 1518, 1327–1329.*) This patient has signs of *disseminated intravascular coagulation* (*DIC*) secondary to meningococcemia. She should be treated with *FFP* for elevated coagulation times (INR and PTT) with signs of active bleeding (oozing gums). FFP will provide lost clotting factors and help to control the bleeding.

Studies involving heparin therapy (a) are inconclusive regarding increased survivability in DIC and therefore can be held until further discussion with the appropriate consultants. Cryoprecipitate (**b**) contains concentrated Factor VIII and fibrinogen. It is helpful in DIC when the fibrinogen is less than 150 mg/dL. Platelets (**d**) should be transfused when the count is below 20,000/μL or below 50,000/μL in patients with active bleeding. Red blood cells (**c**) can be transfused if the anemia is causing symptoms.

235. The answer is d. (*Tintinalli, pp 1315–1318.*) This patient is in *septic shock* from pneumonia and also has *adrenal crisis*. Initial treatment with IV fluids, antibiotics, and dopamine is appropriate. Continued hypotension in a patient on maintenance steroid therapy should make you think of adrenal crisis. Exogenous glucocorticoids suppress hypothalamic release of corticotropin-releasing hormone (CRH) and subsequently anterior pituitary release of adrenocorticotropic hormone (ACTH). The adrenals subsequently atrophy from lack of stimulation. The patient is now faced with an acute stress from pneumonia and sepsis. His adrenals have atrophied and are unable to respond with increased cortisol secretion. Laboratory clues to adrenal crisis include hyponatremia and hyperkalemia due to a lack of aldosterone. The treatment of adrenal crisis in the face of septic shock is *hydrocortisone*.

Mineralcorticoids, such as fludrocortisone (**c**), are not needed. Additional fluids (**a**) and pressors (**b**) and (**e**) are appropriate critical care management for sepsis and should be administered after glucocorticoids.

236. The answer is c. (*Tintinalli, pp 1036–1037, 1105–1108.*) Toxic ingestions must always be considered, especially in suicidal patients. The patient regularly takes atenolol for hypertension and may have taken an overdose. *β-blocker toxicity* classically causes bradycardia and hypotension. Antidotes for β-blocker toxicity, such as *glucagon,* should be given to this patient immediately. Glucagon is thought to work through a separate receptor that is not blocked by β-adrenergic antagonists, ultimately enhancing inotropy and chronotropy. Other medications that may be useful are phosphodiesterase inhibitors, which block cAMP breakdown and maintain intracellular calcium levels. Insulin is a promising experimental treatment for β-blocker toxicity. Ultimately, the patient may require the other treatment options, but glucagon should be the first line of therapy.

You should administer an IV bolus of fluids (**a**) may attempt to administer atropine, and place external cardiac pacers on the patient. However, because this is a β-blocker overdose, the administration of glucagon should treat the patient. (**d**) Epinephrine should be administered if the patient loses his pulse.

237. The answer is d. (*Tintinalli, pp 1605–1607.*) Patients with penetrating trauma to the chest with possible cardiac injury and signs of hemodynamic instability need immediate *operative thoracotomy.* This patient has signs of cardiac tamponade, a collection of blood surrounding the heart and interfering with the heart's ability to contract. He has Beck's triad of hypotension, distended neck veins, and muffled heart sounds. His CXR also shows an enlarged heart. An echocardiogram would be helpful in confirming the diagnosis, but since this patient is unstable and echocardiogram may not be readily available, the treatment is immediate thoracotomy in the OR.

While pericardiocentesis (**c**) may help relieve tamponade, it is not the optimal procedure for traumatic tamponade. Pericardiocentesis may be difficult when clots fill the pericardium and may therefore give false negative results. The procedure may also injure the heart and delay definitive treatment. Some clinicians perform bilateral tube thoracostomy (**b**) prior to thoracotomy to rule out a hemo- and pneumothorax. However, with equal breath sounds, midline trachea, and no evidence of pneumothorax or consolidation on radiograph, chest tubes are low yield in this patient. The patient is not in respiratory distress. Intubation (**a**) should be performed in the OR to prevent additional delays in definitive surgical care. IV fluids and blood transfusion (**e**) increase venous return to the heart and are excellent supportive measures prior to definitive thoracotomy.

238. The answer is d. (*Tintinalli, pp 1876–1877, 383–385.*) This patient has *cardiac tamponade* from metastatic breast cancer. Bedside ultrasound is often diagnostic. The echo-free area around the heart is a *pericardial effusion.* It is important to realize that the presence or absence of pericardial effusion is not diagnostic of tamponade. However, *right atrial* and *ventricular collapse* is *more specific ultrasound signs for tamponade.* Clinical findings should always be considered in making the diagnosis. Patients with tamponade usually have tachycardia, low systolic BP, and narrow pulse pressure. Tamponade must always be considered with trauma to the chest, as well as patients with metastatic malignancy, pericarditis, uremia, and those patients on anticoagulation.

Echocardiogram in congestive heart failure (**b**) will show decreased contractility or ejection fraction. Years of experience with ultrasound are necessary to accurately and reliably interpret ejection fraction. Myocardial infarctions (**c**) will typically show evidence of wall motion abnormalities or global hypokinesis. Dehydration (**e**) will make the heart hyperdynamic with decreased size of the right atria and ventricles from decreased preload.

239. The answer is b. *(Tintinalli, pp 343–359.)* This patient is in *cardiogenic shock* from a right ventricular infarction. The ECG shows ST-segment elevation in leads II, III, and aVF indicating the patient is having an *inferior wall myocardial infarction.* Approximately 30% of inferior MIs involve the *right ventricle (RV).* A right-sided ECG would confirm the diagnosis. RV infarction results in reduced right ventricular end-systolic pressure ultimately leading to decreased cardiac output. Patients with RV infarctions are therefore dependent on preload to maintain cardiac output. In this case, nitroglycerin, a powerful preload reducer, pushed this patient into cardiogenic shock. Patients with RV infarction and hypotension should be treated with IV normal saline to support preload. Dobutamine may also be necessary to support the BP. Furthermore, this patient is having an acute ST-segment elevation myocardial infarction and may be a candidate for percutaneous coronary intervention or fibrinolytics.

(**a**) It is imperative to remember the relationship of inferior MI and RV failure and not discount hypotension after nitroglycerin and morphine to medication side effects alone. Papillary muscle rupture (**c**) is also associated with inferior wall myocardial infarction, but occurs 3–5 days after the primary infarction. Patients present with new-onset dyspnea, exercise intolerance, and new murmur on exam. Free wall rupture (**d**) is a serious complication of myocardial infarctions occurring 1–5 days after the primary event. Patients complain of sudden onset of tearing, severe chest pain and usually present in cardiogenic shock secondary to cardiac tamponade. Rupture of the interventricular septum (**e**) is more common in patients with recent anterior wall infarctions. These patients present with chest pain, shortness of breath, and a new murmur.

240. The answer is b. *(Tintinalli, pp 658–664.)* This patient is in *hypovolemic shock* due to a *ruptured ectopic pregnancy* with bleeding into her abdomen evidenced by fluid in Morrison's pouch. Any female with a positive β-hCG and abdominal pain must be ruled out for an ectopic pregnancy. The pregnant patient should undergo either a transvaginal or abdominal ultrasound to confirm an intrauterine pregnancy. In the case of this patient who is complaining of abdominal pain, is hemodynamically unstable with fluid in her abdomen, has a positive β-hCG and does not have evidence for an intrauterine pregnancy, she *must be taken to the OR by OB/GYN* to treat her for a presumed ectopic pregnancy. No further diagnostic testing is necessary on this patient.

(**a**) The surgery service, although useful in many other abdominal emergencies, is not the appropriate consult for this patient. If the

OB/GYN service determines that the patient is bleeding into her abdomen from a cause other than an ectopic pregnancy, then the surgery service should bring the patient to the OR to perform an exploratory laparotomy. (c) A paracentesis has no role in the workup of a hemodynamically unstable patient with a presumed ruptured ectopic pregnancy. (d) A culdocentesis is a procedure that checks for abnormal fluid in the space just behind the vagina. It is not necessary since the ultrasound is positive for fluid in the abdomen. (e) The patient is hemodynamically unstable and should not undergo a CT scan at this time. Although appendicitis is on the differential diagnosis for RLQ pain, a ruptured ectopic pregnancy is much more likely in this situation.

241. The answer is e. (*Tintinalli, pp 247–252.*) This patient was stung by a yellow jacket, a member of the Hymenoptera order, leading to an IgE-mediated hypersensitivity *anaphylactic reaction* causing *respiratory compromise*. Management in the ED begins with administering oxygen, placing on a cardiac monitoring, and obtaining large-bore IV access. Further intervention depends on the severity of the reaction and affected organ system. The physician must rapidly *assess airway patency* in patients. The first-line treatment for severe anaphylactic reaction with signs of respiratory compromise is IV *epinephrine*. Epinephrine may rapidly reverse airway compromise. If the patient does not respond to the IV epinephrine, an epinephrine drip can be started. Patients with less severe symptoms can be given the intramuscular form of epinephrine in the thigh. If respiratory collapse is imminent, bag-valve-mask ventilation may be effective until the patient can be intubated.

(a) and (b) Diphenhydramine (Benadryl) is an antihistamine that usually works very well in allergic reactions. It should be administered to this patient, however, in hemodynamically compromised patients epinephrine is the first-line treatment. (c) Methylprednisolone is also a useful adjunct medication for allergic reactions; however its delayed onset of action limits its effectiveness in the acutely decompensating patient. (d) Dopamine is a pressor agent that can be used in the setting of hemodynamic comprise. However, it is rarely used in anaphylaxis because epinephrine is the first-line agent that also acts as a pressor.

242. The answer is e. (*Tintinalli, p 1596.*) This patient has a *tension pneumothorax*. Air has entered the pleural space, secondary to the gunshot, and caused the right lung to collapse. This air cannot escape and pressure continues to increase, pushing the right lung into the mediastinum, causing the trachea to shift to the left. If this process is not corrected, *venous return and cardiac output can be compromised* and the patient will die. Classic symptoms of tension pneumothorax include dyspnea, tachypnea, tracheal deviation to the uninjured side, absent breath sounds on the injured side, and hypotension. Treatment of a tension pneumothorax is immediate *needle decompression* using a large 14- or 16-gauge IV catheter inserted into the pleural space. Air should come out of the catheter and the patient's clinical condition should improve. A tube thoracostomy should be performed after the needle decompression.

(a) Tension pneumothorax is a clinical diagnosis and if suspected should be treated immediately, without waiting for a chest x-ray. While intubation (b) is generally helpful for patients in respiratory distress, it can be dangerous in the setting of a tension pneumothorax. Positive pressure ventilation worsens the tension pneumothorax leading to further cardiovascular compromise. This patient will likely require surgical management and the surgical team (d) should be called; however needle decompression and tube thoracostomy are core emergency medicine skills and should be performed immediately by the emergency physician. ED thoracotomy (c) is indicated in penetrating trauma patients who have witnessed loss of pulse in the field or in the ED.

243. The answer is c. (*Tintinalli, pp 501–505.*) Abdominal pain in the elderly can be challenging for many reasons, including poor histories and deviation from classic presentation of diseases. However, abdominal pain in patients over 65 must be taken seriously since 25–44% requires surgical intervention and more than 50% require admission to the hospital. This chest radiograph reveals *free air under the right diaphragm,* likely from a perforated viscous. This is a *surgical emergency* and the surgical service should be contacted.

Antibiotics (a) and a central venous line (d) are appropriate and can be started after the surgical team has been notified. It is important to obtain large-bore IV access for this patient. If peripheral lines are not obtained, then a central venous line should be inserted. A CT scan (b) is not necessary in this patient, especially with her low BP. She should be taken directly to the OR for an exploratory laparotomy. Although the patient has a benign abdominal exam, the caretakers report and her low BP is worrisome and sending the patient home (e) prior to a complete workup would be a mistake.

Altered Mental Status

Questions

244. A 69-year-old woman with a past medical history of hypertension, hypercholesterolemia, and diabetes mellitus type 1 is brought to the emergency department (ED) by her daughter who states that her mom has been acting funny over the last hour. She states that the patient did not know where she was despite being in her own house. She also did not recognize her family and was speaking incomprehensibly. Her blood pressure (BP) is 150/80 mm Hg, heart rate (HR) is 90 beats per minute, temperature is 98.9°F, and his respiratory rate (RR) is 16 breaths per minute. She appears diaphoretic. The rest of her physical exam is unremarkable. Electrocardiogram (ECG) is sinus rhythm with normal ST segments and T waves. Which of the following is the most appropriate course of action for this patient?

a. Call the cardiac catherization lab for potential stent placement
b. Activate the stroke team and bring the patient directly to the CT scanner
c. Get a stat fingerstick and administer dextrose if her blood sugar is low
d. Give a 500 cc intravenous (IV) bolus of normal saline to treat her confusion
e. Administer haloperidol for sedation

245. A 74-year-old lethargic woman is brought to the ED by her family. Her daughter states that the patient has been progressively somnolent over the last week and could not be woken up today. The patient takes medications for diabetes, hypertension, hypothyroidism and a recent ankle sprain, which is treated with a hydrocodone/acetaminophen combination. In the ED, the patient is profoundly lethargic, responsive only to pain, and has periorbital edema and delayed relaxation of the deep tendon reflexes. Her BP is 145/84 mm Hg, HR is 56 beats per minute, temperature is 94.8°F, and RR is 12 breaths per minute. Her fingerstick glucose is 195 mg/dL. Which of the following is the most likely diagnosis?

a. Hypoglycemia
b. Myocardial infarction
c. Stroke
d. Myxedema coma
e. Depression

246. A 79-year-old man presents to the ED by paramedics with the chief complaint of agitation and confusion over the previous 12 hours. He has a past medical history of schizophrenia and is not taking any of his antipsychotics. His BP is 135/85 mm Hg, HR is 119 beats per minute, RR is 18 breaths per minute, O_2 saturation is 97% on room air, and fingerstick glucose is 135 mg/dL. Due to his agitation at triage, he was placed in wrist restraints. At this time, he is calm but confused. Examination reveals warm and clammy skin and 4 mm pupils that are equal and reactive. His cardiac exam reveals tachycardia and no murmurs. His lungs are clear to auscultation and his abdomen is soft and nontender. He is able to move all of his extremities. Which of the following is the most appropriate next step in management?

a. Administer haloperidol or lorazepam
b. Arrange for a psychiatry consult to treat his agitation
c. Order a CT scan
d. Draw his blood for various lab testing
e. Obtain a rectal temperature

247. A 25-year-old man is brought to the ED by emergency medical service (EMS) accompanied by his girlfriend who reports that the patient had a seizure 30 minutes ago and is still confused. The girlfriend reports that the patient is a known epileptic who has been doing well on his latest medication regimen. The exact seizure medications are unknown. On arrival to the ED, the patient develops continuous clonic movements of his upper and lower extremities. The patient's vital signs are BP of 162/85 mm Hg, HR of 110 beats per minute and pulse oximetry of 91% on room air. Capillary glucose level is 95 mg/dL. Which of the following is the most appropriate next step in management?

a. Place the patient in a lateral decubitus position
b. Administer lorazepam
c. Administer phenytoin
d. Perform rapid sequence intubation on the patient
e. Look up the patient's medical records and administer his current antiepileptic regimen

248. A 19-year-old college student presents to the ED complaining of headache, sore throat, myalgias, and rash that developed over the previous 12 hours. Her BP is 95/60 mm Hg, HR is 132 beats per minute, temperature is 103.9°F, RR is 19 breaths per minute, and O_2 saturation is 98% on room air. She is confused and oriented only to person. Physical exam is remarkable for pain with neck flexion, a petechial and purpuric rash on her extremities, and delayed capillary refill. Which of the following best describes the emergency physicians' priority in managing this patient?

a. Collect two sets of blood cultures prior to antibiotic administration
b. Call the patient's parents and have them come immediately to the hospital
c. Call her roommate to gather more information
d. Begin fluid resuscitation, administer intravenous antibiotics, and perform a lumbar puncture (LP)
e. Administer acetaminophen to see if her headache and fever resolve

249. A 14-year-old girl is brought to the ED by her mother stating that her daughter has been very sleepy today. The patient does not have any medical problems or takes any medications. Her BP is 95/61 mm Hg, HR is 132 beats per minute, temperature is 99.7°F, and RR is 20 breaths per minute. Her fingerstick glucose is 530 mg/dL. Which of the following choices most closely matches what you would expect to find on her arterial blood gas with electrolytes and urinalysis?

a. pH 7.38, anion gap 5, normal urinalysis
b. pH 7.47, anion gap 21, presence of glucose and leukocytes in urine
c. pH 7.47, anion gap 12, presence of glucose and ketones in urine
d. pH 7.26, anion gap 12, presence of glucose and ketones in urine
e. pH 7.26, anion gap 21, presence of glucose and ketones in urine

250. A 65-year-old actively seizing woman is brought to the ED by EMS. She was found slumped over at the bus stop bench. EMS personnel state that when they found the woman she was diaphoretic and her speech was garbled. In route to the hospital, she started to seize. As you wheel her to a room, the nurse gives you some of her vital signs which are a BP of 150/90 mm Hg, HR of 115 beats per minute, and O_2 saturation of 96%. Which of the following is the next best step in management of this patient?

a. Request a rectal temperature to rule out meningitis
b. Call the CT technologist and tell them you are bringing over a seizing patient
c. Ask for a stat ECG and administer an aspirin
d. Check the patient's fingerstick blood glucose level
e. Intubate the patient

251. A 48-year-old man presents to the ED with ethanol intoxication. His BP is 150/70 mm Hg, HR is 95 beats per minute, temperature is 97.9°F, RR is 14 breaths per minute, and O_2 saturation is 93% on room air. The patient is somnolent and snoring loudly with occasional gasps for air. On exam, the patient's gag reflex is intact, his lungs are clear to auscultation, heart is without murmurs, and abdomen is soft and nontender. He is arousable to stimulation. A head CT is negative for intracranial injury. His ethanol level is 270 mg/dL. Which of the following actions is most appropriate to assist the patient with respirations?

a. Nasal airway
b. Oral airway
c. Bag-valve mask ventilation
d. Laryngeal mask airway
e. Tracheoesophageal airway

252. A 52-year-old woman is brought to the ED by her husband for altered mental status for 1 day. The patient has hypertension and diabetes but has not been taking her medications for the last 5 days since she lost her insurance and could not afford her prescriptions. Her BP is 168/91 mm Hg, HR is 125 beats per minute, temperature is 99.8°F, and RR is 18 breaths per minute. Her fingerstick glucose is 900 mg/dL. There is glucose in her urine but no ketones. Which of the following is the most appropriate next step in management?

a. Administer IV fluids and insulin
b. Obtain head computed tomography (CT)
c. Obtain ECG
d. Obtain chest radiograph and urine culture
e. Administer broad coverage antibiotics

253. A 45-year-old man is brought to the ED by his coworkers after collapsing to the floor while at work. A coworker states that the patient mistakenly took several tablets of his oral diabetic medications a few hours ago. The patient is unresponsive and diaphoretic. His BP is 142/78 mm Hg, HR is 115 beats per minute, temperature is 98.9°F, and RR is 12 breaths per minute. A bedside glucose reads 42 mg/dL. Which of the following is the most appropriate management of this patient?

a. Administer IV dextrose, obtain a repeat fingerstick glucose, and, if normal, discharge the patient home
b. Administer IV dextrose and continue monitoring his blood sugar for at least 24 hours
c. Administer IV fluids and insulin
d. Administer IV fluids
e. Administer activated charcoal and IV fluids

254. A 59-year-old man is brought into the ED accompanied by his son who states that his father is acting irritable and occasionally confused. The son states that his father has a history of hepatitis from a transfusion he received many years ago. Over the past 5 years, his liver function slowly deteriorated. His vital signs are 145/80 mm Hg, a HR of 78 beats per minute, RR of 16 breaths per minute, O_2 saturation of 98%, and temperature of 98°F. Laboratory results are all within normal limits, except for an ammonia level that is significantly elevated. Which of the following is the best therapy?

a. Vancomycin and gentamycin
b. Lactulose and neomycin
c. Ampicillin and gentamycin
d. Levofloxacin
e. Ciprofloxacin

255. A 40-year-old man who is an employee of the hospital is brought to the ED actively seizing. A coworker states that the patient has a known seizure disorder and currently takes phenytoin for the disorder. He also tells you that the patient has been under stress recently and may not have taken his last few doses of medication. You call for the nurse to place a face mask with 100% O_2 and gain intravenous access. You then ask for a medication to be drawn up. Which is the most appropriate initial medication you should administer in this actively seizing patient?

a. Phenytoin
b. Diazepam
c. Phenobarbital
d. Valproic acid
e. Lithium

256. A 32-year-old G_1P_1 who gave birth by normal vaginal delivery at 38 weeks gestation 2 days ago presents to the ED complaining of bilateral hand swelling and severe headache that started 2 hours ago. Her BP is 187/110 mm Hg, HR is 85 beats per minute, temperature is 97.5°F, and RR is 15 breaths per minute. Urinalysis reveals 3+ protein. As you are examining the patient, she proceeds to have a generalized tonic-clonic seizure. Which of the following is the most appropriate next step in management?

a. Administer magnesium sulfate intravenously
b. Administer labetolol to reduce her BP and morphine sulfate to address her headache
c. Administer sumatriptan and place the patient into a dark quiet room
d. Administer a loading dose of phenytoin, order a head CT scan, and call for a neurology consult
e. Administer diazepam and normal saline intravenously

257. An unconscious 51-year-old woman is brought to the ED by EMS. A friend states that the patient was complaining of feeling weak. She vomited and subsequently "blacked out" in the ambulance. The friend states that the patient has no medical problems and takes no medications. She also states that the patient smokes cigarettes and uses cocaine, and that they were snorting cocaine together prior to her blacking out. The patient's BP is 195/80 mm Hg, HR is 50 beats per minute, temperature is 98.6°F, and RR is 7 breaths per minute. What is the eponym associated with her vital signs?

a. Cushing syndrome
b. Cushing reflex
c. Cullen's sign
d. Charcot's triad
e. Chvostek's sign

258. A 32-year-old man is found unresponsive on the street by paramedics. In route to the ED, he becomes responsive and states that he probably had a seizure since he is noncompliant with his seizure medications. In the ED, he is complaining of severe pain in his left shoulder. His BP is 142/85 mm Hg, HR is 125 beats per minute, temperature is 98.7°F, and RR is 18 breaths per minute. On exam, the patient has significantly limited range of motion of his shoulder, which is held in adduction and internally rotated. What likely seizure complication does this patient have?

a. Anterior shoulder dislocation
b. Posterior shoulder dislocation
c. Humerus fracture
d. Clavicle fracture
e. Todd's paralysis

259. A 47-year-old man is brought to the ED by EMS after being persistently agitated at a business meeting. The patient's coworkers state that he has been working nonstop for a day and a half and that he always seemed like a healthy guy who frequented bars every night. EMS administered 25 g of dextrose and thiamine with no symptom improvement. In the ED, the patient is anxious, confused, tremulous, and diaphoretic. He denies any medical problems, medications, and drug ingestions. His BP is 182/92 mm Hg, HR is 139 beats per minute, temperature is 100.4°F, and RR is 18 breaths per minute and fingerstick glucose is 103 mg/dL. An ECG reveals sinus tachycardia. Which of the following is the next best step?

a. Administer acetaminophen
b. Administer folate
c. Administer diazepam
d. Recheck fingerstick glucose
e. Administer labetalol

260. A 62-year-old man with known type 1 diabetes is brought into the ED by his family who states the patient is having a stroke. They report that the patient became diaphoretic, confused, and had difficulty moving. His BP is 150/85 mm Hg, HR is 97 beats per minute, temperature is 99.3°F, and RR is 16 breaths per minute, and fingerstick is 39 mg/dL. On exam, the patient is difficult to arouse, diaphoretic, confused, and speaking with slurred speech. Which of the following is the most appropriate next step in management?

a. Administer antibiotics and perform a lumbar puncture
b. Give aspirin, O_2, nitroglycerin, and a β-blocker
c. Order an emergent brain CT scan
d. Give the patient a glass of orange juice to drink
e. Place an IV line and administer 50 g of dextrose

261. A 65-year-old man presents to the ED with a headache, drowsiness, and confusion. He has a history of long-standing hypertension. His BP is 220/120 mm Hg, pulse 87 beats per minute, RR 18 breaths per minutes, and O_2 saturation 97% on room air. On exam, you note papilledema. A head CT scan is performed that is normal. Which of the following is the most appropriate method to lower his BP?

a. Intubate the patient and hyperventilate
b. Administer mannitol
c. Administer a high-dose diuretic
d. Administer labetolol until his BP is 120/40 mm Hg
e. Administer labetolol until his BP is 180/100 mm Hg

262. A 74-year-old woman is brought to the ED by EMS for altered mental status. Her BP is 138/72 mm Hg, HR 91 beats per minute, RR 17 breaths per minute, and temperature 100.9°F. A head CT is normal. Lumbar puncture results revealed the following:

> WBC 250/μL with 90% polymorphonuclear cells
> Glucose 21 mg/dL
> Protein 81 g/L

Which if the following is the most likely diagnosis?

a. Subarachnoid hemorrhage
b. Bacterial meningitis
c. Viral meningitis
d. Multiple sclerosis (MS)
e. Encephalitis

263. A 67-year-old man presents to the ED for worsening confusion. His wife states that he received his first dose of chemotherapy for lung cancer 2 days ago. Over the last 24 hours, the patient became confused. His BP is 130/70 mm Hg, HR 87 beats per minute, and temperature 98.9°F. While in the ED, the patient seizes. You administer an antiepileptic and the seizure immediately stops. You compare his current electrolyte panel to one taken 2 days ago.

	Two days ago	Today
Sodium (mEq/L)	139	113
Potassium (mEq/L)	4.1	3.9
Chloride (mEq/L)	105	98
Bicarbonate (mEq/L)	23	20
BUN (mg/dL)	13	17
Creatinine (mg/dL)	0.4	0.7
Glucose (mg/dL)	98	92

Which of the following is the most appropriate treatment?

a. 0.45% saline
b. 0.9% saline
c. 3% saline
d. 5% dextrose
e. 50% dextrose

264. A 31-year-old woman with a history of schizophrenia presents to the ED for altered mental status. A friend states that the patient is on multiple medications for her schizophrenia. Her BP is 150/80 mm Hg, HR 121 beats per minute, RR 20 breaths per minute, and temperature 104.5°F. On exam, the patient is diaphoretic with distinctive "lead-pipe" rigidity of her musculature. You believe the patient has neuroleptic malignant syndrome. After basic stabilizing measures, which of the following medications is most appropriate to administer?

a. Haloperidol
b. Droperidol
c. Dantrolene
d. Doxycycline
e. Acetaminophen

265. A 56-year-old man is brought in from the homeless shelter for strange, irrational behavior and unsteady gait for 1 day. A worker at the shelter reports that the patient is a frequent abuser of alcohol. On exam, the patient is alert but oriented to name only and is unable to give full history. He does not appear clinically intoxicated. You note horizontal nystagmus and ataxia. What is the most likely diagnosis?

a. Wernicke's encephalopathy
b. Korsakoff syndrome
c. Normal pressure hydrocephalus
d. Alcohol intoxication
e. Alcohol withdrawal

266. An 18-year-old girl is brought to ED from a party for agitation and attacking her boyfriend with a knife. Her boyfriend admits that she had several liquor shots and used intranasal cocaine at the party prior to becoming agitated, paranoid and attacking him. Her BP is 145/80 mm Hg, HR is 126 beats per minute, temperature is 100.8°F, and RR is 20 breaths per minute. The patient is agitated, screaming, and resisting exam. What is the next best step in the management of this patient?

a. IV metoprolol
b. IV diazepam
c. Acetaminophen
d. Rapid sequence intubation
e. Drug-abuse specialist consult

267. A 78-year-old woman is transferred from a nursing home with altered mental status and fever. The nursing home reports the patient was febrile to 102.3°F, disoriented, confused, and incontinent of urine. Her past medical history includes hypertension, a stroke with residual right-sided weakness, and nighttime agitation for which she was started on haloperidol 3 days ago. Her BP is 215/105 mm Hg, HR is 132 beats per minute, temperature is 102.8°F, and RR is 20 breaths per minute. On exam the patient is oriented to name only, tremulous, diaphoretic and has marked muscular rigidity and 3/5 right upper and lower extremity strength. What is the most likely diagnosis?

a. Urinary tract infection
b. Malignant hyperthermia
c. Neuroleptic malignant syndrome
d. Recurrent stroke
e. Meningoencephalitis

268. A 54-year-old man is brought to the ED by his wife for bizarre behavior. The wife complains that her husband has been acting unlike himself for the last several days without any change in sleep, appetite or activity level. She also recalls him complaining of morning headaches for the last 2 months. The patient is otherwise in good health and does not take any medications. His BP is 135/87 mm Hg, HR is 76 beats per minute, temperature is 98.9°F, and RR is 14 breaths per minute. His exam is unremarkable. Which of the following is the most likely diagnosis?

a. Depression
b. Tension headache
c. Subarachnoid hemorrhage

d. Pseudotumor cerebri
e. Frontal lobe mass

269. A 16-year-old girl is brought from school to the ED after having a generalized seizure 30 minutes prior to arrival. The school nurse reports that the patient has a history of seizures and takes levetiracetam (Keppra). In the ED, her BP is 124/65 mm Hg, HR is 84 beats per minute, temperature is 98.2°F, RR is 16 breaths per minute, and O_2 saturation is 97%. The patient is alert and localizes to pain. Which of the following is the most appropriate next step?

a. Perform rapid sequence intubation
b. Continue monitoring and observation
c. Administer IV lorazepam
d. Obtain a head CT
e. Perform a LP

270. A 55-year-old man is brought to the ED by EMS after being found on the street confused and disoriented. In the ED, the patient is unable to tell you what happened. On exam you notice a left forearm fistula and in his wallet is the phone number of his dialysis center. You call the center and the nurse there tells you the patient was recently started on hemodialysis but missed his last two appointments. Which of the following likely abnormal findings must be addressed immediately in this patient?

a. Encephalopathy
b. Anemia
c. Hyperkalemia
d. Hypocalcemia
e. Fluid overload

271. A 27-year-old woman is brought to the ED by her husband after having a first-time seizure at home. She has no past medical history but just had an uncomplicated vaginal delivery 1 week prior to presentation. In the ED, her BP is 178/95 mm Hg, HR is 92 beats per minute, temperature is 99.2°F, and RR is 16 breaths per minute. On exam she has mild edema of her hands and feet. The patient tells you that she is feeling well now and would like to go home to her baby. Which of the following is the most appropriate diagnostic test?

a. Complete blood count
b. Head CT
c. Lumbar puncture
d. Urinalysis
e. ECG

272. A 46-year-old woman is brought to the ED by her husband for 1 day of worsening confusion. The patient has a history of systemic lupus erythromatosus (SLE) and takes chronic oral steroids. She has not been feeling well for the last few days. Her BP is 167/92 mm Hg, HR is 95 beats per minute, temperature is 100.3°F, and RR is 16 breaths per minute. On exam the patient is oriented to name and has diffuse petechiae on her torso and extremities. Laboratory results reveal hematocrit 23%, platelets 17,000/μL, BUN 38 mg/dL, creatinine 1.9 mg/dL. Which of the following is the most likely diagnosis?

a. Henoch-Schönlein purpura
b. Disseminated intravascular coagulopathy
c. Von Willebrand disease
d. Idiopathic thrombocytopenic purpura
e. Thrombotic thrombocytopenic purpura (TTP)

273. A 63-year-old man presents to the ED complaining of headache, vomiting, and "not being able to think straight" for 1 day. The patient states that he has hypertension and diabetes but ran out of his medications in the last week. His BP is 245/138 mm Hg, HR is 90 beats per minute, temperature is 98.7°F, and his RR is 14 breaths per minute. Fingerstick glucose is 178 mg/dL. On exam the patient appears slightly confused and oriented to name and place only. The neurologic exam is significant for papilledema. Which of the following is the most appropriate next step in management?

a. Nitroprusside IV
b. Magnesium sulfate IV
c. Metoprolol by mouth
d. Hydrochlorothiazide by mouth
e. Obtain head CT

274. A 64-year-old woman is brought to the ED by her sister after a witnessed syncopal episode on the street. Her sister reports that they were walking in the park when the patient complained of not feeling well, fell backward and had to be supported by a man behind them. The patient has a history of hypertension and diabetes and takes multiple medications. Her BP is 168/84 mm Hg, HR is 67 beats per minute, temperature is 97.8°F, and RR is 18 breaths per minute. Her exam is unremarkable. Which of the following is the *least* likely cause of this patient's syncope?

a. Myocardial infarction
b. Pulmonary embolus
c. Transient ischemic attack

d. Medications
e. Situational syncope

275. A 26-year-old man with a long history of epilepsy is brought to the ED for a recent seizure. While in the ED, he is rhythmically moving his right leg and is unresponsive. Which of the following best describes this seizure pattern?

a. Petit mal seizure
b. Generalized tonic-clonic seizure
c. Partial seizure with secondary generalization
d. Simple partial seizure
e. Complex partial seizure

276. A 19-year-old man is brought in by a friend who reports that he found the patient passed out on a chair, wearing only shorts in his apartment. The patient is arousable upon arrival to the ED with a HR of 70 beats per minute, a BP of 115/66 mm Hg, a RR of 12 breaths per minute, and an O_2 saturation of 98% on 2 L oxygen nasal cannula. He describes feeling nauseated and having a mild, generalized headache. The friend states that he went to check on the patient because he had missed his classes that day. A roommate, who subsequently presents later on to visit, states that he has had similar, but milder, symptoms as well. Based on the history given and his clinical status, what is the most likely reason for this patient's presentation to the ED?

a. Seizure
b. Cardiac tamponade
c. Carotid sinus sensitivity
d. Orthostatic hypotension
e. Carbon monoxide poisoning

277. A 58-year-old woman is brought in to the ED after a witnessed syncopal event. Upon arrival, the patient appears confused and agitated. Her vitals include a HR of 89 beats per minute, a BP of 145/70 mm Hg, a RR of 16 breaths per minute, and an O_2 saturation of 98% on room air. Within a few minutes, the patient is more alert and oriented. She denies any chest pain, headache, abdominal pain, or weakness preceding the event and is currently asymptomatic. She also states that she has not taken her antiepileptic medications in 2 days. The patient's exam is unremarkable including a nonfocal neurological exam. Given this patient's history and evolving examination, what is the most likely etiology of this patient's syncopal event?

a. Cerebrovascular accident
b. Transient ischemic attack
c. Seizure
d. Aortic dissection
e. Pulmonary embolus

278. A 53-year-old woman presents to the ED lethargic. She states that she has been a diabetic for many years and is compliant with her medications, which include an oral hypoglycemic agent. She also states that she was confused earlier in the day and may have taken too many of her diabetic pills but denies any other ingestions. Her vitals include a HR of 88 beats per minute, a BP of 135/70 mm Hg, and a RR of 18 breaths per minute with an O_2 saturation of 96% on room air. Her fingerstick glucose level is below normal. Her physical examination reveals a middle-aged woman that appears tachypneic and in mild distress. Upon auscultation, her chest is clear and she has normal bowel sounds. She is not tender to palpation and her neurological exam is nonfocal. A blood gas reveals a pH of 7.3 with normal CO levels and lowered bicarbonate level. A urinalysis is negative for ketones. What is the underlying mechanism for this patient's symptoms?

a. Diabetic ketoacidosis
b. Lactic acidosis
c. Respiratory alkalosis
d. Metabolic alkalosis
e. Uremia

Altered Mental Status

Answers

244. The answer is c. *(Rosen, pp 1748–1750.)* The patient never got a *fingerstick* at triage. *Hypoglycemia* can mimic a cerebrovascular accident or seizure. Therefore, it is critical that all patients who present with altered mental status get a fingerstick glucose. It should be considered a vital sign. Hypoglycemia is a common problem in patients with type 1 diabetes. The clinical presentation of hypoglycemia is caused by increased secretion of epinephrine and central nervous system (CNS) dysfunction. They include diaphoresis, nervousness, tremor, tachycardia, hunger, and neurologic symptoms ranging from confusion, bizarre behavior to seizures and coma.

(a) The patient's ECG is normal. The catherization lab is not indicated. (b) The stroke team should be activated in patients who present with signs and symptoms of a stroke that are not due to hypoglycemia. Therefore, these patients need a fingerstick glucose. (d) Saline and haloperidol are not indicated.

245. The answer is d. *(Tintinalli, p 1314.)* *Myxedema coma* is a life-threatening *complication of hypothyroidism.* Mortality in myxedema coma approaches 20–50% even with appropriate management. The patient exhibits classic signs and symptoms of the disease: lethargy or coma, hypothermia, bradycardia, periorbital and nonpitting edema, and delayed relaxation phase of deep tendon reflexes (areflexia in more severe cases). Myxedema coma can be triggered by sepsis, trauma, surgery, congestive heart failure, prolonged cold exposure, or use of sedatives or narcotics.

(a) The patient is actually hyperglycemic. Abnormal reflexes, hypothermia, and periorbital edema are inconsistent with the diagnosis of hypoglycemia as well as that of myocardial infarction (b). Stroke (c) should be on the differential in this case but the patient's signs and symptoms are more consistent with abnormal metabolic state than with purely neurovascular change. Depression (e) is an often forgotten diagnosis in the elderly and may present with a wide variety of signs and symptoms. Severe depression may appear as lethargy. It is unlikely, however, to have associated hypothermia and abnormal reflexes.

246. The answer is e. (*Roberts and Hedges, pp 19–24.*) Patients frequently present to the ED with agitation. It is important to discern what is causing their agitation; the range of etiologies is expansive from ethanol intoxication to intracerebral bleeding. The approach to the emergency patient always begins with the ABCs (*airway, breathing, and circulation*). In addition, the *vital signs* must be obtained early in a patient's assessment in order *to reveal potentially life-threatening conditions*. The patient in the vignette presents with agitation and tachycardia. Although it is tempting to attribute his agitation to his untreated schizophrenia, doing this without investigating medical causes of agitation can be disastrous. Finding out that the patient's temperature is 103.1°F will lead you down a different clinical path than if his temperature was 98°F. This patient was ultimately diagnosed with meningitis.

(**a**) Administering a medication to control agitation or psychotic behavior is appropriate even when there are coexistent medical problems. However, it is important to rule out potential life threats that may be causing the agitation. (**b**) A psychiatry consultation should be obtained once life-threatening conditions are excluded or in the case of the patient above, when he is stable and communicative as an inpatient. (**c and d**) A head CT and blood work will need to be obtained in this patient; however, all of the vital signs should be obtained first.

247. The answer is a. (*Tintinalli, p 1412.*) The initial approach to a seizing patient should involve protecting them from injury. Seizing patients should be immediately *placed in a lateral decubitus position to prevent aspiration of gastric contents*. Other initial measures are O_2, pulse oxymetry, glucose level determination, and an IV line.

Benzodiazepines (i.e., lorazepam) (**b**) are the first-line agents of an actively seizing patient. Benzodiazepines are sedative hypnotics which increase gamma-aminobutyric acid (GABA) activity. Phenytoin (**c**) is a second-line anticonvulsant in a continuously seizing patient. It requires a loading dose and has to be administered slowly because rapid administration may cause hypotension and cardiac dysrhythmias. Rapid sequence intubation (RSI) (**d**) should not be performed at this time. The patient's pulse oximetry is 92% on room air and can be improved by supplemental O_2 and a nasopharyngeal airway if necessary. RSI should be done if the patient becomes apneic or his O_2 saturation drops despite O_2 supplementation. (**e**) Once the acute seizure is controlled, levels of the patient's anticonvulsant medications should be checked and supplemented if subtherapeutic.

248. The answer is d. (*Hamilton, p 5.*) The first question an emergency physician asks for each patient is whether a life-threatening process is causing the patient's complaint. Emergency medicine is primarily a complaint-oriented rather than disease-oriented specialty. Its emphasis rests on anticipating and recognizing a life-threatening process, rather than seeking the diagnosis. The goal is to think about and plan to prevent the life-threatening things from happening or progressing in the patient. The patient in the vignette may have meningitis, a life-threatening condition, or a viral syndrome with dehydration. *The initial approach is stabilization and treatment or prevention of a life-threatening process.* This patient requires fluid resuscitation for her BP, altered mental status, and delayed capillary refill. Antibiotics should be started immediately and a lumbar puncture performed once increased intracranial pressure is evaluated by fundoscopic exam or CT scan. She should be placed in isolation. Her disposition is directed by her response to initial resuscitation and results of the LP.

(a) It is important to collect blood cultures, however initial stabilization and treatment is priority. **(b)** The patient's parents should be contacted if the patient cannot do it herself, but treatment should proceed in the mean time. **(c)** Gathering more information is invaluable; however, this should be done after initial stabilization and treatment. **(e)** Observation in a patient with a life-threatening condition is not recommended.

249. The answer is e. (*Tintinalli, p 1288.*) This patient presents with an anion gap metabolic acidosis, glucosuria, and ketonuria, which is consistent with *diabetic ketoacidosis (DKA)*. DKA is an acute, life threatening disorder occurring in patients with insulin insufficiency. It results in hyperglycemia, ketosis and osmotic diuresis and clinically presents with gastrointestinal (GI) distress, polyuria, fatigue, dehydration, mental confusion, lethargy, or coma. When the diagnosis of DKA is clinically suspected and hyperglycemia is confirmed by elevated fingerstick glucose, the results of a blood gas and urinalysis confirm the diagnosis. In DKA the liver metabolizes free fatty acids into ketone bodies for alternative fuel in the setting of cellular glucose underutilization. The result is *ketonuria* and *anion gap metabolic acidosis.* *Glucosuria*, the result of hyperglycemia-related osmotic diuresis, is another manifestation of DKA.

The anion gap is calculated by subtracting Cl^-, and HCO_3^- from Na^+.

$$Anion\ gap\ (AG) = [Na^+] - ([Cl^-] + [HCO_3^-])$$

A normal anion gap is 8–12 mEq/L. An elevated gap is due to an increased concentration of unmeasured anions. In DKA, the elevated anion gap is due to the production of ketones.

Other answers (a, b, c, and d) are incorrect choices in the DKA presentation.

250. The answer is d. (*Rosen, pp 1748–1750.*) In a patient who is *actively seizing*, it is essential to check the *blood glucose* level. *Hypoglycemia* is an easily *reversible* cause of seizure and is corrected with the administration of *dextrose*, not the usual anticonvulsants. Patients at both extremes of age are particularly susceptible to glucose stress during acute illness.

If the blood glucose level is normal then requesting a rectal temperature (a) is appropriate. However, this should be done concomitantly with addressing airway protection, gaining IV access and administering, and anticonvulsant. A CT scan (b) may be necessary in a seizure patient; however, this should occur once the patient is stabilized. An ECG and aspirin (c) is usually the initial management for patients with chest pain. In an actively seizing patient, nothing should be administered by mouth because there is an increased risk for aspiration and the patient may not have a gag reflex. Intubating (e) the patient may be necessary if the patient is not protecting his or her airway or is in status epilepticus. In the above patient, her O_2 saturation is 96%.

251. The answer is a. (*Tintinalli, pp 103–104.*) A *nasal airway* is made of a pliable material that allows it to be placed into the nostril of a somnolent patient with an *intact gag reflex*. The nasal airway is an excellent device that can be placed in a patient who may have decreased pharyngeal muscle tone and an obstructing soft palate and tongue. It allows air to bypass such obstructions. The patient in the vignette is intoxicated and appears to have episodes of transient obstruction.

(b) An oral airway is a rigid instrument that is used to prevent the base of the tongue from occluding the hypopharynx. It should be used to maintain the airway only in a patient with an absent gag reflex. (c) Bag-valve mask ventilation is typically used to oxygenate a patient in preparation for a definitive airway such as orotracheal intubation. (d and e) Tracheoesophageal and laryngeal mask airways are devices typically used in the ED as rescue devices in failed intubation or in the prehospital setting when orotracheal intubation is not a viable option. These devices are designed to be placed in apneic, unconscious patients.

252. The answer is a. (*Tintinalli, p 1307.*) Profound hyperglycemia, absence of ketonuria, and diabetes medication noncompliance should raise your suspicion for *nonketotic hyperosmolar crisis (NKHC)* in this patient. This condition is a syndrome of hyperglycemia without ketoacidosis as small amounts of insulin protect against adipose tissue metabolism. This syndrome is more common in type 2 diabetics. Causes of NKHC are similar to those of DKA and include *diabetes medication noncompliance, infection, stroke, and myocardial infarction.* Patients are profoundly dehydrated due to osmotic diuresis. The mainstay of NKHC therapy consists of *replacing fluid losses.* Electrolyte deficiencies should be replaced and insulin administered. Fluid deficit in NKHC is significant and needs to be slowly corrected, as rapid correction may lead to cerebral edema. Insulin requirements in NKHC are usually less than in DKA.

Further diagnostic tests are important to obtain depending on the patients presentation and suspicion of an underlying etiology of NKHC. In this case, medication noncompliance is most likely. In other cases, head CT for workup of intracranial pathology (**b**), ECG for evaluation of myocardial infarction (**c**), or chest radiograph and urine culture for infectious etiology workup (**d**) might be necessary. Broad coverage antibiotics (**e**) are not necessary in this patient.

253. The answer is b. (*Tintinalli, p 1283.*) This is a case of *hypoglycemia* due to *oral hypoglycemic medication overdose.* Diabetic oral agents that cause hypoglycemia work by increasing pancreatic insulin secretion. This group includes sulfonylureas (glyburide, glipizide) and nonsulfonylurea secretagogues (repaglinide, nateglinide). Other common causes of hypoglycemia are insulin overdose, alcohol abuse (inhibition of gluconeogenesis) and sepsis. The presentation of a hypoglycemic patient generally involves signs and symptoms of CNS dysfunction due to the release of counterregulatory hormones secondary to the unavailability of glucose. These include anxiety, diaphoresis, palpitations, and confusion. Don't be fooled by improved blood glucose levels after dextrose administration in overdose with oral hypoglycemic agents. *Hypoglycemia can last more than 24 hours due to long-lasting pancreatic effects* and will recur after dextrose infusion. Patients need to be observed in the hospital with frequent bedside glucose checks. They can be placed on a dextrose drip. Octreotide, an inhibitor of insulin release can also be administered.

Choice (**a**) is inappropriate since hypoglycemia will recur after administration of a single bolus of dextrose. Intravenous fluids and insulin (**c**) are treatments for hyperglycemia. IV fluid without dextrose (**d**) is not helpful in hypoglycemia management. Activated charcoal administration (**e**) is recommended within an hour after certain toxic ingestions or when there may be a coingestion of an unknown toxin.

254. The answer is b. (*Rosen, p 1260.*) The patient has *hepatic encephalopathy*, which is a clinical state of disordered cerebral function occurring secondary to acute or chronic liver disease. Laboratory tests may be normal in patients, but the *serum ammonia level is usually elevated. Lactulose and neomycin* represent the main therapeutic agents. Lactulose is a poorly absorbed sugar metabolized by colonic bacteria that traps ammonia and helps excrete it in the stool. Neomycin is a poorly absorbed aminoglycoside that is believed to act by reducing colonic bacteria that are responsible for producing ammonia.

255. The answer is b. (*Rosen, pp 1445–1455.*) Generally, the *first-line* pharmacologic treatment in an actively seizing patient is a parental *benzodiazepine* such as diazepam (Valium), lorazepam (Ativan), or midazolam (Versed). Benzodiazepines are effective in terminating ictal activity in 75–90% of patients. Diazepam can be administered intravenously, intramuscularly, or down an endotracheal tube. Lorazepam and midazolam can be given intravenously or intramuscularly. All three have similar efficacy in terminating seizures.

Phenytoin (**a**) is a second-line agent that can be administered intravenously. Although the cause of the patient's seizure may be due to subtherapeutic levels of phenytoin, benzodiazepines are still the first-line therapy due to their rapid onset. The onset of diazepam is 2–5 minutes while phenytoin's is 10–30 minutes. In addition, phenytoin requires at least 20 minutes for administration due to its potential to cause hypotension and cardiac dysrhythmias. Phenobarbital (**c**) is a third-line agent. Its onset of action is 15–30 minutes. Valproic acid (**d**) is rarely used in the acute seizure setting. There is no role for lithium (**e**) in acute seizure management.

256. The answer is a. (*Rosen, pp 2421–2424.*) This patient has *postpartum eclampsia*, which needs to be managed with *magnesium sulfate* and admission to the obstetrical service. Preeclampsia is defined as new-onset hypertension (>140/90 mm Hg) and proteinuria (1 g/L in random specimen or > 3 g/L over 24 hours). Some clinicians also use generalized edema as a requirement. Preeclampsia is most common in the third trimester. Eclampsia occurs with the development of seizures or coma in a patient with preeclampsia. A preeclamptic woman may worsen after delivery and develop late postpartum eclampsia, which usually occurs in the first 24–48 hours postpartum but may present several weeks after delivery. Management of eclamptic seizures in the ED involves administering magnesium sulfate, which is believed to act as a membrane stabilizer and vasodilator, reducing cerebral ischemia. Although magnesium sulfate is not a direct antihypertensive, the hypertension associated with eclampsia is often controlled adequately by treating the seizure.

(b) Treating the seizure will most likely also lower the patient's BP. Less than 10% of eclamptic patients require specific antihypertensive therapy. **(c)** This is the treatment for migraines, which this patient does not have. **(d & e)** This patient's seizure is secondary to eclampsia. The first-line treatment is with magnesium sulfate. If the seizure is not treated despite appropriate magnesium sulfate then a benzodiazepine can be administered and etiologies of seizure should be sought other than eclampsia.

257. The answer is b. *(Rosen, p 290.)* The patient has a triad of *hypertension, bradycardia,* and *respiratory depression,* which is called *Cushing reflex.* This is observed in a third of patients with a potentially lethal *increase in intracranial pressure (ICP).* Increased ICP may result from traumatic brain injury or, as in this patient's case, from hemorrhagic stroke and subsequent brain edema. Tobacco and cocaine use are known risk factors for hemorrhagic stroke. Increasing ICP can result in cerebral herniation, which has a mortality rate close to 100%. For any chance of survival, it must be rapidly controlled by intubation, elevation of the head of the bed, hyperventilation, mannitol, and definitive neurosurgical intervention.

Cushing syndrome **(a)** describes the hyperadrenal state associated with increased production of cortisol, leading to hypertension, truncal obesity, abdominal striae, and hirsutism. Cullen's sign **(c)** is purplish discoloration around the umbilicus that results from intraperitoneal hemorrhage. Charcot's triad **(d)** constitutes fever, right upper quadrant (RUQ) pain, and jaundice and is associated with cholangitis. Chvostek's sign **(e)**, associated with hypocalcemia, is twitching of the nose or lips with tapping of the facial nerve.

258. The answer is b. *(Rosen, p 596.)* Although anterior shoulder dislocations are more common, *posterior shoulder dislocations* are classically associated with generalized tonic-clonic seizures. Other causes include electrocution and falling on an outstretched arm. During a sudden muscle contraction seen with seizures, the stronger internal rotator muscles cause a posterior humeral head dislocation. In posterior shoulder dislocations the arm is generally held *adducted and internally rotated,* as opposed to an abducted and externally rotated arm position in anterior shoulder dislocations.

(a) Anterior shoulder dislocations do occur in patients with seizures. In this particular case, the patient's arm is held in adduction and is internally rotated, which is more consistent with a posterior shoulder dislocation. (b & d) Humeral and clavicular fractures are not commonly seen after a seizure. Todd's paralysis (e) is a transient focal neurological deficit persisting after a seizure.

259. The answer is c. *(Tintinalli, p 1415.)* This patient presents with *alcohol withdrawal.* Signs and symptoms of this condition occur along a continuum ranging from simple shakes to delirium tremens following a reduction or cessation of alcohol. Early symptoms usually appear 6–8 hours after cessation of drinking and involve tremulousness, anxiety, mild hypertension, and tachycardia. In more severe withdrawal, these symptoms worsen and paranoia, auditory, and visual hallucinations may develop proceeding to delirium tremens (DTs) with severe autonomic hyperactivity and profound altered mental status. DTs usually occur 3–5 days after alcohol cessation and carries 5–15% mortality even with supportive care. Additionally, alcohol withdrawal seizures may occur anywhere from 6 to 48 hours after cessation of alcohol. *Benzodiazepines* are the mainstay of therapy in alcohol withdrawal as well as in sympathomimetic overdose and sedative-hypnotic withdrawal.

Acetaminophen (a) and labetalol (e) would treat the symptoms of low-grade fever and hypertension/tachycardia, respectively, without addressing the underlying etiology. Folate (b) should be given to all potentially undernourished patients, especially alcoholics, to prevent folate-deficient anemia. Dextrose was just administered by EMS without symptom improvement; however, fingerstick glucose levels are important to check in all patients with altered mental status.

260. The answer is e. *(Rosen, pp 1748–1749.)* Symptomatic *hypoglycemia* occurs in most adults at a blood glucose level of 40–50 mg/dL. Hypoglycemia is a common problem in patients with type 1 diabetes. Patients who are very young or very old are also at risk. Signs and symptoms of hypoglycemia are caused by CNS dysfunction and excessive secretion of epinephrine. Neurologic symptoms include bizarre behavior, confusion, seizures, and coma. Patients also exhibit sweating, tremor, tachycardia, and nervousness. Fingerstick glucose should be considered a vital sign and is required on all altered patients. Management of these patients includes administering one to three ampules (25–75 g) of 50% dextrose in water intravenously while you address the ABCs. Most patients normalize immediately after administration of glucose. **(a)** This would be correct if you suspected meningitis. **(b)** This is a good regimen for patients with chest pain and suspicion for cardiac ischemia, which is unlikely in this patient. **(c)** If the patient doesn't improve after administration of glucose, then an emergent CT scan is needed to diagnose a possible stroke. Symptoms of hypoglycemia can mimic symptoms of an acute stroke; therefore it is necessary to obtain blood glucose levels early in the workup of the patient. **(d)** If the patient was more alert, giving a glass of orange juice is appropriate. However, in this patient there is an increased risk of aspiration because he is altered.

261. The answer is e. *(Rosen, pp 1161–1162.)* The patient has *hypertensive encephalopathy*, which is defined by a rapid *rise in BP* that is accompanied by *neurologic changes.* Patients typically present with a systolic BP > 220 mm Hg and diastolic BP > 110 mm Hg. Neurologic findings include severe headache, vomiting, drowsiness, confusion, seizure, blindness, focal neurologic deficits, or coma. Hypertensive emergency is a medical emergency. The goal is to *carefully reduce the BP* avoided dropping the pressure too low or too rapidly as this may lead to cerebral ischemia. The immediate goal is to reduce the mean arterial BP by 25%. This can be accomplished by *labetolol,* a β_1- and β_2-receptor blocker and α_1-receptor blocker. Another useful medication is nitroprusside.

(a and b) Intubation and hyperventilation and mannitol are used in the acute setting to lower intracranial pressure if there are signs of herniation, such as a unilateral dilated pupil. **(c)** Diuretics are not useful to acutely lower BP, but may be started as a maintenance antihypertensive. **(d)** Lowering the BP to 120/40 mm Hg can cause cerebral ischemia. The mean arterial pressure should only be lowered by 25% in the first hour.

262. The answer is b. *(Rosen, pp 1527–1538.)* The CSF analysis in *bacterial meningitis* typically shows an *elevated white blood cell count* with predominant *polymorphonuclear leukocytes. Protein is elevated and glucose is low.* A Gram stain may show bacteria. The most specific marker for the diagnosis is a positive culture.

(a) The CSF in a subarachnoid hemorrhage is grossly bloody. However, the blood count should be analyzed on the first and last tubes to avoid a false positive from a bloody tap. **(c)** In viral meningitis, the cerebrospinal fluid (CSF) white cell count is made up of lymphocytes or monocytes, but early in the disease polys may predominate. CSF glucose is normal and protein is elevated in viral meningitis. A Gram stain will be negative and culture will show no growth. (**d**) The CSF in multiple sclerosis (MS) may have a mild lymphocytosis with an increased protein concentration. CSF protein electrophoresis in MS shows discrete bands of immunoglobulin G (IgG) called oligoclonal bands. (**e**) Encephalitis is diagnosed by CSF culture or serology. CSF analysis may reveal blood.

263. The answer is c. *(Tintinalli, pp 169–171.) Hyponatremia* is defined as a measured serum sodium less than 135 mEq/L. However, the development of symptoms secondary to hyponatremia is related more to the rate of change in the serum sodium than to the absolute value. Levels less than 120 mEq/L tend to cause symptoms regardless of the rate to reach this value. Symptoms can include confusion, lethargy, nausea, vomiting, anorexia, muscle cramps, and seizures. There are many causes of hyponatremia including renal or GI losses, third-spacing, endocrine abnormalities, syndrome of inappropriate antidiuretic hormone release (SIADH), cirrhosis, CHF, and nephrotic syndrome. Many medications cause SIADH, in addition to pulmonary and CNS disease. This patient, in particular, just started chemotherapy for lung cancer. The treatment for hyponatremia is guided by the cause of the process. However, if a patient is symptomatic (i.e., seizing), *hypertonic saline (3%)* should be carefully administered to raise the serum sodium to 120 mEq/L.

(**a and b**) 0.45% and 0.9% do not provide adequate amounts of sodium to raise the serum level and can actually cause a drop in serum sodium in certain conditions. (**d and e**) Dextrose is the treatment of choice for hypoglycemic patients.

264. The answer is c. *(Tintinalli, p 1046.) Neuroleptic malignant syndrome (NMS)* is a rare, but potentially fatal reaction commonly associated with the use of *antipsychotic drugs.* The classic triad for its clinical presentation includes *altered mental status, hyperthermia, and muscle rigidity.* The cornerstone of treatment is supportive care with rapid cooling, fluid and electrolyte repletion, and monitoring. *Dantrolene,* a nonspecific skeletal muscle relaxant, generally used in the treatment of malignant hyperthermia, is also effective for NMS. In addition, benzodiazepines are useful in the treatment of NMS.

(**a and b**) These are both antipsychotic medications that can worsen the symptoms of NMS and should not be administered. (**c**) Doxycycline is an antibiotic that is not useful in this situation. (**e**) Acetaminophen, an antipyretic, may help with lowering the temperature. However, NMS is a centrally mediated process. External cooling is more effective.

265. The answer is a. *(Tintinalli, p 1015.)* This patient exhibits the classic triad of *Wernicke's encephalopathy (WE): confusion, ataxia and ophthalmoplegia.* WE is a result of *thiamine deficiency* leading to decreased glucose metabolism and neuronal destruction, primarily in the cerebellum, hypothalamus, vestibular system and memory. It is typically found in *chronic alcoholics* due to nutritional deficiency, but can also occur in other malnutrition states, pregnancy, persistent vomiting or dialysis. WE can mimic acute stroke symptoms and can lead to permanent nystagmus and ataxia. It carries 10–20% mortality if untreated.

Eye exam findings in WE include horizontal nystagmus, vertical gaze palsy or CN VII palsy. Cerebellar destruction presents with ataxic, wide-based gait. WE is a clinical diagnosis. Thiamine deficiency can also lead to the development of high-output cardiac failure and Korsakoff syndrome. The treatment is parenteral thiamine supplementation.

Korsakoff syndrome **(b)** is another sign of thiamine deficiency and involves disorientation and confabulation. Normal pressure hydrocephalus **(c)** presents with dementia, ataxic gait and urinary incontinence. Head CT shows large ventricles. Alcohol intoxication **(d)** may cause ataxia and apparent confusion, but is unlikely to produce nystagmus. Alcohol withdrawal **(e)** typically presents with sympathetic and CNS overactivity.

266. The answer is b. *(Tintinalli, p 1113.)* The patient has *cocaine-induced autonomic and CNS hyperactivity* causing agitation, paranoia, and hyperadrenergic state. More severe CNS manifestations of cocaine poisoning include hyperthermia, intracranial hemorrhage, seizures, spinal cord infarctions and acute dystonic reactions. The CNS effects of cocaine are managed with *benzodiazepines,* which decrease sympathetic tone and prevent hyperthermia and seizures.

Metoprolol **(a)**, a β-adrenergic receptor blocker, decreases HR and BP. In this case, however, metoprolol administration does not address the underlying cause of the adrenergic hyperactivity. More importantly, β-adrenergic receptor blockade in cocaine poisoning leaves unopposed stimulated α-adrenergic receptors, thus worsening vasoconstriction. Therefore, β-receptor blocker use in cocaine poisoning is contraindicated. Fever or hyperthermia in cocaine poisoning is due to hypothalamic stimulation and not due to inflammatory mediators. Hyperthermia should be treated with cooling methods such as cool mist spray or ice-bath immersion. Acetaminophen **(c)** is not helpful in this situation. Rapid sequence intubation **(d)** is not appropriate at this time. In any poisoned patient airway is to be assessed and managed first, but this patient does not exhibit any signs of respiratory compromise. Drug abuse specialists (e) should be consulted when the patient is medically cleared.

267. The answer is c. (*Tintinalli, p 1046.*) The patient presents with a rare but potentially life-threatening NMS. *Antipsychotic drugs (i.e., haloperidol)* are the most common offending agents in the development of NMS, causing *central dopamine depletion*. The disorder is typically characterized by *hyperthermia, muscle rigidity, altered mental status,* and *autonomic instability*. Since NMS carries a high mortality, it is important to aggressively treat it with muscle relaxers, such as IV benzodiazepines, dantrolene, and dopamine agonists.

Urinary tract infection (a) in a debilitated or nursing home patient can easily lead to altered mental status and sepsis. The patient's muscular rigidity, however, does not fit this diagnosis. The presentation of malignant hyperthermia (b) is similar to NMS, also involving hyperthermia and muscle rigidity. It is caused by anesthetic agents, which this patient did not receive. Dantrolene is also used for muscle relaxation in malignant hyperthermia. Recurrent stroke (d) is unlikely in this presentation with hyperthermia and muscle rigidity. Right-sided motor findings on exam are residual deficits from the old stroke. Meningoencephalitis (e) is certainly high on the differential in this patient but is unlikely to cause generalized muscular rigidity. It typically presents with fever, headache, nuchal rigidity, altered mental status, and focal neurologic signs.

268. The answer is e. (*Tintinalli, p 1378.*) The most likely diagnosis in this patient is a *space-occupying lesion* in the *frontal lobe of the brain*. Brain tumors can present with *morning headaches associated with nausea and vomiting.* Neurologic exam is normal in most patients. Papilledema might provide an important clue of increased intracranial pressure and the presence of a brain mass. Frontal lobe tumors typically involve *personality changes* as seen in this patient.

Depression (a) is characterized by pervasive sad mood or loss of interest in usual activities for at least 2 weeks which this patient does not exhibit. The diagnosis of depression in the elderly population may involve atypical complaints of generalized pain, headaches or lethargy and may not be recognized in the ED. Persistent morning headaches and personality changes in this case are inconsistent with the diagnosis of tension headache (b). Tension headache is described as bilateral pressure-like pain, not worsened with activity and associated with stress. Headaches in patients over 50 years of age are unusual and should be taken seriously and well evaluated. Subarachnoid hemorrhage (c) typically presents with severe headache of acute onset, classically described as "the worst headache of my life," with associated nausea and vomiting. Pseudotumor cerebri (**d**) or benign intracranial hypertension is a disorder seen in young obese females complaining of chronic headaches.

269. The answer is b. (*Tintinalli, p 1413.*) This patient is obtunded due to the *postictal state,* which is a *transient neurological deficit following a seizure.* Postictal deficits may include altered mental status, blindness or focal motor weakness (i.e., Todd's paralysis). The symptoms usually resolve spontaneously within an hour after seizure and definitely should resolve within 48 hours. As long as their postictal deficits are improving, patients should be observed through this period. Routine labs should be sent to check sodium, glucose, calcium, and creatinine levels in a patient with new-onset seizure, but in this case of an epileptic patient with a break-through seizure, only a blood anticonvulsant level is helpful.

Rapid sequence intubation (**a**) is not necessary in this patient. She is oxygenating and ventilating well based on her vital signs. Intravenous lorazepam (**c**) is a good choice for treating actively seizing patients. The patient in the case, however, is recovering from a seizure or is postictal and benzodiazepines at this time are unnecessary. Head CT (**d**) should be obtained in patients with a new-onset seizure, change in seizure pattern, history of head trauma leading to or causing a seizure, and those not recovering appropriately in the postictal period. In a patient with known epilepsy with a single seizure, head CT is unnecessary. Lumbar puncture (**e**) should be obtained in any patient with a suspected CNS infection.

270. The answer is c. (*Tintinalli, p 600.*) This patient presents with altered mental status in the setting of renal failure and missed hemodialysis. The most immediate threat in this case is *hyperkalemia* due to decreased potassium excretion in renal failure. The potassium level must be rapidly determined and aggressively managed with agents that stabilize the myocardium (calcium gluconate or calcium chloride), shift potassium to the intracellular space (insulin/glucose, sodium bicarbonate, albuterol) and promote GI excretion of potassium (Kayexalate).

Uremic encephalopathy (**a**) is a possible cause of this patient's altered mental status. Uremic encephalopathy improves with dialysis but can lead to coma and death if not addressed. Normochromic normocytic anemia (**b**) in renal failure patients is a common chronic problem in part due to decreased erythropoietin production by the kidneys. Hypocalcemia (**d**) in renal failure develops secondary to low calcitriol levels, which is produced by the kidneys, leading to decreased intestinal calcium absorption. It is chronically managed by calcium and calcitriol supplementation. The state of total-body fluid overload (**e**) develops secondary to poor sodium and free water excretion in renal failure. It is controlled by proper dialysis or additional use of loop diuretics.

271. The answer is d. (*Tintinalli, p 678.*) One more piece of evidence, *proteinuria* on *urinalysis,* is required for the diagnosis of *eclampsia* in this previously healthy postpartum patient with peripheral edema, hypertension and a new-onset seizure. Preeclampsia (hypertension, proteinuria, peripheral edema) and eclampsia complicate 5–10% of pregnancies and occur most commonly in the *third trimester* but may persist or *present up to 3 weeks postpartum.* The patient needs to be admitted and treated with magnesium sulfate and antihypertensive medications.

A complete blood count (**a**) and lumbar puncture (**c**) are helpful if there is concern for an infectious etiology of the seizure, such as meningitis. The patient, however, is afebrile and has no complains of headache, meningismus, or altered mentation. Obtaining a head CT (**b**) should be considered to exclude structural causes of a new-onset seizure. ECG (**e**) is likely to be normal and noncontributory in this case.

272. The answer is e. (*Tintinalli, p 1346.*) This patient presents with four of the five symptoms classically associated with *TTP.* These include *thrombocytopenia, hemolytic anemia, neurologic deficits, renal impairment, and fever.* TTP develops with fibrin-strand deposition in small vessels that attract platelets leading to platelet thrombi and thrombocytopenia. Passing RBCs get sheared in occluded vessels resulting in microangiopathic hemolytic anemia. Renal and neurologic impairment occur due to the lodging of thrombi in respective circulations. Plasmaphoresis decreases TTP mortality from 90% to 10%. Adjunct therapies include fresh frozen plasma infusion and steroids. It is important to realize that although patients may be severely thrombocytopenic, platelet infusion is contraindicated since it exacerbates the underlying cycle of thrombogenesis. Risk factors for TTP include pregnancy, autoimmune disorders, drugs, infection, and malignancy. Hemolytic-uremic syndrome (HUS) is a closely related entity usually seen in children. There is pronounced renal dysfunction without altered mentation.

Henoch-Schönlein Purpura (HSP) (**a**) is a small-vessel vasculitis mostly seen in children and associated with a preceding upper respiratory illness in about 50% of patients. It is characterized by purpura, usually lower extremities, abdominal pain, and hematuria. Disseminated intravascular coagulation (DIC) (**b**) is a coagulopathic state triggered by major trauma, infection, malignancy, drugs, or pregnancy complications. The underlying process activates the coagulation cascade which leads to diffuse thrombosis and coagulopathy as platelets and coagulation factors are consumed. Patients with DIC have profuse GI or puncture site bleeding, markedly prolonged PT/PTT times, thrombocytopenia and elevated fibrin split products. DIC management involves treatment of the underlying disorder and replacement of depleted coagulation cascade components. Von Willebrand disease (**c**) is the most common bleeding disorder and involves deficiency or defect in von Willebrand factor, which normally aids in platelet adherence and carries factor VIII in plasma. Von Willebrand disease presents clinically with GI bleeding, epistaxis, easy bruising, and prolonged bleeding. Idiopathic thrombocytopenic purpura (ITP) (**d**) is a disorder of antibody-mediated platelet destruction. It is acute in children, usually following a viral infection, and is chronic in adults who often require splenectomy for definitive treatment.

273. The answer is a. (*Tintinalli, p 397.*) This patient presents with headache and altered mental status in the setting of severe hypertension leading to the diagnosis of *hypertensive encephalopathy*. A hypertensive emergency is defined by severe hypertension with evidence of organ dysfunction. The BP needs to be aggressively, but carefully lowered to prevent cerebral bleeding and progression to coma and death. Patients also can present with seizures, focal neurological deficits, visual acuity changes or coma. Patients with hypertensive encephalopathy are managed with *short-acting titratable IV antihypertensive medications* such as IV *nitroprusside* or labetalol. The BP should not be significantly lowered since it can result in brain hypoperfusion and infarction. Typically, the mean arterial pressure (MAP) is lowered by 20–25% in the first hour of treatment.

Magnesium sulfate (**b**) is used in the management of hypertension and seizures in eclampsia. It is not useful in other hypertensive emergency situations. Metoprolol (**c**) is a useful agent for hypertension but is not helpful in situations requiring rapid and precise BP control. Hydrochlorothiazide (**d**) is a good agent for chronic hypertension control. It does not offer rapid and precise BP control required in this case. Obtaining a head CT (**e**) should be considered in this patient since intracranial hemorrhage and brain tumor are in the differential diagnosis.

274. The answer is e. (*Tintinalli, p 359.*) All of the choices above are etiologies of syncope. Situational syncope, however, is the least likely culprit in the patient having a syncopal episode while walking. Situational and vasovagal syncope are types of reflex-mediated syncopal episodes. Cerebral hypoperfusion in situational syncope is a result of an abnormal automatic reflex response to a physical stimulus. Triggers of the abnormal response include coughing, swallowing, defecation, and micturition.

275. The answer is e. (*Tintinalli, p 1409.*) This is a *complex partial seizure*, also known as temporal seizure; although it does not necessarily originate in temporal lobe. It is characterized by *focal electrical discharges* (partial seizure), such as clonic leg activity, and *alteration of consciousness*.

Petit mal seizures (**a**), also known as absence seizures, involve sudden brief loss of consciousness without the loss of postural tone. Patients appear detached or withdrawn and do not respond to stimulation. The seizures might be frequent and classically occur in children. A generalized tonic-clonic seizure (**b**) involves both hemispheres and loss of consciousness (generalized component) and clonic activity of the extremities. Partial seizure with secondary generalization (**c**) starts with focal abnormal activity which spreads to involve bilateral cortex and mimics a generalized seizure. A simple partial seizure (**d**) is focal abnormal activity and intact consciousness.

276. The answer is e. (*Rosen, pp 172–178.*) It is difficult to obtain an adequate depiction of what occurred in this patient, given that there were no direct witnesses. There are details in the history, however, that lend to the diagnosis. This mainly includes the similar but milder symptoms seen in the roommate, which explains the event to be of a more environmental nature. A simple cooximetry panel measuring both O_2 and *CO* levels may be drawn. Patients with CO poisoning may have headache, general malaise, nausea, vomiting, seizures, or present unresponsive. Given that this patient was initially unresponsive, he warrants a more extensive workup and possible transfer to a hyperbaric oxygen unit to decrease his CO levels.

Seizure (**a**) is a possibility given that there were no witnesses to this patient's syncopal event; however, a quick blood gas may help delineate the etiology before further testing is taken. This patient's vitals put cardiac tamponade (**b**) lower on the differential. Patients in tamponade usually present with muffled or distant heart sounds, hypotension and jugular venous distention due to right ventricular collapse. Carotid sinus sensitivity (**c**), also known as necktie or shaving syncope, occurs when there is an external force or pressure applied to the carotid sinus producing a vagal stimulation. This stimulation reduces HR and lowers BP causing a hypotensive response that lifts when the force is no longer applied. The nature in which this patient was found renders this diagnosis unlikely. Orthostatic hypotension (**d**) is an entity that occurs when not enough blood flow is perfusing the brain, whether it be hypovolemic or postural in nature. Orthostatic vital signs include a BP drop of ≥ 20 mm Hg upon standing for 1 minute with a pulse rise of 30 beats per minute or greater. These measurements should be taken lying supine, sitting, and then standing.

277. The answer is c. *(Rosen, pp 172–178.)* The emergency medicine physician is often faced with differentiating whether the cause of a patient losing consciousness is due to syncope or a *seizure*. The most likely etiology of this patient's symptoms is in the history that she gives. She tells you that she has *not taken her antiseizure medications* in 2 days. Also given her evolving mental status and improvement in alertness, this patient most likely presented in a postictal state after she has seized. Without any focal deficit and further improvement in her mental status, one might be comfortable with this diagnosis. Serum testing of her antiepileptic drug levels must be performed to further investigate this suspicion. A CT of the head, ECG and further investigation is warranted if these levels are normal and do not explain her loss of consciousness.

Other neurological causes such as a cerebral vascular accident (CVA) **(a)** and transient ischemic attack (TIA) **(b)** should also be in the differential. Typical TIA symptoms include any neurological symptom which improves within 30 minutes. In this case, however, her history and presentation most likely precludes this diagnosis. The possibility of her having a stroke is further diminished by her normal neurological exam. This patient did not complain of any chest or abdominal symptoms **(d and e)**, which place aortic dissection and pulmonary embolus further down on the differential list.

278. The answer is b. *(Rosen, pp 1714–1723.)* This patient is on an oral hypoglycemic agent, most likely a biguanide, which causes a *lactic acidosis* if taken in excessive amounts. The mechanism of toxicity includes an increased sensitivity to insulin and a suppression of gluconeogenesis, creating an acidotic state. The symptoms seen in this clinical presentation are early, but may progress to delirium, coma, or a focal neurologic deficit. A lactic acidosis is typically seen in these types of ingestions. Treatment includes glucose monitoring as severe hypoglycemia may occur, charcoal, and admittance to the hospital as effects may typically be exhibited over the course of 24 hours.

DKA **(a)** is ruled out with a lower glucose level and lack of ketones in the urine. Given the pH, this patient does not have an alkalosis **(c and d)**. She also does not have a history of renal failure or symptoms of uremia **(e)**.

Headache

Questions

279. A 21-year-old college student is brought by her roommate to the emergency department (ED). The roommate states that earlier in the day the patient complained of a severe headache, stiff neck, and photophobia. On their way to the ED, the roommate states that the patient was confused. Her vital signs are blood pressure (BP) 110/80 mm Hg, heart rate (HR) 110 beats per minutes, respiration rate (RR) 16 breaths per minute, and temperature 102°F. What is the next step in the management of this patient?

a. Start empiric antibiotics, noncontrast head CT prior to performing lumbar puncture (LP)
b. Order a noncontrast head CT and start antibiotics once the results are back
c. Give 1 g of acetaminophen, start fluid hydration, and perform an LP
d. Perform an LP and start antibiotics once the results are back
e. Order a noncontrast head computed tomography (CT), perform an LP, then start antibiotics

280. A 29-year-old woman presents to the ED complaining of a generalized headache over the last 2 months. She has seen many doctors for it but has yet to get a correct diagnosis. She describes the headache as moderate in intensity and worse with eye movement. Occasionally, it awakes her from sleep and is worse when tying her shoes. She is scared because her vision gets blurry for a few minutes everyday. Her only medication is acetaminophen and an oral contraceptive. Her BP is 140/75 mm Hg, HR is 75 beats per minute, temperature is 98.9°F, and RR is 16 breaths per minute. On physical exam you appreciate papilledema. Which of the following is the most appropriate next step in management?

a. Call a neurosurgeon for immediate surgery
b. Administer 2 g of ceftriaxone, and place her in isolation
c. Order an magnetic resonance imaging (MRI) to look for a carotid artery dissection
d. Tell her she probably has a migraine and prescribe her a triptan
e. Perform a CT scan and if negative perform an LP specifically to measure the opening pressure

281. A 67-year-old woman presents to the ED complaining of a 2-day history of general malaise, subjective fevers, chills, diffuse headache, and right-sided jaw pain. Her symptoms are minimally relieved with acetaminophen. She denies any sick contacts. The patient's vitals include an oral temperature of 100.6°F, HR is 95 beats per minute, BP is 130/75 mm Hg, and RR is 16 breaths per minute with O_2 saturation of 99% on room air. After a complete history and physical examination, what is the diagnostic test of choice?

a. Influenza A/B assay
b. Rapid strep test
c. Erythrocyte sedimentation rate (ESR)
d. Complete blood count
e. Temporal artery biopsy

282. A 25-year-old stockbroker presents to the ED complaining of 6 weeks of daily headaches. Her headaches are band-like in distribution and are not associated with nausea, vomiting, visual phenomena, or neurologic symptoms. Normally they respond to acetaminophen, but they have increased in frequency in the past week as she stopped taking a medication that had been prescribed to prevent them. What type of primary headache syndrome is the patient likely experiencing?

a. Migraine headaches
b. Cluster type headaches
c. Trigeminal neuralgia
d. Postherpetic neuralgia
e. Tension headache

283. A 22-year-old woman presents to the ED complaining of headache. She states that while at home she experienced a headache that was associated with blurry vision in both eyes with a shimmering line in her vision. She subsequently lost her vision and felt uncoordinated, followed by increased pain at the base of her skull. Upon arrival in the ED, her vision returned to normal. A head CT scan and LP are both negative. She now complains of a persistent, severe, pulsatile headache. She has had two similar episodes in the past year with the headache refractory to over the counter medications. Which of the following is likely to relieve her symptoms?

a. Diazepam 2 mg
b. High flow O_2

c. Sumatriptan injected
d. Acetaminophen
e. LP with removal of 15 cc cerebrospinal fluid (CSF)

284. A 25-year-old man presents to the ED complaining of headache for 2 days. He describes the pain as pulsatile and occipital. The patient had an LP 3 days prior and was diagnosed with viral meningitis after 4 days of symptoms. Noncontrast head CT at that time was normal. He improved shortly thereafter with defervescence of his fever and resolution of his constitutional and nuchal symptoms. He states that his new headache is different than his previous in that it is exacerbated by standing or sitting upright and is relieved by sitting down and is not associated with photophobia or neck stiffness. The headache is not relieved by over the counter pain medications. He is afebrile and nontoxic appearing. Which of the following is definitive therapy for this patient's headache?

a. A 1-L bolus of intravenous (IV) normal saline
b. Treatment with standard pharmacologic agents for migraine
c. Treatment with meclizine
d. Consultation with anesthesia for a blood patch
e. Repeat LP to improve symptoms

285. A 27-year-old woman with known idiopathic intracranial hypertension presents to the ED complaining of a bifrontotemporal headache several times a day for 6 weeks after running out of her medications. She complains of occasional pulsatile tinnitus but no visual disturbances. Fundoscopic exam reveals no papilledema and normal venous pulsations. Which of the following factors determines the need for urgent treatment in patients with idiopathic intracranial hypertension?

a. The presence of papilledema on fundoscopic exam
b. A history of pulsatile tinnitus
c. Presence of an empty sella on CT scan
d. Complaint of visual loss or visual disturbances
e. A history of concomitant minocycline use

286. A 57-year-old man with a past medical history of hypertension and migraines presents to the ED complaining of a headache that started 2 days ago. He states the headache began suddenly with peak intensity while he was defecating. The pain is continuous particularly in the occipital region and is associated with mild nuchal rigidity and mild photophobia. He denies having a recent fever. A noncontrast head CT is obtained and is normal. Which of the following is the most appropriate next step in management?

a. Administer metoclopramide for nausea relief and ketorolac for pain control
b. Diagnostic LP
c. Empiric treatment for meningitis with IV antibiotics
d. IV mannitol to lower intracranial pressure (ICP)
e. Angiography to evaluate for an aneurysm

287. A 27-year-old woman presents to the ED complaining of headache lasting approximately 1 hour in length that is unrelieved by aspirin and acetaminophen. She states the headache was not preceded by any visual phenomena, is left sided, pulsatile, and has occurred nearly monthly coinciding with her menstrual period for the past 6 months. She also complains of nausea and sensitivity to sound and light. Which of the following is the most appropriate therapy for this patient at the time of presentation?

a. IV morphine sulfate
b. Another trial of aspirin and acetaminophen
c. Sumatriptan injected intramuscularly
d. Topiramate given by mouth
e. Hydromorphone and acetaminophen

288. A 55-year-old woman presents to the ED complaining of 1 day of a left-sided headache that is associated with scalp and ear pain. She describes the pain as gradual in onset, dull, and constant. She describes a week of constitutional symptoms prior to the onset of her headache syndrome including joint pain, tenderness of the muscles of her lower extremities, and fatigue. She is afebrile with no nuchal symptoms, photophobia, or phonophobia. Physical exam reveals a tender scalp and a thickened, painful temporal artery. Which of the following is the most appropriate next step in management?

a. Initiation of corticosteroid therapy
b. LP to rule out subarachnoid hemorrhage (SAH)
c. Injection of lidocaine at the base of the occiput
d. Initiation of antibiotic therapy
e. C-reactive protein to evaluate etiology

289. A 28-year-old male military recruit presents to the ED complaining of headache, fever, and neck stiffness. His temperature is 39°C and he refuses to move his neck. He is somewhat lethargic appearing and winces when the lights are turned on in the examining room. He has a nonfocal neurologic exam and you proceed with LP. Which of the following is the most specific finding for suspected bacterial meningitis?

a. The presence of phonophobia and photophobia
b. Fever higher than 39°C
c. Elevated polymorphonuclear white blood cell (WBC) count on CSF analysis
d. Elevated protein on CSF analysis
e. Increased glucose on CSF analysis

290. A 55-year-old man presents to the ED with headache for 1 hour. He describes the headache as boring, constant, and located behind his right eye. He has tried 600 mg of ibuprofen and 650 mg of acetaminophen without relief. He states he had identical headaches a year ago every day for 2 weeks for which he was evaluated by a neurologist. Noncontrast CT of the head is obtained and is normal. His appearance is shown below. What is the most appropriate next step in managing this patient?

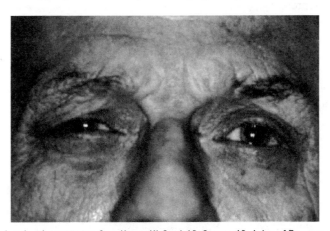

(Reproduced, with permission, from Knoop KJ, Stack LB, Storrow AB. Atlas of Emergency Medicine. New York, NY: McGraw-Hill, 2002: 65. (Courtesy of Frank Birinyi, MD))

a. Administer thrombolytics to treat an ischemic stroke
b. LP to rule out SAH
c. Administer aspirin
d. Administer diazepam
e. Provide high-flow oxygen via nasal cannula

291. As a senior resident in the ED, an intern calls you over to see a patient he treated for a migraine headache. The patient is a 21-year-old woman with a history of poorly controlled migraines. The patient was using a number of migraine medications at home and several were administered intravenously. As you approach the patient, you note her tongue is protruding and her head is tilted to the left. She is grimacing. The intern is concerned that the patient is having an acute stroke and would like to obtain a head CT scan. You advise the intern that the symptoms are likely the result of a medication side effect. Which of the following medications is likely to have caused the patient's symptoms?

a. Morphine sulfate
b. Acetaminophen
c. Metoclopramide
d. Caffeine
e. Sumatriptan

292. A 63-year-old man who lives in a homeless shelter presents to the ED complaining of headache with photophobia for 6 hours. Upon arrival to the ED, the triage nurse places him in an isolation room. The triage note states that the patient was alert and conversant during the nursing interview. You enter the isolation room and attempt to speak to the patient but he is lethargic and combative. You note that his temperature is 103°F. He is unwilling to move his neck and winces when you attempt to check his pupillary reflexes with a pen light. The nurse informs you that laboratory analyses are delayed this evening due to staffing issues. Which of the following is the most appropriate next step in management?

a. Diagnostic LP
b. Initiation of IV antibiotic therapy
c. A loading dose of IV corticosteroids
d. Aggressive antipyretic therapy
e. Sedation of the patient and noncontrast head CT

293. A 22-year-old woman with known idiopathic intracranial hypertension who is scheduled for a ventriculoperitoneal shunt in 2 weeks presents to the ED complaining of severe headache. She states the headache is similar to the normal headaches associated with her condition except that it is refractor to her regular medications, including triptans, and opiates. Her neurologist increased her dose of acetazolamide, but this also did not help. Her noncontrast head CT is unchanged from previous and she does not have papilledema. Which of the following is likely to provide prompt relief?

a. IV corticosteroids
b. Infusion of mannitol
c. LP with removal of 15 cc of CSF
d. IV metoclopramide
e. NSAIDs

294. A 55-year-old woman with a past medical history of diabetes presents to the ED with fevers, headache, vision complaints, and right-sided weakness. She was treated for otitis media 2 weeks ago with amoxicillin as an outpatient. You obtain the CT scan seen below. What is the most likely diagnosis?

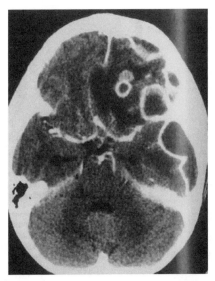

(Reproduced, with permission, from Schwartz DT, Reisdorff EJ. Emergency Radiology. *New York, NY: McGraw-Hill, 2000: 430.)*

a. Central nervous system (CNS) toxoplasmosis
b. Subdural hygroma
c. Glioblastoma multiforme
d. Brain abscess
e. SAH

295. A 35-year-old woman presents to the ED for the second time. She is complaining of fever, neck stiffness, and photophobia. She was seen in your ED 2 days ago for the same symptoms. At that time, she had a normal neurologic exam, was otherwise well-appearing, and underwent diagnostic LP. The results of her CSF analysis were as follows:

Glucose	82
Protein	60
WBC	150 (98% lymphocytes)
Gram stain	No organisms seen

The patient was sent home after a period of observation with presumed viral meningitis. She was told to return if her symptoms were not better in 48 hours. Since then, her fever increased (38–39°C). What is the next most appropriate step in management?

a. Administration of acyclovir
b. Aggressive antipyretic therapy and observation
c. CT scan of the sinuses
d. CT of the head and, if no contraindication, repeat LP
e. Viral cultures and polymerase chain reaction (PCR) from previously obtained CSF

296. A 75-year-old man presents to the ED with right-sided headaches for several months and blurry vision. He was treated with nonsteroidal anti-inflammatory drugs (NSAIDs) and triptans for his headaches which were initially mild but are now excruciating. His ESR is 110 mm/hr. Noncontrast head CT is normal and the patient's neurologic exam is nonfocal. The patient is depicted below. What do you expect to find on physical exam of this patient?

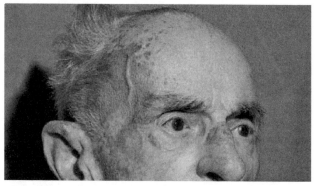

(Reproduced, with permission, from Wolf K, Johnson RA, Suurmond D. Color Atlas and Synopsis of Clinical Dermatology. New York, NY: McGraw-Hill, 2005: 417.)

a. Bilateral retinal hemorrhages on fundoscopy
b. Papilledema
c. Resolving vesicular rash
d. A focal neurologic deficit
e. A tender, pulseless temporal artery

297. A 34-year-old woman presents to the ED complaining of headaches for 3 weeks. She is obese but otherwise healthy. She describes the headaches as pulsatile and exacerbated by bending over to pick up objects. You suspect idiopathic intracranial hypertension. Which of the following is consistent with the diagnosis of idiopathic intracranial hypertension?

a. A markedly decreased CSF glucose level
b. Multiple focal neurologic deficits
c. Lack of papilledema on fundoscopic exam
d. Ventricular enlargement on noncontrast head CT
e. An LP opening pressure in excess of 200 mm H_2O

298. A 68-year-old man presents to the ED complaining of a daily headache for almost a month. He describes the headache as being dull, difficult to localize, most intense in the morning, and abating in the early afternoon. He also noticed progressive weakness of his right upper and lower extremity. Which of the following headache syndromes are the signs and symptoms most consistent with?

a. Headache caused by a mass lesion
b. Cluster headache
c. Tension-type headache
d. Headache from intracranial hypertension
e. Waking or morning migraine

299. A 75-year-old man presents to the ED with a depressed level of consciousness. His wife is at the bedside and states he was stacking heavy boxes when he complained of a sudden intense headache. He subsequently sat down on the couch and progressively lost consciousness. She states that he had a headache the previous week that was also sudden but not as intense. He had gone to visit his primary care physician who sent him to have a CT scan of the brain, which was normal. Over the course of the past week, he complained of intermittent pulsating headaches for which he took sumatriptan. In the ED, you intubate the patient and obtain the noncontrast head CT seen below. The scan is most consistent with which diagnosis?

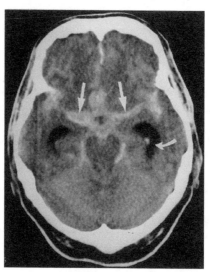

(Reproduced, with permission, from Tintinalli J, Kelen G, and Stapczynski J. Emergency Medicine A Comprehensive Study Guide. New York, NY: McGraw-Hill, 2004: 1445.)

a. Meningoencephalitis
b. SAH
c. Normal pressure hydrocephalus
d. Epidural hematoma
e. Subdural hematoma

300. A 43-year-old homeless man presents to the ED with fever and nuchal rigidity. His mental status is depressed but his neurologic exam is otherwise nonfocal. Noncontrast head CT is normal. You obtain an LP for diagnostic purposes and initiate empiric antibiotic treatment for bacterial meningitis with ceftriaxone and ampicillin. The result of the CSF analysis is complete after 1 hour. The protein and glucose are within normal range but the WBC count consists of 220 mononuclear cells. The Gram stain is negative. The patient was recently purified protein derivative (PPD) negative and had a normal chest x-ray. In addition to the treatment already initiated, what is the next most appropriate step in this patient's management?

a. Empiric treatment with isoniazid
b. Empiric treatment with antiviral medications for herpes virus
c. Empiric treatment with antifungals
d. Antibiotic coverage for *Bartonella sp.*
e. Addition of vancomycin to the antibiotic regimen

301. A patient presents to the ED complaining of fever and headache. The patient is a 65-year-old man who is otherwise healthy. He does not have any gross neurologic complaints but is febrile to 102°F and has neck stiffness. He also states he has lost approximately 25 lb in the last 3 months. A LP is obtained to rule out meningitis. Approximately 1 hour later, after you have given the patient antibiotics and are awaiting CSF results, a nurse calls you to the bedside stating that the patient is not responsive and is apneic. You go to examine the patient and note asymmetry in his pupils with the right being dilated. Despite resuscitative efforts, the patient expires. Postmortem examination reveals a large glioblastoma multiforme. CSF analysis shows meningitis caused by *Haemophilus influenza*. Which of the following criteria should be met in order to ensure that a patient can have an LP to rule out meningitis without neuroimaging?

a. Age <60
b. No history of seizures in the patient's lifetime.
c. Focal neurologic deficit limited to one extremity or cranial nerve
d. Glasgow coma scale >13
e. CNS disease in remission

302. A 53-year-old man presents to your ED stating he has had an excruciating right-sided headache since leaving the movie theater. He states that the headache is unilateral, severe, and associated with nausea and vomiting. His vision is blurry and notes seeing halos around objects. He denies trauma or a history of headaches in the past. Physical exam reveals right conjunctival injection and a pupil that reacts only marginally. Which exam is likely to yield the correct diagnosis?

a. Measurement of intraocular pressure
b. Fundoscopic exam
c. Fluorescein examination
d. LP with cell count
e. Visual acuity testing

303. A 78-year-old man presents to triage of your ED complaining of gradual onset of headache over the course of the day. The headache is present almost everyday and wonders if it is related to the unusually cold temperatures this winter. He describes the headache as bounding and constant. You notice that his face is very ruddy in appearance. He is afebrile but looks rather lethargic and seems somewhat short of breath. He is afebrile and saturating 100% on pulse oximetry. One of your coworkers informs you that the patient's wife is in another part of the emergency room with a similar presentation. Two more ambulances arrive, one with a patient complaining of a similar headache and another with a patient who is obtunded. All live in the same building. What is the next most appropriate step in the management of these patients?

a. Place the patient in respiratory isolation for presumed *Neisseria meningitidis* infection
b. Draw a blood gas and send it for cooximetry
c. Start antibiotic therapy and perform a LP
d. Treatment for migraine with triptans or IV antiemetics
e. Transfer of all three patients to the nearest hyperbaric facility

304. A 35-year-old man presents to the ED complaining of a headache over the previous 4 weeks. He was assaulted with a bat 4 weeks ago and was admitted to the hospital for observation in the setting of a small traumatic subdural hematoma. Repeat noncontrast CT scan of the head 2 weeks ago was normal with resolution of the hematoma. He states he has headaches several times each day. They last from 5 minutes to several hours. They are sometimes band-like, other times they are localized to the site where he was struck. They can be pulsating or constant and are associated with sensitivity to sound. A head CT scan today is normal. Which of the following is the most likely diagnosis?

a. Postconcussive syndrome
b. Posttraumatic hydrocephalus
c. Subdural hygroma
d. Cluster headache
e. Posttraumatic stress disorder

305. A 35-year-old woman presents to the ED complaining of headache and blurry vision. She has had daily headaches for 3 months associated with blurry vision. She is afebrile, not losing weight, and has a normal neurologic exam, including fundoscopy. You ask when her last menstrual period was and she states she has not menstruated for 5 months and is not taking oral contraceptive pills. She also complains of galactorrhea. Noncontrast head CT is normal. An LP is performed and reveals a normal opening pressure. Which of the following is the most appropriate next step in managing the patient's headaches?

a. Repeat head CT with administration of IV contrast.
b. Initiation of therapy with bromocriptine
c. Evaluation of CSF for xanthrochromia and RBCs
d. Treatment of her headache with analgesia and referral for a MRI
e. Repeat LP with removal of 15 mL CSF for therapeutic benefit

306. A 37 year-old woman with a history of migraines presents to the ED complaining of crampy lower abdominal pain for 3 days. Workup reveals an intrauterine pregnancy and early prenatal care is arranged with obstetrics as an outpatient. You are concerned because her headaches are controlled with a significant number of medications. She uses medications for both abortive therapy and for prophylaxis. Which of the following classes of medications do you advise she discontinue while pregnant?

a. Antiepileptics
b. β-Blockers
c. Triptans
d. Acetaminophen
e. Antiemetics

Headache

Answers

279. The answer is a. *(Rosen, pp 1527–1541.)* This patient presents with symptoms consistent with *meningitis. Antibiotics* are administered *empirically* as diagnostic workup proceeds. The best choice in this patient is *ceftriaxone,* which has good CNS penetration. In order to avoid transtentorial herniation in this patient with a *neurologic deficit (confusion),* a *noncontrast head CT* should be performed *prior to LP.* It is controversial whether or not a head CT needs to be performed prior to all LPs. However, if there is papilledema or a neurologic deficit, then head CT is mandatory.

(**b**) It is not prudent to wait for results from a head CT. This will only delay treatment of a potentially fatal disease. (**c**) Although this patient can benefit from acetaminophen and hydration, starting antibiotics empirically is more important. In addition, this patient requires a head CT prior to LP. (**d & e**) As previously stated, antibiotics should be started early in management and not be delayed while waiting for results.

280. The answer is e. *(Rosen, pp 1463–1464.)* The patient most likely has *idiopathic intracranial hypertension (pseudotumor cerebri),* a neurologic disease seen primarily in *young obese women* of *childbearing age.* Clinically, patients complain of a generalized headache of gradual onset and moderate severity. It may worsen with eye movements or with the Valsalva maneuver. Visual complaints are common and may occur several times a day and can become permanent in 10% of patients. Patients typically have papilledema and visual field defects on physical exam. Diagnosis is made by a normal neuroimaging scan and an *elevated intracerebral pressure (>200 mm H_2O)* measured by the opening pressure from a LP.

This patient does not require immediate surgery (**a**), but may require a ventricular shunt in the future if she exhibits impending vision loss. Two grams of ceftriaxone (**b**) is therapy for meningitis, which this patient does not have. Carotid artery dissections (**c**) present classically with the triad of unilateral headache, ipsilateral partial Horner's syndrome, and contralateral hemispheric findings such as aphasia, visual disturbances, or hemiparesis. Migraines (**d**) tend to be unilateral and pulsating and associated with nausea, vomiting, photophobia, phonophobia, blurred vision, and light-headedness. Patients should not exhibit papilledema.

281. The answer is e. *(Rosen, pp 1613–1614.)* This patient's clinical picture is consistent with *temporal arteritis (TA)*. Patients are usually *middle-aged females* who present with malaise, fevers, and headache. A complete physical examination would have revealed temporal artery tenderness to palpation. This patient also complains of symptoms consistent with *polymyalgia rheumatica,* a general achiness that may become confused with influenza. Carbon monoxide (CO) poisoning must also be on the differential in any patient that presents with vague flu-like symptoms, headache, and nausea with report of similar symptoms in coinhabitants. Temporal or giant-cell arteritis is a granulomatous inflammation that involves the large and medium-sized arteries of the body, commonly the carotid artery and its branches. The mesenteric system may also be involved. Symptoms are produced as a result of ischemia to the organs fed by the branches of the artery. Visual loss in one eye, transient diplopia and jaw claudication are common symptoms when the branches of the internal and external carotid are affected. A *temporal artery biopsy* is the *diagnostic test of choice.* Treatment up until the time of biopsy should include the *glucocorticoids,* namely Prednisone. This does not alter biopsy results and may prevent progression of the disease. Hospitalization is warranted in patients with severe debilitation or impending visual loss and may require high-dose steroids.

(a) Symptoms of influenza closely mimic those of polymyalgia rheumatica, were it not for the specific eye/jaw symptoms. **(b)** Patients with Strep pharyngitis may present with profound general malaise, however, they are typically more febrile and have a history of sick contacts and dry cough. Tonsillar exudates and anterior cervical adenopathy might be evident upon physical examination.

(c) An ESR >100 mm/h is a good initial test to further the suspicion of TA, however, it is not the diagnostic test of choice. An elevated C-reactive protein may also be present. **(d)** A CBC may indicate anemia, which results from the arterial inflammation that furthers the breakdown of red blood cells (RBCs). However, this and an elevated white blood cell count are nonspecific findings.

282. The answer is e. *(Lange: Clinical Neurology, Ch 2 Headache syndromes)* *Tension headaches* are typically often occur *daily,* and classically cause bilateral occipital pain that is described as a *band tightening* around the head. In general, people experience a constant, dull pain that is nonthrobbing and without the ancillary features associated with migraines (visual phenomena, aura, neurologic complaints, nausea, vomiting). There is often secondary contraction of the neck and scalp musculature. First line treatment includes NSAIDs and acetaminophen. If the headaches occur frequently enough to cause dysfunction in daily activities, patients may benefit from preventive therapy such as amitriptyline, desipramine, or propranolol.

Migraine headaches (**a**) classically begin with visual phenomena or another aura and are pulsatile, unilateral, associated with nausea, vomiting, photophobia, and phonophobia. They may also have associated neurologic phenomena. Cluster headaches (**b**) are more common in men and are unilateral, boring, and may be associated with neurologic phenomena or autonomic activation. They are short lived and generally recur daily at the same time for days or weeks before the patient has remission of their symptoms. Trigeminal neuralgia (**c**) is thought to result from microvascular compression of the trigeminal nerve roots. It presents as shooting facial pain, in the distribution of the fifth cranial nerve, particularly the second and third nerve roots. In less than 5% of cases, it involves the first division of the trigeminal nerve and patients will present complaining of headache. Treatment includes carbamazepine or other antiepileptic drugs. Postherpetic neuralgia (**d**) is pain that continues after an eruption of herpes zoster. It is often described as a burning or stabbing pain that is constant in the dermatome originally affected by the zoster outbreak. In 50% of patients it subsides after 6 months. In some patients it lasts for years. Treatment is with gabapentin, phenytoin, or amitriptyline.

283. The answer is c. (*Tintinalli, pp 1379–1381.*) The patient is experiencing a *migraine* variant known as a *basilar migraine*. Its onset is similar to other migraines in that it can begin with scotomata or aura. The visual symptoms are often bilateral and followed by a brief period of cortical blindness. Symptoms related to the basilar circulation then predominate including incoordination, dysarthria, vertigo, and numbness and tingling in the arms or legs. These symptoms generally last 10–30 minutes then resolve. Occasionally, transient coma or quadriplegia can develop but can persist for several hours. The resulting headache is occipital and pulsating. The symptoms may mimic a vertebrobasilar ischemic event. Treatment with first-line agents for migraine is recommended. Threshold should be low to seek neurologic consultation unless the diagnosis is certain.

Diazepam (**a**) is useful for treating cervical muscle spasm and torticollis. At high doses, it has the principle side effect of respiratory depression.

It is unlikely to relieve the pain associated with a migraine although it may be useful for associated scalp and trapezius spasm. High flow O_2 (**b**) is beneficial to migraine patients but is not the mainstay of treatment. Other adjuncts to pharmacotherapy include decreasing ambient light and noise and putting a cool cloth over the forehead. Acetaminophen (**d**) is a useful first-line treatment with NSAIDs for migraine and tension type headaches. They represent a safer first line to triptans which are contraindicated in patients with dysrhythmias, poorly controlled hypertension, or coronary artery disease. Therapeutic removal of CSF (**e**) is indicated in cases of idiopathic intracranial hypertension.

284. The answer is d. (*Rosen, p 1464. Candido, pp 451–469.*) The patient has a *post-LP headache*. The headache is thought to be due to removal of CSF during LP with a continued leakage of CSF. It is exquisitely *sensitive to position* and many patients will experience complete relief of pain after being placed in Trendelenberg position. A *blood patch* is placed by injecting an aliquot of the patient's blood in a sterile fashion just external to the dura mater at the same interspace where the LP occurred. The majority of patients have relief of symptoms with this procedure. Prevention of the post-LP headache includes using a 22-gauge or smaller needle, removing as little fluid as possible, and facing the bevel up when the patient is in the lateral position.

Administering IV fluids (**a**) is thought to increase intravascular volume and CSF production, thereby reducing symptoms. It is not, however, definitive treatment. Standard migraine treatments (**b**) are often ineffective in treating the post-LP headache. The headache often responds well to caffeine based therapy. Meclizine (**c**) is a medication used to treat peripheral vertigo and is ineffective in the treatment of the post-LP headache. Repeat LP (**e**) is unlikely to yield new diagnostic information and is likely to exacerbate the headache. Headaches that improve after dural puncture are those typically associated with idiopathic intracranial hypertension. There are case reports of spontaneous subdural hematoma post-LP caused by relative descent of the brain in the setting of decreased CSF with stretch on bridging veins. If this is a diagnostic consideration, a head CT scan should be obtained.

285. The answer is d. (*Goetz, pp 1797–1798.*) *Idiopathic intracranial hypertension (IIH),* formerly *pseudotumor cerebri,* requires urgent treatment when there is a history of visual phenomena, particularly transient vision loss. Agents used to lower ICP in this setting include carbonic anhydrase inhibitors (i.e., acetazolamide) and loop diuretics (i.e., furosemide). Transient visual loss, pain, or blurring occurs frequently and can be permanent in up to 10% of patients. Treatment of the headache itself often employs the same agents used to treat migraines; ergots, antiemetics, and occasionally steroids. The headache is often refractory and difficult to manage. The condition is associated with obesity and weight loss is sometimes helpful.

Papilledema (**a**) in the setting of intermittent frontotemporal headaches and an otherwise normal neurologic exam is consistent with IIH. Its presence does not rule in or out other intracranial pathology. It is not by itself a risk factor in patients with IIH for neurologic deterioration. A history of pulsatile tinnitus (**b**) is often associated with IIH but its prognostic significance is unclear. An empty sella (**c**) is frequently seen on CT scan of IIH patients. It is likely caused by herniation of arachnoid CSF into the sellar space and is sometimes reversible with lowering of CSF pressure. Another finding to look for on CT scan is an occluded venous sinus which indicates a secondary cause of elevated ICP. Minocycline, oral contraceptive pills, vitamin A, and anabolic steroids (**e**) have been associated with the development of IIH.

286. The answer is b. (*Manno, pp 347–366.*) The patient presents with a clinical history that is consistent with a *SAH*. Noncontrast computed tomography is approximately 90–100% sensitive in the first 24 hours after the onset of a SAH; its sensitivity beings to decline thereafter. Diagnostic LP with confirmed presence of xanthrochromia (yellow color of supernatant in a centrifuged specimen of CSF) indicates the presence of bilirubin in CSF and is diagnostic of a SAH. Patients who present late in the course of their headache who have a clinical history consistent with SAH but with a nondiagnostic CT and LP (the sensitivity is minimal for both after approximately 2 weeks) should be referred for outpatient angiography to evaluate for the presence of an aneurysm.

Administration of metoclopramide and ketorolac (**a**) is useful in managing pain due to a migraine syndrome. Because of their antiplatelet activity, ketorolac (Toradol) and other NSAIDs are contraindicated in patients who may be actively bleeding. Treatment of meningitis (**c**) with IV antibiotics should not be delayed if the diagnosis is suspected. However, the patient's clinical history is inconsistent with this diagnosis (he is afebrile and without constitutional symptoms) and LP is readily available. Infusion of IV mannitol (**d**) lowers ICP acutely via osmotic diuresis. It is indicated in patients displaying symptoms of increased ICP or when impending herniation is suspected. Angiography (**e**) is the gold standard for diagnosis of a cerebral aneurysm but LP should be performed to confirm the presence of intracranial bleeding prior to contrast-based imaging. If bleeding has stopped, cerebral angiography will not help diagnose the approximately 20% of SAHs that are due to drug intoxication, dural arteriovenous fistulas, or pituitary apoplexy.

287. The answer is c. (*Tintinalli, pp 1379–1381.*) The headache described is a *menstrual migraine,* a common *variant of the migraine headache syndrome.* Appropriate abortive therapies (this headache is just starting) are diverse and include IV ergot, triptans, and antiemetics. Sumatriptan (Imitrex) is an injectable triptan which acts by blocking the 5-hydroxytryptamine (5-HT, serotonin)1D receptor. It also has less associated nausea and vomiting than ergots. It may have a higher incidence of minor side effects (flushing, injection site reaction) and a higher relapse rate than ergots. Contraindications to triptans or ergots include pregnancy, hypertension, coronary artery disease, or use of either class of agent within the last 24 hours.

Opioid analgesics **(a)** and **(e)** are reserved for failed abortive therapy or when there are contraindications to readily available abortive drugs. Opioids decrease the pain associated with headache syndromes, but fail to interrupt the neurochemical dysfunction. Frequent use of opioids for primary headache syndromes is associated with poor outcomes. **(b)** NSAIDs and acetaminophen are appropriate first-line therapy for patients with minor migraine symptoms. If a patient has tried these in the past and they have been ineffective, there is little utility in trying again. **(d)** Topiramate (Topamax) is an antiepileptic drug that is used for migraine prevention in patients with frequent and difficult to control headache syndromes.

288. The answer is a. (*Goldman, pp 1693–1695.*) In a case of suspected *TA, initiation of corticosteroid therapy is indicated emergently* to prevent irreversible complications. *Loss of vision* is known to occur and prompt initiation of corticosteroid therapy decreases this possibility. TA, also referred to as giant cell arteritis, is a granulomatous inflammation of the proximal great vessels and its carotid bifurcations. It has an overlapping clinical syndrome with *polymyalgia rheumatica.*

The description of this headache syndrome is inconsistent with a SAH **(b)**, which classically presents with sudden onset of pain and is associated with nausea, photophobia, and nuchal rigidity. It is rarely preceded by constitutional symptoms. Injection of lidocaine at the base of the occiput is an effective treatment for cervical neuralgia **(c)** but has no place in the treatment or diagnosis of TA. The patient's clinical history is inconsistent with meningitis. Laboratory analysis is sometimes helpful in diagnosing TA, but waiting for serum analysis inappropriately delays treatment (**e**). ESR is normally elevated to the 50–100 range, but a mildly elevated sedimentation rate does not rule out the diagnosis.

289. The answer is c. (*Rosen, pp 1716–1719.*) The normal number of WBCs in the cerebrospinal fluid is 5 or fewer with 1 or less *polymorphonuclear neutrophils (PMN)*. Numbers greater than these should be taken as evidence for CNS infection. In cases of *acute bacterial meningitis,* cell counts of 1000–20,000 WBCs are observed, often with neutrophil predominance. In cases of aseptic (viral) meningitis, cell counts are generally lower with lymphocyte predominance. Initial treatment with antibiotics prior to LP is unlikely to affect the cell count, after 6 hours though, the culture is less likely to return positive. It should be noted that a subset of patients with bacterial meningitis may present with lymphocytic predominance. Therefore, lymphocytic predominance does not rule out bacterial meningitis and antibiotics should be given.

The classic clinical presentation of bacterial meningitis includes photophobia, headache, fever, and nuchal rigidity. None of these symptoms are specific (**a**) and LP must be obtained. The classic clinical presentation is altered in states of immunocompromise (human immunodeficiency virus [HIV], corticosteroid use), so clinical suspicion should be higher in these patients. Fevers (**b**) are generally thought to be high in bacterial meningitis, but there is no number that is specific for its diagnosis. CSF protein level (**d**) generally ranges from 15 to 45 mg/dL. Levels greater than 150 mg/dL are often seen in acute bacterial meningitis, but can result from many other conditions including CNS abscesses, encephalitis, and fungal infections. Fungal infections often have CSF proteins that are markedly elevated, often greater than 1000 mg/dL. Glucose levels are generally depressed (**e**) in cases of bacterial meningitis.

290. The answer is e. (*Capobianco, pp 242–259.*) The patient is exhibiting *unilateral Horner's syndrome* in the setting of a *cluster headache.* Cluster headaches present as unilateral, constant, and intense headaches lasting from several minutes to 2 hours. Conjunctival injection, lacrimation, and nasal stuffiness are also common. The most appropriate treatment for this headache is *high flow oxygen,* which provides partial or complete relief in 75% of patients. Injected *triptans* and ergotamine are similarly effective but should be avoided in patients with contraindications, such as heart disease and severe hypertension.

Treatment with thrombolytics (**a**) is appropriate for patients with ischemic stroke. The neurologic symptoms associated with different headache syndromes can mimic ischemic or hemorrhagic strokes. The clinician must have a firm understanding of these entities to ensure diagnostic accuracy. LP (**b**) is used to diagnose SAH when clinical suspicion is high and noncontrast CT of the head is negative. The presence of red cells or xanthrochromic fluid is indicative of SAH. Aspirin (**c**) is no more affective than other NSAIDs. (**d**) Diazepam is not used in treating cluster headaches.

291. The answer is c. (*Goetz, pp 1192–1194. Rosen, pp 1456–1459.*) *Dystonic reactions* may occur with the use of dopamine blocking agents. Medications classically associated with dystonic reactions are typical antipsychotics (e.g., haloperidol) but can also occur with the antiemetics used to treat migraines. They are generally not life-threatening and respond almost immediately to administration of diphenhydramine (Benadryl) given intravenously or intramuscularly. Common dystonic reactions include oculogyric crises (eyes deviating in different directions), torticollis, tongue protrusion, facial grimacing, and difficulty speaking.

Morphine sulfate (**a**) has the principal side effect of respiratory depression. This effect and the drug's analgesic properties are reversed by naloxone. Localized reactions including erythema, swelling, and pruritis are common after intramuscular or subcutaneous injection. Anaphylaxis has been described but is rare. Acetaminophen (**b**) has the principal side effect of hepatotoxicity. In patients using it chronically without following dose-based guidelines, liver damage is possible. (**d**) Caffeine is a methylxanthine. Side effects include palpitations, anxiety, tremulousness, and dry mouth. Sumatriptan (**e**) has side effects related to the cardiovascular system. They include hypertension and coronary artery vasospasm. Several cases of myocardial infarctions have been observed after its use.

292. The answer is b. (*Tintinalli, pp 1431–1434.*) The clinical presentation is consistent with *meningitis*. The patient's mental status has declined between initial nursing assessment and the physician's interview. Delay of antibiotic therapy in order to first confirm the diagnosis with CSF analysis may lead to increased mortality.

LP (**a**) performed even several hours after initiation of antibiotic therapy is often still culture positive for the causative organism. Administration of IV corticosteroids prior to antibiotic administration (**c**) has been shown in some studies to reduce the mortality of patients with bacterial meningitis. Their use in the ED for undifferentiated cases of meningitis has not been sufficiently studied. Antipyretics (**d**) are used to reduce fever but will not stop the primary pathologic process. Noncontrast head CT (**e**) should be obtained prior to LP when question of mass effect or increased ICP might lead to herniation from CSF removal. Antibiotic therapy should not be delayed in cases of suspected meningitis for neuroimaging.

293. The answer is c. (*Rosen, pp 1463–1464.*) IIH is an idiopathic elevation of ICP. In the setting of a normal CT, the diagnosis is made by LP with an elevated opening pressure often between 250 and 450 mm H_2O. Patients often experience complete relief of their symptoms with LP and return of their ICP to levels <200 mm H_2O.

Corticosteroids **(a)** are controversial in the management of headache in IIH, but many neurologists use them routinely. Mannitol **(b)** is an osmotic diuretic that is used to acutely lower ICP, often in the setting of trauma to prevent impending herniation. Its use is not recommended in the setting of IIH. It should not be confused with acetazolamide, a carbonic anhydrase inhibitor that works as a diuretic and is part of maintenance treatment for IIH. Metoclopramide **(d)** is normally used as an antiemetic but is also highly effective in the treatment of migraines. Ketorolac and other NSAIDs **(e)** are the mainstays of treatment for many headache syndromes including tension headaches, migraines, cluster headaches, and others. Their use should be avoided when there is suspicion that the patient has an intracranial bleed because they have antiplatelet effects and can exacerbate bleeding.

294. The answer is d. (*Cohen & Powderly, pp 279–283.*) *Brain abscesses* are uncommon and their incidence has decreased over the past several years as a result of better antibiotic treatment of the remote infections that cause them. Today, the majority of brain abscesses in developed countries are the result of contiguous spread from otitis media, mastoiditis, paranasal sinusitis, or meningitis. They can also occur after trauma, classically after a basilar skull fracture. Presentation is often nonspecific, with almost half present with headache alone. Focal weakness, fevers, and nausea are other common presenting complaints. Antibiotic choice should be guided by suspected source and ability to penetrate the CNS. On this CT with IV contrast, the abscess appears with an *enhancing wall containing fluid.*

(a) CNS toxoplasmosis is uncommon in the developed world outside the setting of advanced HIV or other immunocompromised states. Patients often present with altered mental status, neurologic deficits, or seizures. On contrast enhanced CT, there are often multiple, small, ring enhancing lesions. **(b)** Subdural hygromas are fluid-filled subdural pockets containing xanthrochromic fluid. They are often the result of trauma and present with signs and symptoms of increased ICP or with neurologic deficits. They are thought to result from tears in the arachnoid with fluid accumulation. **(e)** Spontaneous SAHs present as severe headaches associated with nausea, vomiting, nuchal rigidity, and can have neurologic deficits associated with them. It appears on noncontrast CT as hyperdense fluid that may fill the cisterns and subarachnoid space.

295. The answer is d. *(Tintinalli, pp 1434–1435.)* Patients with CSF analysis consistent with viral meningitis can be managed as outpatients with close follow up. These patients must be reliable for follow up, not immunocompromised and otherwise well-appearing. They should be told to return for reevaluation if their symptoms do not improve within 48 hours. If they have not improved, *reevaluation* including *neuroimaging, repeat LP,* and treatment with antibiotics is indicated.

Administration of acyclovir **(a)** is indicated in patients with presumed meningoencephalitis due to Herpes virus. Antipyretic therapy **(b)** is indicated for patient comfort, but repeat diagnostic evaluation is essential. Sinus pain **(c)** can often present as a frontal, pulsating headache. Patients may be febrile and can seed the CSF from direct extension of sinusitis. Nevertheless, meningitis must still be ruled out and treated, even if there is CT confirmation of sinus opacification. Analyzing CSF already in the lab **(e)** from a previous LP is not recommended.

296. The answer is e. *(Tintinalli, p 1378.)* The above picture depicts a prominent *superficial temporal artery* in an elderly man complaining of unilateral headaches and vision change. This is consistent with temporal (giant cell) arteritis. Loss of vision in these cases is a later complication but can occur rapidly and is prevented with prompt treatment with corticosteroids. It is due to occlusion of the ophthalmic arteries with granulomatous infiltrate. Definitive diagnosis through temporal artery biopsy is rarely made in the ED, but this should not delay initiation of treatment. Early in the disease, the *temporal artery* will be *tender and pulsatile.* As the disease progresses, middle size arteries fill with granulomatous infiltrate and lose their pulses. Other complications include arteritis of the aorta and its branches. It is an illness that overlaps in clinical presentation with polymyalgia rheumatica and may presents with malaise, arthralgias, low-grade fever, weight loss, and mild leukocytosis.

Papilledema **(b)** may occur but is exceedingly rare in cases of TA. Papilledema should also lead the clinician to search for other causes of increased ICP. A resolving vesicular **(c)** rash is consistent with varicella zoster. Postherpetic neuralgia can give persistent pain in the dermatomal distribution of the original outbreak, but this patient has no history of prior zoster. Vision loss can also be associated with zoster involving the first branch of the trigeminal nerve if the patient develops a keratitis. If trigeminal zoster is suspected, the patient should receive a slit lamp examination with fluorescein to evaluate for the classic branching dendritic pattern associated with keratitis. Focal neurologic deficits (d) as the result of an ischemic stroke are incredibly rare in the setting of TA. Because the intracranial arteries have minimal elastic intima, they are rarely affected. Only a few cases of ischemic stroke have been described, likely due to occlusion of vertebral or carotid circulation with poor collateral flow.

297. The answer is e. *(Rosen, pp 1463–1464.)* Diagnosis of IIH is made according to clinical criteria, neuroimaging and LP. An *opening pressure of greater than 200 mm H_2O is consistent with IIH.* IIH has a predilection for women, is most prevalent between ages 20 and 40 years, and is often associated with obesity. There seems to be a greater incidence of the disease in patients with a prior history of head trauma.

Examination of the CSF shows normal glucose (a) but there may be mildly decreased protein. Elevation of protein or alterations in CSF glucose should steer the diagnosis away from IIH. The hallmark of IIH is headache and signs of increased ICP without focal neurologic symptoms (b). Focal neurologic deficits merit further investigation. Papilledema is often present on neurologic exam regardless of whether the patient is complaining of visual deficits or loss. IIH has been described with and without papilledema, but its presence or absence neither confirms nor rules out the diagnosis (c). Non-contrast head CT is required to rule out other causes of headache with signs of increased ICP. Empty sella is a common finding that is thought to arise from herniation of CSF into the arachnoid space of the sella. The ventricles should appear normal (d) and no sign of mass effect should be present.

298. The answer is a. *(Tintinalli, pp 1375–1381.)* Headaches due to a *mass lesion* are classically described as *worse in the morning,* associated with *nausea and vomiting,* and *worse with position.* Rarely do patients present with focal neurologic symptoms. When they do, imaging is a necessary adjunct prior to leaving the ED. If a mass lesion is part of the differential diagnosis, LP should be deferred until neuroimaging has been performed due to the risk of herniation.

Cluster headaches (b) are rare, generally occur in males, last less than 2 hours, and present as unilateral eye or temporal pain. There is often unilateral tearing, swelling, or nasal congestion. In contrast to the migraine patient, patients with cluster headaches are typically restless. Cluster headaches respond to ergots, triptans, and often high-flow oxygen. Tension-type (c) headaches are bilateral, not pulsating, not worsened by exertion, and should not be associated with nausea or vomiting. They generally respond to NSAIDs or acetaminophen. Headaches associated with intracranial hypertension (d) are exacerbated by changes in position (e.g., squatting), are often frontotemporal, and may be associated with disturbances of gait and incontinence. They are difficult to control. Migraines (e) are generally unilateral, pulsating, associated with phonophobia or photophobia, nausea, and vomiting. They are slow in onset and generally last 4–72 hours. There is considerable heterogeneity in their presentation. Most patients who are chronic migraneurs can describe their headache syndrome and are able to differentiate between their normal migraine and another headache. Change in the character, intensity, location, or duration of a migraine should prompt suspicion of another cause.

299. The answer is b. (*Tintinalli, pp 1389–1390.*) The CT depicts subarachnoid arachnoid blood. This patient may have had a sentinel bleed, a small SAH, the previous week. Noncontrast CT misses a small percentage of SAH and therefore, in cases of high suspicion, an LP must be obtained to exclude the diagnosis.

Irritation of the meninges or inflammation of the brain (a) may not appear at all on noncontrast CT of the brain. If contrast is used, meningeal or cerebral enhancement may be apparent, but diagnosis of these conditions is not based on imaging. High clinical suspicion must be present for either condition and LP is used to confirm the diagnosis. Hydrocephalus (c) appears as dilated ventricles on CT scan. If all of the ventricles are patent and dilated, it is termed communicating hydrocephalus. If part of the ventricular system is collapsed and the others dilated, an obstructive cause of hydrocephalus is present. Epidural hematomas (d) are the result of brisk arterial bleeds into the space between the dura and the calvarium. They are classically caused by trauma and are associated with a "lucid period" during which level of consciousness is normal prior to neurologic deterioration. On noncontrast CT, they appear as hyperdense intracranial collections of blood that are bilenticular in shape. Subdural hematomas (SDH) (e) are intracranial blood collections that result from tearing of the bridging veins between the dura and the brain. Risk factors for SDH include advanced age and chronic alcohol use. Both conditions are associated with decreased brain volume and provide stretch on these delicate veins. On noncontrast CT, SDHs appear as crescent shaped collections of hyperdense blood.

300. The answer is b. (*Tintinalli, pp 1434–1435.*) The CSF analysis in this patient is consistent with a *viral or atypical cause of meningitis.* Although patients may have a mononuclear predominance and still have bacterial meningitis, viral causes should be considered. CSF should be sent for PCR analysis and empiric treatment initiated for *herpes encephalitis.* The mortality of meningoencephalitis due to herpes simplex virus (HSV) is exceptionally high if untreated.

Tuberculosis (TB) meningitis **(a)** should be considered in this undomiciled patient. Other risk factors for TB include immunocompromise and living in an endemic region. However, the patient is recently PPD and chest x-ray (CXR) negative, making this possibility less likely. In an immunocompromised patient PPD may be less reliable so a CSF acid fast stain and mycobacterial culture should still be sent. Fungal causes **(c)** of CNS pathology are also a diagnostic consideration but are less likely than viral causes. In this patient, fungal cultures are recommended in addition to CSF cryptococcal antigen. *Bartonella sp.* **(d)** and other rare causes of meningitis are not considered until other first and second tier analyses are conducted. Vancomycin **(e)** is used when methicillin resistant gram positive organisms are suspected. In patients who have been recently hospitalized, have repeated instrumentation, have been treated with antibiotics for other causes, or have reasons to seed their bloodstream with potentially resistant organisms (i.e., IV drug abuse), vancomycin should be administered.

301. The answer is a. (*Hasbun, p 1727.*) The case illustrates one of the catastrophic *complications of LP.* The patient had an *uncal herniation* due to increased ICP from his tumor. Patients often present with multiple comorbidities. Patients greater than 60 years of age are at greater risk for all causes of increased ICP.

Patients could have seizures in their lifetime **(b)** but if one has taken place in the past week, they should have neuroimaging prior to LP. Any focal neurologic deficit **(c)** is an indication to image prior to LP. Similarly, a patient should have full sensorium and be free of known CNS disease **(d and e)** prior to LP.

302. The answer is a. (*Tintinalli, pp 1459–1460.*) The patient presents with *acute angle closure glaucoma* which results from obstruction of aqueous outflow of the anterior chamber of the eye with a resulting *rise in intraocular* *pressure*. It is the result of a shallow anterior chamber or a chamber distorted by the development of a cataract. Classically, it occurs when a patient leaves a prolonged dimly lit situation. When the iris becomes mid-dilated, it maximally obstructs the trabecular meshwork occluding aqueous humor flow. Intraocular pressures may rise from normal (10–21 mm Hg) to levels as high as 50–100. *Visual acuity is usually decreased* in the affected eye due to resulting corneal edema. Treatment is aimed at lowering intraocular pressure with acetazolamide, ophthalmic β-blockers, prostaglandin analogues, and pilocarpine to induce miosis. Ophthalmologic consultation and follow-up is indicated. Patients may present complaining of headache, nausea, and vomiting, but will often endorse that the symptoms began with acute eye pain.

Fundoscopic exam (b) is occasionally abnormal in acute glaucoma, but associated papilledema rarely develops acutely. Corneal examination with fluorescein (c) is used to diagnose corneal abrasions or other corneal pathology (i.e., ulcers, keratitis, foreign body, corneal rupture). The cornea may appear normal or "steamy" in the setting of acute glaucoma as the edges accumulate edema from the increase pressure of the anterior chamber. The cornea should not take up fluorescein. LP (d) is used to diagnose intracranial pathology. The acute unilateral pain of glaucoma may make the clinician consider a SAH, but glaucoma should always be considered. A change in visual acuity (e) is nonspecific and should not diagnostic for glaucoma.

303. The answer is b. *(Kao, pp 985–1018.)* The patients are experiencing symptoms of *CO poisoning*. CO is *colorless* and *odorless*. Patients often present with mild nonspecific symptoms including headache, malaise, and fatigue. Severe toxicity manifests as neurologic and cardiac toxicity. Severe cases may manifest as disseminated intravascular coagulation, circulatory shock, multiorgan failure, ischemic cardiac disease, renal failure, or noncardiogenic pulmonary edema. Although there is decreased blood oxygen content, patients will not exhibit cyanosis as there is not enough deoxyhemoglobin present to cause it. Common sources of CO include fossil fuel burning engines, fumes from coal or gas burning stoves, and smoke from accidental fires. CO intoxication is more prevalent during the winter when potentially faulty heating systems are in use or when patients attempt to supplement their home heat using their oven. Initial therapy is aimed at increasing arterial oxygen content by providing supplemental oxygen. Mild intoxication can be managed with supplementary oxygen alone. Elevated carboxyhemoglobin levels require treatment with hyperbaric oxygen.

Respiratory isolation (a) is indicated in cases of suspected bacterial meningitis where *N. meningitidis* is thought to be the causative organism.

Antibiotics and LP (**c**) are appropriate if you suspect meningitis. Triptans and antiemetics (**d**) are first-line treatments for migraine headaches. Transfer to a hyperbaric facility (**e**) is indicated for persistent altered mental status, loss of consciousness, seizure, stroke, myocardial ischemia, or pregnancy with a documented carboxyhemoglobin level greater than 15%.

304. The answer is a. (*Evans, pp 237–249.*) After head trauma, 30–90% of patients complain of headache during their convalescence. *Postconcussive headaches* are notable for their *variability* in frequency, location, and associated symptoms. They are often exacerbated by physical activity or changes in position and may be clinically difficult to distinguish from other headache syndromes. In patients with preexisting migraines, increased frequency of their normal migraine syndrome is often noted. Most patients have resolution of their headaches after 4 weeks. In 20% of patients, their postconcussive headache persists for longer than a year. Headache may be one feature of a larger postconcussive syndrome including nervous system instability. This may include fragmentation of sleep, emotional lability, inability to tolerate crowds, restlessness, inability to concentrate, and anxiety.

Posttraumatic hydrocephalus (**b**) is a rare complication of minor head trauma. It presents with signs and symptoms of increased ICP including headache, gait instability, dizziness, nausea, and vomiting. It is often transient and may appear as a mild dilatation of the ventricles. Subdural hygromas (**c**) can occur in the weeks following a trauma or may appear as incidental findings. They occasionally increase in size causing symptoms due to mass effect. Cluster headaches (**d**) happen daily at the same time for days or weeks. They are unilateral, short, and boring in quality. The autonomic instability of posttraumatic nervous instability overlaps considerably with posttraumatic stress disorder (**e**), which has led some researchers to postulate that they share a similar mechanism.

305. The answer is d. (*Harrison, pp 2033–2034.*) The patient presents with symptoms consistent with a *prolactin-secreting pituitary adenoma*. The appropriate imaging modality to diagnose a pituitary adenoma is with high resolution MRI with thin cuts through the sella. Women often present with amenorrhea, infertility, and galactorrhea. Men will present with decreased libido. In both cases, extension beyond the sella may present with visual field defects or other mass-related symptoms.

(**a**) Noncontrast and contrast enhanced CT are not particularly sensitive for these lesions that sit in the sella turcica. Bromocriptine (**b**) or other centrally acting dopamine agonists are used to treat pituitary macro- and microadenomas. The presence of RBCs or xanthrochromia in the CSF (c) is diagnostic for a SAH. The clinical presentation is inconsistent with SAH. (e) Removing CSF is treatment for idiopathic intracranial hypertension.

306. The answer is a. (*Scheinfeld N, Teratology and Drug Use during Pregnancy, eMedicine 2006.*) *Antiepileptic medications* are sometimes used as prophylaxis for migraines. Phenytoin, valproic acid, phenobarbitol, and topiramate are among the antiepileptics commonly used to prevent migraines. Phenytoin causes *fetal hydantoin syndrome,* a constellation of birth defects including growth retardation, cleft palates, hand deformities, and structural cardiac defects. Valproic acid has similar effects with the addition of *neural tube defects.* Phenobarbitol, declining in its use for migraine prevention, causes cardiac defects, facial clefts, and urinary tract abnormalities. Early data on topiramate reveals teratogenicity in animal models.

β-Blockers (b) are generally safe during pregnancy. There is significant controversy over the safety of using triptans (c) during pregnancy. The concern is that their vasoconstrictive properties might cause uterine vessels to constrict, limiting fetal blood flow. Most research has shown infants born to mothers taking triptans during pregnancy have rates of birth defects no higher than background. Hypertension and cardiac conditions are primary contraindications to triptan therapy, and the drug should be discontinued if early preeclampsia is suspected. Acetaminophen and antiemetics (d and e) are generally safe to take during pregnancy.

Weakness and Dizziness

Questions

307. A 78-year-old man presents to the emergency department (ED) complaining of left arm weakness that started 10 minutes ago in the clinic. The patient states that he has a history of hypertension and diabetes, but has never had similar symptoms in the past. He is feeling well otherwise. His blood pressure (BP) is 157/85 mm Hg, heart rate (HR) is 87 beats per minute, temperature is 98.8°F, and respiratory rate (RR) is 14 breaths per minute. His neurologic exam is unremarkable and the patient embarrassingly states that his left arm is no longer weak. Which of the following is the most likely diagnosis?

a. Thrombotic stroke
b. Hemorrhagic stroke
c. Migraine with focal neurological deficit
d. Transient ischemic attack (TIA)
e. Todd's paralysis

308. A 56-year-old man presents to the ED complaining of intermittent lightheadedness and nausea throughout the day. He believes it started after eating leftover shrimp salad in the morning. On further questioning, he reports that during the lightheadedness episodes the room is spinning around him and the episodes are triggered by turning his head to the right. He denies hearing loss, tinnitus or other associated symptoms. His BP is 137/85 mm Hg, HR is 67 beats per minute, temperature is 98.5°F, and RR is 14 breaths per minute. The patient reproduces the symptoms by turning his head to the right. Which of the following is the most likely diagnosis?

a. Benign positional vertigo (BPV)
b. Food poisoning
c. Meniere's disease
d. Labyrinthitis
e. TIA

309. A 29-year-old woman presents to the ED complaining of double vision for 3 days. She states that she has been feeling very tired lately, particularly at the end of the day, when even her eyelids feel heavy. She feels better in the morning and after lunch when she is able to rest for an hour. Her BP is 132/75 mm Hg, HR is 70 beats per minute, temperature is 98.4°F, and RR is 12 breaths per minute. On exam you find ptosis and proximal muscle weakness. What is the most appropriate diagnostic test?

a. Perform an edrophonium test
b. Send blood to check the hematocrit
c. Order a head computed tomography (CT) scan
d. Send blood to check the electrolytes
e. Perform a lumbar puncture

The next two questions are based on the following vignette.

310. A 40-year-old woman is brought to the ED by the paramedics complaining of bilateral foot weakness and numbness that started a few hours ago and is progressively worsening. She denies similar episodes in the past. On the review of systems, she describes having abdominal cramps with nausea, vomiting, and diarrhea 2 weeks ago that resolved after 2-3 days. Her BP is 124/67 mm Hg, HR is 68 beats per minute, temperature is 98.8°F, and RR is 12 breaths per minute. On exam, you elicit 2/5 strength, decreased sensation, and loss of deep tendon reflexes in the lower extremities below the hips. Which of the following is the most likely diagnosis?

a. Middle cerebral artery (MCA) occlusion
b. Guillain-Barré syndrome
c. Peripheral vascular disease
d. Tetanus
e. Brain abscess

311. What life-threatening complication is associated with this disease process?

a. Permanent paralysis
b. Thrombocytopenia
c. Respiratory failure
d. Need for surgery
e. Kidney failure

312. A 58-year-old man presents to the ED complaining of generalized weakness for the last 2 days. He states that a few days ago he had abdominal cramps, vomiting, and diarrhea when his whole family got sick after a picnic. These symptoms resolved a day and a half ago but he has not been eating well and now feels weak all over. The patient has a history of hypertension for which he takes hydrochlorothiazide (HCTZ), which was recently increased. His BP is 144/87 mm Hg, HR is 89 beats per minute, temperature is 98.7°F, and RR is 12 breaths per minute. The physical exam reveals hyporeflexia. His electrocardiogram (ECG) is shown below. Which of the following is the most likely diagnosis?

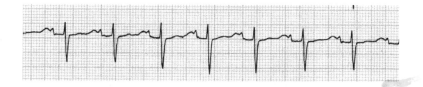

a. Hypernatremia
b. Hyponatremia
c. Hyperkalemia
d. Hypokalemia
e. Hypercalcemia

313. A 69-year-old man is brought to the ED by his son, who states that his father developed left arm and leg weakness this afternoon and now has difficulty walking. The patient states that he has a history of heart palpitations and recently stopped taking his blood thinning medicine because it was giving him an upset stomach. His BP is 165/90 mm Hg, HR is 97 beats per minute, temperature is 98.9°F, and RR is 16 breaths per minute. You suspect the patient is having a stroke and rush him to the CT scanner. The result of the head CT is seen below. What percentage of all stroke patients will have this type of stroke?

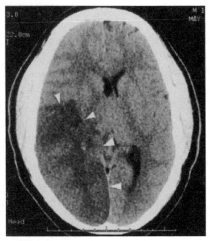

(Reproduced, with permission, from Brunicardi CF et al. Schwartz's Principles of Surgery. New York, NY: McGraw-Hill, 2005: 1616.)

a. 20%
b. 40%
c. 60%
d. 80%
e. 95%

The next two questions are based on the following vignette.

314. A 35-year-old woman presents to the ED complaining of left arm weakness and right facial pain for 1 day. She denies any past medical history, but on the review of systems remembers having pain and decreased vision in her left eye approximately 4 months ago that has since resolved. She attributed it to being stressed and tired and did not see a physician at the time. Her BP is 126/75 mm Hg, HR is 76 beats per minute, temperature is 98.8°F, and RR is 12 breaths per minute. The physical exam is unremarkable except for 3/5 strength in the left upper extremity. Which of the following is the most likely diagnosis?

a. Anxiety
b. Multiple sclerosis (MS)
c. Vertebrobasilar artery occlusion
d. Encephalitis
e. Varicella zoster

315. Which of the following is the most appropriate next step in management?

a. Obtain white blood cell count
b. Obtain an ECG
c. Perform a lumbar puncture and send cerebrospinal fluid (CSF) for culture
d. Obtain a head CT
e. Obtain a head magnetic resonance imaging (MRI)

316. A 52-year-old woman is brought to the ED by emergency medical service (EMS) complaining of weakness, dizziness, and mild confusion for the last hour. Per EMS report, the patient's coworkers called 911 soon after lunch when the patient started to complain of weakness and lightheadedness and became confused. The patient has a medical history of hypertension and diabetes, and was recently started on insulin. The patient's BP is 158/85 mm Hg, HR is 73 beats per minute, temperature is 98.7°F, and RR is 14 breaths per minute. The patient appears weak, pale, and confused. Which of the following is the most appropriate next step?

a. Send arterial blood gas with electrolytes
b. Send cardiac enzymes
c. Check capillary glucose level
d. Obtain ECG
e. Administer aspirin

317. A 58-year-old woman is brought to the ED by paramedics complaining of worsening left leg weakness for 1 hour. She reports a history of hypertension, diabetes, and smoking. She denies any past surgeries. Her BP is 165/83 mm Hg, HR is 110 beats per minute, temperature is 98.4°F, RR is 18 breaths per minute, pulse oxymetry is 98% on room air, and capillary glucose is 147 mg/dL. On exam, the patient appears anxious and has 2/5 strength and decreased sensation in left lower extremity. The patient's head CT is normal. It has been 100 minutes since the onset of symptoms. Which of the following is the most appropriate next step in management?

a. Perform rapid sequence intubation
b. Administer nitroprusside
c. Administer heparin
d. Administer fibrinolytic therapy
e. Administer aspirin 325 mg

318. A 37-year-old woman presents to urgent care complaining of general weakness and blurry vision over the last month. She states that she feels great in the morning, but by dinner she has trouble cooking and complains of double vision. Her husband notices that her eyelids sometimes look droopy in the evening. On physical exam, her cranial nerves are intact, pupils are equal and reactive, extraocular muscles are intact; however, you notice slight ptosis. What is the most likely diagnosis of this patient?

a. Botulism
b. Lambert-Eaton myasthenic syndrome
c. Tick paralysis
d. Guillian-Barre syndrome
e. Myasthenia gravis

319. A 63-year-old woman accompanied by her husband is brought to the ED by EMS with worsening right arm weakness that started 90 minutes ago at the opera. Her husband states that she has a history of hypertension and a long smoking history. She has no surgical history. The husband states that his wife was fine when going to the opera. The patient's BP is 215/118 mm Hg, HR is 97 beats per minute, temperature is 99.3°F, and RR is 14 breaths per minute. On exam, the patient is anxious, mildly aphasic, has 2/5 strength and diminished sensation in the right upper extremity. An emergent head CT scan is normal. It has been 2 hours since the onset of symptoms. Which of the following is the most appropriate next step in management?

a. Administer labetalol
b. Administer fibrinolytic therapy
c. Administer aspirin 325 mg
d. Administer phenytoin
e. Administer mannitol

320. A 46-year-old woman presents to the ED with her husband complaining of flu-like symptoms, headache, vomiting, and dyspnea. She states that she never had similar symptoms in the past and that her husband is getting sick with similar symptoms as well but refuses to see a doctor. She reports feeling well yesterday and even helped her husband set up a home generator in their garage. Her BP is 142/85 mm Hg, HR is 97 beats per minute, temperature is 100.6°F, and RR is 20 breaths per minute. On exam the patient is slow to respond to questions. Which of the following is the most appropriate diagnostic test?

a. Send blood to check the white blood cell count
b. Order a head CT scan
c. Send blood to check the carboxyhemoglobin level
d. Perform a lumbar puncture
e. No testing is necessary at this point

321. An 82-year-old right-handed woman is brought to the ED by her daughter stating that her mother has not been able to walk after waking up from a nap 30 minutes ago. The patient has a history of hypertension and diabetes. Her BP is 179/76 mm Hg, HR is 91 beats per minute, temperature is 98.9°F, and RR is 14 breaths per minute. On exam, you elicit neurological deficits and emergently bring her to the CT scanner. The radiologist tells you there is an abnormality in the left parietal lobe and a likely MCA stroke. Which of the following motor deficits are you likely to find in this patient?

a. Right sensorimotor deficit in arm greater than leg and aphasia
b. Left sensorimotor deficit in arm greater than leg and aphasia
c. Right sensorimotor deficit in leg greater than arm, slowed response to questions, and impaired judgment
d. Right motor deficit and left facial droop
e. Right leg hemiplegia only

322. A 67-year-old man is brought to the ED by his wife who states that her husband's face looks different and that he has been nauseated, vomiting, and unsteady on his feet since yesterday. The patient also states that he has been having blurry vision and difficulty swallowing, in addition to feeling like the room is tilting from side to side. The patient attributes this to eating leftover salmon last night. The patient's past medical history is notable for obesity and hypertension. His BP is 187/89 mm Hg, HR is 86 beats per minute, temperature is 99.3°F, and RR is 13 breaths per minute. On exam, you find a right facial droop, diplopia, vertical nystagmus, and severe ataxia. Which of the following is the most likely diagnosis?

a. Gastroenteritis
b. BPV
c. Labyrinthitis
d. Basilar artery occlusion
e. Vertebrobasilar artery occlusion

323. A 45-year-old man presents to the ED complaining of recurrent episodes of lightheadedness and nausea overnight. He describes the episodes as a room swaying from side-to-side when he lies on his left side. He reports mild headache now and denies tinnitus, hearing loss, fevers, or vomiting. He has no medical problems and takes no medications except for occasional acetaminophen. His BP is 123/65 mm Hg, HR is 69 beats per minute, temperature is 98.5°F, and RR is 12 breaths per minute. The patient is asymptomatic now and the exam is unremarkable. Which of the following is the most appropriate diagnostic test?

a. Dix-Hallpike maneuver
b. Caloric stimulation testing
c. Orthostatic vital signs
d. Head CT scan
e. ECG

324. A 9-month-old boy is brought to the ED by EMS. His mother states that for the last 2 days he had several episodes of vomiting, has been eating poorly and is now lethargic, drooling, and whimpering. The patient has not had fevers, diarrhea, cough, or runny nose. His mother mentions that she expanded his diet recently, with the latest addition of honey rice cakes to the food. The patient was born at term by a vaginal delivery, without any complications. All immunizations are up-to-date. His BP is 100/60 mm Hg, HR is 120 beats per minute, temperature is 99.1°F, and RR is 8 breaths per minute. On exam you find a lethargic, well-developed boy with poor muscle tone, weak cry, drooling, and droopy eyelids. Which of the following is the most likely diagnosis?

a. Sepsis
b. Tetanus
c. Guillain-Barré syndrome
d. Botulism
e. Dehydration

325. A 23-year-old woman presents to the ED complaining of dizziness and weakness for 2 days. She complains that she does not have energy to perform her duties at work and even gets short of breath going up the stairs to her third-floor apartment. She denies shortness of breath at rest, fevers, nausea, vomiting, diarrhea, chest pain, headache, recent travel, or other associated symptoms. She does not have any medical problems and takes no medications. On further questioning, she reports that she is on day 9 of her menstrual period, which has been heavy. Her periods are regular and last about 10 days. Her BP is 122/75 mm Hg, HR is 108 beats per minute, temperature is 98.7°F, and RR is 12 breaths per minute. Physical exam is unremarkable except for pale conjunctiva and mild tachycardia. Which of the following is the most appropriate initial diagnostic test?

a. Basic metabolic panel
b. Complete blood count
c. Obtain ECG
d. Obtain chest x-ray
e. Obtain chest CT with contrast

326. A 57-year-old man presents to the ED with generalized weakness and pain, abdominal discomfort, and nausea for 2 days. On the review of systems he also admits to recent polydypsia, polyuria, and a 10 lb weight loss. His medical history includes hypertension for which he takes no medications. He has a 20-pack-year smoking history. The vital signs are remarkable for mild tachycardia and hypertension. Laboratory results reveal a calcium level of 12.6 mEq/L. Which of the following is the most appropriate next step in management?

a. Administer calcitonin
b. Start 0.9% normal saline intravenous (IV) bolus
c. Administer furosemide IV
d. Obtain chest radiograph
e. Obtain ECG

327. A 46-year-old woman presents to the ED with left-sided arm and leg weakness for half an hour. She has no medical problems except for chronic neck pain after a motor vehicle collision 5 years ago. On exam she has right eye miosis, partial ptosis, and 3/5 strength in her left upper and lower extremities. Which of the following is consistent with the patient's ocular findings?

a. Homan's sign
b. Bell's palsy
c. Horner syndrome
d. Kehr's sign
e. Nikolsky's sign

328. On further questioning, the patient above states that earlier in the day she saw a chiropractor for her neck pain. After the session she developed severe right-sided neck pain. About an hour later she noticed difficulty using her left side of her body. Which of the following is the most likely diagnosis?

a. Internal carotid artery dissection
b. Cavernous sinus syndrome
c. MS
d. Lung neoplasm
e. Herpes zoster infection

329. A 64-year-old man presents to the ED complaining of an episode of vertigo he experienced while exercising in the gym today. He states that he has been having similar episodes with exercise for a week. His routine consists of running on a treadmill, lifting weights, and doing leg presses. The vertigo usually occurs mid-routine when he is lifting weights and resolves with cessation of exercise. He also noticed unusual left arm pain during these episodes. He has hypertension for which he takes antihypertensive medication and had a myocardial infarction 6 years ago. He decreased his smoking from 1 pack-per-day to 5 cigarettes per day over the last 6 years. His BP in the right arm is 148/80 mm Hg and 129/74 mm Hg in the left arm. Which of the following is the most likely diagnosis?

a. Musculoskeletal pain
b. BPV
c. Subclavian steal syndrome
d. Angina pectoris
e. Vestibular neuronitis

330. A 3-year-old girl is brought to the ED by her mother for fever and weakness over the last 4 days. Mom states that the child has been having high fevers at home and was diagnosed with a viral syndrome by her pediatrician 2 days ago. Since then, the child feels weak, is complaining of diffuse aches, and is eating poorly. She also developed a rash and her eyes are red. On exam the patient appears dehydrated, with red cracked lips, strawberry-like tongue, conjunctival injection, edematous hands, and a diffuse papular rash. Which of the following is the most likely diagnosis?

a. Botulism
b. Rocky Mountain spotted fever (RMSF)
c. Scarlet fever
d. Kawasaki disease
e. Niacin deficiency

331. For the patient in the previous clinical scenario, which of the following is the most appropriate management?

a. High-dose aspirin and IV immunoglobulin
b. Doxycycline IV
c. Ibuprofen and IV steroids
d. Vancomycin IV and ceftriaxone IV
e. Plasmaphoresis

332. A 36-year-old woman presents to the ED complaining of worsening weakness over the past few weeks. She states that initially she attributed it to being overworked but for the last few days she has been having unusual difficulty getting out of chair or walking the steps to her fourth-floor apartment. She has no prior medical history and takes no medications. Her vital signs are unremarkable. On exam she has 5/5 strength in her bilateral upper and lower extremities distally but 3/5 strength proximally. Sensory exam and reflexes are normal. You also notice a red confluent macular rash on her eyelids. Which of the following is the most likely diagnosis?

a. Myasthenia gravis
b. MS
c. Dermatomyositis
d. Rhabdomyolysis
e. Disseminated gonococcal infection

333. A 32-year-old woman presents to the ED complaining of sudden onset of left facial weakness that began half an hour ago that was noticed by her coworker. She denies having medical problems or taking medications. On the review of systems she admits to subjective fevers, fatigue, and arthralgias for the last week, which she attributed to the flu. She also reports having a rash on the back of her thigh a month ago, around the time she was hiking in Rhode Island. On exam she has left facial paralysis. Which of the following is the most likely diagnosis?

a. Bell's palsy
b. Lyme disease
c. Ramsay Hunt syndrome
d. Brain tumor
e. RMSF

334. A 24-year-old woman presents to the ED complaining of dizziness and numbness and tingling in her fingertips with decreased range of motion. Her initial vitals include a HR of 100 beats per minute, a RR of 30 breaths per minute with an oxygen saturation of 100% on room air. The patient denies any other symptoms. Upon physical examination, the patient appears anxious, tachypneic with a clawed appearance to both hands which are difficult to range. An arterial blood gas is drawn that shows a pH of 7.55 with a decreased carbon dioxide level and normal bicarbonate level. Which of the following underlying metabolic disturbances is responsible for this patient's symptoms?

a. Metabolic acidosis
b. Metabolic alkalosis
c. Respiratory acidosis
d. Respiratory alkalosis
e. Hyperthyroidism

Weakness and Dizziness

Answers

307. The answer is d. *(Rosen, p 1435.)* The patient had a *TIA*, which involves *neurological deficits that resolve within 24 hours of onset.* TIAs often precede ischemic stroke; up to 50% of patients with a TIA will have a stroke in the next 5 years, with the highest incidence in the first month. It is important to recognize TIAs and to evaluate patients for *cardiac or carotid arterial sources of emboli.* Although the symptoms often resolve, many patients with a TIA will have evidence of infarction on CT/MRI.

The patient did not have a thrombotic **(a)** or hemorrhagic **(b)** stroke. Neurologic deficits are not transient in a cerebral vascular accident. Although migraine auras can include focal neurological deficits **(c)**, the patient in the vignette does not have a history of migraines and is not complaining of a headache. Todd's paralysis **(e)** is a transient focal neurological deficit that persists after a seizure.

308. The answer is a. *(Tintinalli, p 1404.)* BPV is a transient positional vertigo associated with nystagmus. The problem occurs secondary to the creation and movement of canaliths (free-moving densities) in the semicircular canals of the inner ear with a particular head movement. Neurologic deficits are absent in BPV. Note that horizontal, vertical, or rotary *nystagmus* can occur in BPV. It is important to pay special attention to a patient with vertical nystagmus because it may be associated with a brainstem or cerebellum lesion. BPV is treated with the *Epley maneuver* (a series of head and body turns that reposition the canalith), antiemetics, and antihistamines.

Food poisoning **(b)** would not cause vertigo. If it is associated with vomiting and diarrhea, it can lead to dehydration and lightheadedness but not vertiginous symptoms. Meniere's disease **(c)**, is an inner ear disease of unclear etiology. It presents with recurrent attacks of vertigo and tinnitus, with deafness of the involved ear between attacks. Labyrinthitis **(d)** presents with hearing loss and sudden, brief positional vertigo attacks. TIAs **(e)** involving the vertebrobasilar system can present with vertigo but is an unlikely diagnosis in this case of recurrent positional vertiginous symptoms.

309. The answer is a. *(Rosen, p 1522.)* High clinical suspicion in this case is for *myasthenia gravis,* an autoimmune condition in which *acetylcholine receptor antibodies* block acetylcholine binding and prevent normal neuromuscular conduction. The disease typically affects young women and older men and presents with *generalized weakness worsening with repetitive muscle use that is usually relieved with rest.* Ptosis and diplopia are usually present. The *edrophonium test* is used to help diagnose myasthenia gravis. It involves administering edrophonium, a short-acting anticholinesterase, which prevents acetylcholine breakdown. With the increased acetylcholine levels at the neuromuscular junction, the patient experiences a brief return of strength.

310. The answer is b. *(Rosen, pp 120–122.)* The patient has a *progressive ascending peripheral neuropathy,* also known as *Guillain-Barré syndrome.* Patients can usually remember a preceding viral illness, usually gastroenteritis. *Deep tendon reflexes are typically absent.*

MCA occlusion **(a)** would present with contralateral, not symmetric, findings. Peripheral vascular disease **(c)**, a common complication of long-standing diabetes, causes paresthesias in the distal lower extremities and not acute paralysis. Tetanus **(d)** manifests as muscular rigidity due to the *Clostridium tetani* toxin preventing release of inhibitory neurotransmitters. Lockjaw is a common complaint in generalized tetanus. A brain abscess **(e)** typically presents with fever, headache, and focal neurologic findings and is usually caused by an associated trauma, surgery, or infectious spread from another site.

311. The answer is c. *(Rosen, pp 120–122.)* Progressive paralysis in Guillain-Barré syndrome can rapidly ascend to the respiratory system and cause *respiratory failure.* Patients need to be monitored and provided ventilator support as necessary.

(a) Guillain-Barré syndrome is a transient, not permanent, condition. **(b, d, and e)** are not complications of the syndrome.

312. The answer is d. *(Tintinalli, p 172.)* This patient presents with *hypokalemia,* secondary to increased potassium losses through vomiting and diarrhea as well as reduced oral intake. Potassium deficiency results in hyperpolarization of the cell membrane and leads to *muscle weakness, hyporeflexia, intestinal ileus, and respiratory paralysis.* Characteristic ECG findings include flattened T waves, U waves, and prolonged QT and PR intervals.

Hyponatremia **(a)** and hypernatremia **(b)** mainly affect the central nervous system, resulting in headache, anorexia, lethargy, and confusion. In more severe cases, hyponatremia causes seizures, coma, and respiratory arrest; whereas patients with profound hypernatremia develop ataxia, tremulousness, and spasms. Hyperkalemia (c) can lead to cardiac dysrhythmias and typically exhibits distinctive ECG findings including peaked T waves, prolonged QT and PR intervals, and widened QRS complex that can progress to a sine wave pattern. Signs of hypercalcemia (e) include bony and abdominal pain, renal stones, and altered mental status (remembered by: "bones, stones, groans, and psychiatric overtones"). In addition, cardiac effects include bradycardia, heart blocks, and shortened QT interval on ECG.

313. The answer is d. *(Rosen, pp 1434–1435.)* The CT image shows a large hypodensity in the right parietal-occipital region representing an *ischemic stroke*. Ischemic strokes comprise *80%* of all strokes, with hemorrhagic strokes accounting for the other 20%. Ischemic events include *thrombotic* (thrombus forming at the site of an ulcerated atherosclerotic plaque), *embolic* (thrombus embolized to a distal site), and *lacunar* (small terminal artery occlusion) strokes. This patient likely had a cardioembolic secondary to atrial fibrillation. Atrial fibrillation is an important risk factor for an embolic stroke, particularly when patients are noncompliant with anticoagulation therapy, as the patient in the vignette. Intracranial bleeding secondary to a hemorrhagic event appears hyperdense on CT scan. The diagram below illustrates the cerebral circulation.

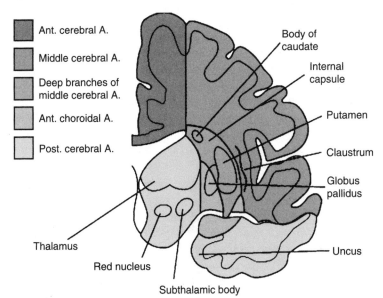

(Reproduced, with permission, from Kasper DL et al. Harrison's Principles of Internal Medicine. New York, NY. McGraw-Hill, 2005: 2381.) (Courtesy of CM Fisher, MD.))

314. The answer is b. (*Rosen, pp 253–254.*) Consider MS as a diagnosis in presentations of various neurological symptoms that are difficult to explain by a single CNS lesion, particularly those occurring in a female in her third decade of life. MS is a *multifocal demyelinating CNS disease* that in 30% of cases initially presents with *optic neuritis* (unilateral eye pain and decreased visual acuity).

Anxiety (**a**) is a diagnosis of exclusion and would not explain the objective arm weakness. Vertebrobasilar insufficiency (**c**) presents with cerebellar and brainstem symptoms, such as vertigo, dysphagia, and diplopia, none of which are present in this patient. Encephalitis (**d**) is an infection of brain parenchyma and presents with altered mental status that may be associated with focal neurologic deficits. Patients might present with behavioral and personality changes, seizures, headache, photophobia, and generalized symptoms of fever, nausea, and vomiting. Varicella Zoster (**e**), also known as shingles, is an infection caused by reactivation of latent Varicella virus. It typically occurs in a unilateral dermatomal distribution. The characteristic vesicular rash is often preceded by intense pain, burning, or itching sensation in the affected dermatomes.

315. The answer is e. (*Rosen, pp 2553–2554.*) Demyelinating MS lesions are often well demonstrated on *MRI* but cannot be visualized on CT scan.

White blood cell count (**a**) and ECG (**b**) are not going to contribute to the diagnosis. Performing a lumbar puncture (**c**) is a good idea as CSF can show oligoclonal banding and elevated protein, but there is no utility in sending CSF for culture since you do not suspect anything infectious.

316. The answer is c. (*Tintinalli, p 1283.*) Any patient with symptoms of weakness, dizziness, or confusion should get an immediate bedside check of *capillary glucose level* (fingerstick) to rule out *hypoglycemia*. The suspicion of hypoglycemia is particularly high in this case because the patient uses insulin for diabetes control. It is very important for patients to be educated about correct insulin use as incorrect dosing can have life-threatening consequences.

(**a**, **b**, and **d**) are good steps in the evaluation of this patient if the fingerstick is not diagnostic. They should not be the initial steps, however. Aspirin administration (**e**) is indicated if you suspect acute coronary syndrome.

317. The answer is d. (*Rosen, pp 1440–1442.*) The patient is a good candidate for *fibrinolytic therapy*. She is having an *acute ischemic stroke*, has no contraindications to the therapy and is being evaluated within the 3-hour therapeutic window from the onset of symptoms. Exclusion criteria for the use of thrombolytics include:

- evidence of intracranial hemorrhage on noncontrast head CT (absolute)
- minor or rapidly improving stroke symptoms
- clinical suspicion for subarachnoid hemorrhage
- active internal bleeding within last 21 days
- known bleeding diathesis
- within 3 months of serious head trauma, stroke, or intracranial surgery
- within 14 days of major surgery or serious trauma
- recent arterial puncture at noncompressible site
- lumbar puncture within 7 days
- history of intracranial hemorrhage, A-V malformation
- witnessed seizure at stroke onset
- recent myocardial infarction, or SBP >185 mm Hg or DBP >110 mm Hg

The head CT may initially appear normal and starts to show the extent of injury within 6-12 hours after the onset of symptoms.

Rapid sequence intubation (**a**) is unnecessary in this patient as her tachypnea is likely related to anxiety and not respiratory failure. She is protecting her airway, is alert and oriented, and has a normal lung exam and oxygen saturation on room air. However, if there are any signs of brain herniation, the patient should be intubated. (**b**) Only persistent SBP>220 mm Hg or MAP >130 mm Hg should be treated with labetalol or nitroprusside in an acute stroke. It is important to maintain a BP that is high enough to maintain cerebral perfusion. If fibrinolytic therapy is considered, labetalol should be used to lower BP below 185/110 mm Hg prior to the therapy. The benefit of heparin (**c**) in an ischemic stroke is unproven and it should not be given to the patient. Aspirin (**e**) should not be given within 24 hours of thrombolytic therapy since it increases the risk of hemorrhagic complications. Maintenance therapy with daily aspirin or another antiplatelet agent has been shown to help reduce stroke recurrence after a TIA.

318. The answer is e. (*Rosen, pp 1522–1524.*) *Myasthenia gravis* is an autoimmune disease of the *neuromuscular junction* that is more common in women in their 20s and 30s and men in their 70s and 80s. Myasthenia gravis results from autoantibodies directed against the nicotinic acetylcholine receptor at the neuromuscular junction. This leads to destruction of acetylcholine receptors and competition with acetylcholine for the remaining receptors. *Muscular weakness* and *fatigability* are the hallmarks of myasthenia gravis. Ocular symptoms manifest early and include ptosis, diplopia, and muscle weakness. Symptoms usually worsen as the day progresses. Diagnosis is usually made by the *edrophonium* or *Tensilon test*.

(a) Botulism is a toxin-mediated disease that causes acute weakness by the irreversible binding of botulinum toxin to the presynaptic membrane of nerves subsequently inhibiting the release of acetylcholine. The classic presentation of botulism is a descending, symmetric paralysis. Unlike myasthenia gravis, botulinum toxin decreases cholinergic output, which may lead to anticholinergic signs such as dilated pupils, dry skin, urinary retention, constipation, and increased temperature. (b) Lambert-Eaton myasthenic syndrome is often associated with small-cell carcinoma of the lung. Autoantibodies cause a decreased release of acetylcholine from presynaptic nerves. However, with repeated stimulation, the amount of acetylcholine in the synaptic cleft increases leading to an improvement of symptoms throughout the day. (c) Tick paralysis is due to a tick toxin that diminishes the release of acetylcholine. It classically presents as an ascending, flaccid motor paralysis. (d) Guillian-Barre syndrome is an ascending peripheral neuropathy classically presenting after a history of viral illness. It is associated with loss of deep tendon reflexes and earlier symmetric, distal weakness.

319. The answer is a. (*Rosen, pp 1440–1442.*) This patient's BP of 215/118 needs to be lowered *below 185/110 mm Hg* to make her a good candidate for *thrombolytic therapy*. *Labetalol* is the agent of choice in this case.

Fibrinolytic administration (b) at this level of hypertension carries a risk of intracranial bleed. Daily aspirin (c) has been shown to reduce the incidence of strokes. However, aspirin should not be administered within 24 hours of fibrinolytic use since it increases the risk of postthrombolytic bleed. Antiseizure prophylaxis with phenytoin (d) is not indicated in ischemic strokes although a small percentage of stroke patients will seize within the first 24 hours. Hyperventilation and mannitol (e) are used for temporary management of increased intracranial pressure due to cerebral edema in an ischemic stroke, which peaks at 72-96 hours. There is no role for mannitol in acute stroke in a patient without signs of elevated intracranial pressure.

320. The answer is c. (*Rosen, p 2169.*) Patients with initial flu-like symptoms *from the same household* who were exposed to combustion products (i.e., from a home generator) are at risk for *CO poisoning*. CO binds to hemoglobin with greater affinity than oxygen and shifts the oxygen-hemoglobin dissociation curve to the left, thus decreasing oxygen release. Clinically, patients with mild CO toxicity present with flu-like symptoms, nausea, and vomiting, which progresses to chest pain, dyspnea, confusion, seizures, dysrhythmias, and coma. CO level can be obtained by a *carboxyhemoglobin level* from blood. CO poisoning is treated with *oxygen* and, if severe, with *hyperbaric oxygen* therapy.

An important clue to the diagnosis is the development of similar symptoms in the patient and her husband at the same time. While it is important to consider ordering a white blood cell count (**a**), head CT scan (**b**), and lumbar puncture (**d**) for evaluation of the symptoms, think CO poisoning when there are multiple patients with the same symptoms in the setting of exposure to combustible products. It is not appropriate to do nothing (**e**) since the patient is clearly in need of medical attention.

321. The answer is a. (*Rosen, pp 1436–1437.*) Neurologic abnormalities of a stroke involving the MCA include *contralateral sensorimotor findings more pronounced in upper than lower extremity, aphasia, and ipsilateral hemianopsia.* Aphasia results from the involvement of the dominant hemisphere (left in most patients) in patients with a MCA stroke.

Choice (**b**) is incorrect since the findings are ipsilateral to the area of injury. Choice (**c**) describes deficits in the anterior cerebral artery (ACA) distribution with greater deficits in lower extremity and altered mentation due to frontal lobe involvement. Crossed deficits such as contralateral motor and ipsilateral cranial nerve findings (**d**) occur in brainstem strokes, which are supplied by the posterior circulation. Pure motor (**e**) or sensory loss occurs in lacunar infarcts, which involve small penetrating arteries.

322. The answer is e. (*Rosen, pp 1437–1438.*) Do not get confused with the multiple signs and symptoms in this case! They involve three distinct areas of the brain; the brainstem (facial droop, dysphagia, vertigo, and vertical nystagmus), cerebellum (ataxia, vertigo, and vertical nystagmus), and visual cortex (diplopia). All of these anatomical areas are supplied by the posterior circulation, specifically the *vertebrobasilar artery.* A mnemonic to help remember the presentation of a vertebrobasilar stroke is the "three D's": *dizziness (vertigo), dysphagia, and diplopia.*

(**a**) The patient's neurologic deficits and absence of diarrhea are not consistent with a diagnosis of gastroenteritis. BPV (**b**) is a transient positional vertigo associated with nystagmus. Neurologic deficits are absent in BPV. Note that horizontal, vertical, or rotary nystagmus can occur in BPV; however vertical nystagmus is *always* worrisome as it may indicate a brainstem or cerebellum lesion. Labyrinthitis (**c**), an infection of the labyrinth, presents with hearing loss and sudden brief positional vertigo attacks and does not involve other neurological deficits. Basilar artery occlusion (d) typically presents with quadriplegia, locked-in syndrome, or coma.

323. The answer is a. (*Tintinalli, p 1405.*) You should suspect *BPV* in this patient. BPV is a transient positional vertigo associated with nystagmus. The problem occurs secondary to the creation and movement of canaliths (free-moving densities) in the semicircular canals of the inner ear that is associated with a particular head movement. The *Dix-Hallpike maneuver* is a diagnostic test designed to reproduce transient vertiginous symptoms and nystagmus of BPV. The maneuver involves having the patient go from sitting to a supine position with eyes open and head rotated to the affected side. The test is positive if the maneuver reproduces vertigo and the patient exhibits latent rotary nystagmus. A negative Dix-Hallpike maneuver does not exclude the condition.

Caloric stimulation testing (b) is performed for acoustic nerve evaluation by introducing cold or warm water or air into an ear canal and observing transient nystagmus. It is unnecessary for BPV diagnosis. Orthostatic vital signs (c) should be obtained if you suspect orthostatic hypotension. The patient in this case is symptomatic when he lies down, not when he is standing or sitting up, which is not consistent with this diagnosis. Head CT scan (d) should be ordered if you suspect central, rather than peripheral causes of vertigo. ECG (e) is necessary if you suspect a cardiac cause of dizziness.

324. The answer is d. (*Tintinalli, p 988.*) The patient is exhibiting signs and symptoms of *infant botulism,* a paralytic illness caused by *Clostridium botulinum's toxin.* Infant, food-borne, and wound botulism are three types of the disease. Infant botulism is caused by ingestion of *Clostridium* spores, usually in *honey,* which then germinate and produce toxin in the intestines. The infant's immune system is not fully developed and cannot clear the infection. Botulinum toxin blocks release of acetylcholine at the synapse, resulting in a *flaccid paralysis,* described as a "floppy baby" in infants, consisting of poor muscle tone, weak cry, lethargy, and poor feeding. The symptoms progress to muscle paralysis and respiratory failure that require long-term ventilation and medical care. Children under the age of one should not be fed honey.

Although sepsis (a) should be considered, it is unlikely in an afebrile 9 month old with no clear source of infection. Tetanus (b), or rigid paralysis, results from a wound infection with *Clostridium tetani.* The bacterium produces a neurotoxin that prevents release of inhibitory neurotransmitters and causes muscle rigidity and contractions, essentially the opposite of the flaccid presentation of botulism. Guillain-Barré syndrome (**c**) is an ascending paralysis following an upper respiratory tract infection. Mild dehydration (**e**) could result from a few days of poor feeding and vomiting but does not account for the neurologic symptoms in this patient.

325. The answer is b. (*Rosen, p 1667.*) This woman presents with *iron-deficiency anemia* secondary to *menorrhagia*. A history of chronic heavy menses and pale conjunctiva on exam should make you suspicious of this common disorder. About 20% of women and 3% of men are iron deficient. *Complete blood count* provides *hemoglobin and hematocrit* levels to diagnose anemia. Typically, the mean corpuscular volume (MCV) is low in iron-deficiency anemia. In addition, the patient usually exhibits low serum iron, low serum ferritin, and a high total iron-binding capacity.

Electrolyte or renal function abnormalities (**a**) are unlikely in a young healthy woman. Except for tachycardia, the ECG (**c**) will be normal unless the patient has underlying cardiac disease, which can lead to ischemia in the setting of anemia. Chest x-ray (**d**) is not useful as an initial diagnostic test. It is appropriate to obtain it if you suspect a lung infiltrate, mass, congestive heart failure, or other cardiopulmonary disease. Chest CT with contrast (**e**) would help to diagnose a pulmonary embolism that may present with weakness, dyspnea on exertion, and tachycardia. In this case, however, the patient has no risk factors and has a better alternative diagnosis based on history and physical exam findings.

326. The answer is b. (*Tintinalli, p 176.*) This common presentation of *hypercalcemia* is initially managed with *aggressive isotonic saline IV hydration* to restore volume status. Hypercalcemia impairs renal concentrating ability, and patients typically present with *polyuria, polydypsia,* and *dehydration* and may develop *kidney stones.* Increased calcium levels also cause generalized weakness, bone pain, neurologic symptoms (ataxia, altered mental status), GI dysfunction (abdominal pain, nausea, vomiting, anorexia), and ECG abnormalities (shortened QT interval). A handy mnemonic for symptoms of hypercalcemia is "bones, stones, groans, and psychiatric overtones."

Calcitonin (**a**) decreases calcium levels by reducing bony osteoclast activity and intestinal calcium absorption. It does not produce an immediate effect and is generally not started in the ED. Loop diuretics such as furosemide (**c**) increase renal elimination of calcium but worsen volume depletion. Patients need to be hydrated first. Obtaining a chest radiograph (**d**) is a good idea while the patient is getting IV hydration. This patient has a significant smoking history and recent weight loss which should raise your suspicion of a neoplastic lung process causing hypercalcemia. Malignancy is an important cause of hypercalcemia; others include endocrine abnormalities (hyperparathyroidism, hyperthyroidism, pheochromocytoma, adrenal insufficiency), granulomatous disease (sarcoidosis, tuberculosis), drugs (thiazides, lithium), and immobilization. The patent's ECG (e) may show a shortened QT interval. Very high calcium levels may cause heart block.

327. The answer is c. (*Tintinalli, p 1463.*) Unilateral findings of ptosis and miosis as well as anhidrosis are seen in *Horner syndrome* which results from *interrupted sympathetic nerve supply to the eye.*

Homan's sign (**a**) refers to leg pain with dorsiflexion of the foot sometimes seen in patients with deep venous thrombosis. This sign has poor sensitivity and specificity. Bell's palsy (**b**) involves unilateral facial paralysis due to peripheral involvement of the facial nerve. In patients with a central facial nerve lesion the forehead is spared. Kehr's sign (**d**) refers to left shoulder pain associated with splenic rupture. Nikolsky's sign (**e**) is sloughing of the outer epidermal layer with rubbing of the skin seen in dermatologic diseases such as pemphigus vulgaris and scalded skin syndrome.

328. The answer is a. (*Tintinalli, pp 1387, 1463.*) This patient has an *internal carotid artery (ICA) dissection* secondary to chiropractic neck manipulation. ICA dissection can occur spontaneously or in minor neck trauma and should be considered in a *young patient with acute stroke.* ICA dissection should also be suspected in patients with *neck pain and Horner syndrome* due to the disruption of ipsilateral oculosympathetic fibers. In this scenario, it presents with ipsilateral Horner syndrome and contralateral ischemic motor deficits. Other causes of acute Horner syndrome include *tumors* (i.e., Pancoast tumor), stroke, herpes zoster infection, and trauma.

Cavernous sinus syndrome (**b**) presents with headache, ipsilateral eye findings, and sensory loss in the distribution of CN V-ophthalmic branch. Eye findings include proptosis, chemosis, Horner syndrome, and ophthalmoplegia due to the involvement of CN III, IV, and VI. It does not cause decreased strength in the extremities. MS (**c**) is an inflammatory demyelinating CNS disease resulting in various neurological abnormalities, such as optic neuritis, transverse myelitis, and paresthesias. Lung neoplasm, (**d**) such as Pancoast tumor, can cause ipsilateral Horner syndrome by invading cervical and thoracic ganglia carrying sympathetic fibers. Horner syndrome can be a rare complication of ophthalmic or thoracic herpes zoster infection (**e**), but left-sided motor deficits are inconsistent with the infectious etiology.

329. The answer is c. (*McIntyre KE, Subclavian Steal Syndrome, eMedicine 2006.*) This patient presents with *vertebrobasilar insufficiency* (vertigo) and *claudication* (atypical arm pain with exercise), symptoms consistent with *subclavian steal syndrome.* This phenomenon occurs in patients with subclavian artery occlusion or stenosis proximal to the vertebral artery branch, which causes retrograde blood flow in the vertebral artery with ipsilateral arm exercise. Collateral arteries arising from the subclavian artery distal to the obstruction deliver blood to the arm. During arm exercise these vessels dilate and siphon blood from the head, neck, and shoulder to increase perfusion of ischemic arm muscles. This results in temporary reversal of blood flow in the vertebral artery leading to vertebrobasilar insufficiency and symptoms of vertigo, dizziness, syncope, dysarthria, and diplopia. Arm pain is due to muscle ischemia.

The diagnosis of musculoskeletal pain (**a**) cannot explain the neurologic symptoms that this patient experiences with exercise. BPV (**b**) is a transient positional vertigo associated with nystagmus, nausea, and vomiting due to the movement of canaliths in the semicircular canals of the inner ear. It does not cause motor deficits. Angina pectoris (**d**) refers to myocardial ischemia caused by insufficient coronary blood flow to meet myocardial oxygen demand. It typically presents with symptoms of chest discomfort relieved with rest or nitroglycerin. Patients might complain of arm pain or radiation of pain to the arms, but the presentation does not involve neurologic deficits. Vestibular neuronitis (**e**) refers to acute self-limiting dysfunction of the peripheral vestibular system that causes vertigo.

330. The answer is d. (*Tintinalli, p 887.*) This child has *Kawasaki disease,* a generalized small- and medium-vessel vasculitis. The diagnostic criteria are fever lasting longer than 4 days and at least 4 out of 5 main features:

1. painful erythema and edema of palms and soles
2. polymorphic rash of trunk and extremities
3. lip and oropharyngeal mucosal changes
4. conjunctival injection
5. unilateral nontender cervical lymphadenopathy

This initial stage is followed by desquamation of the digits and development of coronary artery aneurysms which puts the patient at risk for sudden death.

Botulism (**a**) is a paralytic disease due to *Clostridium* neurotoxin. The toxin blocks acetylcholine release at the peripheral cholinergic terminals, and the disease generally presents as bilateral descending paralysis.

RMSF (**b**) is a tick-borne *Rickettsia rickettsii* infection. The disease involves constitutional symptoms of high fever, myalgias, severe headache, and a characteristic blanching erythematous macular rash which spreads from the distal extremities to the trunk. Scarlet fever (**c**) follows a group A β-hemolytic streptococcal infection in 10% of patients. It is mediated by a bacterial exotoxin, with a rash developing 12-48 hours after the onset of fever, sore throat, headache, abdominal pain, and malaise. Niacin deficiency (**e**) or pellagra is classically described as the "3D's": dermatitis, dementia, and diarrhea. The disease presents with weakness and anorexia with later development of erythematous pruritic lesions over sun-exposed skin, confusion, glossitis, abdominal pain, and diarrhea.

331. The answer is a. *(Tintinalli, p 887.)* High-dose aspirin and IV immunoglobulin have been shown to reduce fever, inflammation, and the rate of coronary artery aneurysms.

Doxycycline (**b**) is the antibiotic of choice for RMSF. It can also be given orally. Choices (**c**), (**d**), and (**e**) are incorrect.

332. The answer is c. *(Tintinalli, p 1418.)* This patient presents with *symmetric proximal muscle weakness* and characteristic *heliotrope rash* of *dermatomyositis*. It is an idiopathic inflammatory myopathy with associated dermatitis. The characteristic of the disease is progressive symmetric proximal muscle weakness with possible dysphagia, symmetric heliotrope rash in the periorbital region or neck, elevated creatinine kinase, and abnormal electromyogram and muscle biopsy. There is also an associated risk of malignancy.

Myasthenia gravis (**a**) is an autoimmune disorder of the neuromuscular junction in which antiacetylcholine receptor antibodies compete with acetylcholine at the nicotinic postsynaptic receptors. The disease causes characteristic progressive reduction in muscle strength with repeated muscle use. Bulbar muscles are most commonly involved, and patients report worsening of symptoms at night and improvement with rest or in the morning. MS (**b**) is an inflammatory demyelinating CNS disease resulting in various neurological abnormalities, such as optic neuritis, transverse myelitis, and paresthesias. Rhabdomyolysis (**d**) refers to muscle fiber breakdown due to a variety of etiologies, such as trauma, burns, ischemia, seizures, excessive muscular activities, sepsis, and myopathies. Its complications include hyperkalemia, metabolic acidosis, and acute renal failure. Disseminated gonococcal infection (**e**) is a systemic disease secondary to the presence of *Neisseria gonorrhoeae* in the bloodstream. In the early bacteremic phase patients present with fevers, migratory polyarthritis, and rash; this evolves from disseminated erythematous macules into hemor-rhagic pustular lesions. Serious complications may include meningitis, osteomyelitis, and endocarditis.

333. The answer is b. *(Tintinalli, p 970.)* This patient has *Lyme disease,* the most common vector-borne zoonotic infection in the United States. The spirochete, *Burrelia burgdorferi,* is transmitted to humans by the *deer tick Ixodes,* and although the risk of infection after a bite is about 3% in highly endemic areas (Northeast and Midwest); it increases to 25% if the tick is attached for longer than 72 hours. This patient presents in the second stage of Lyme disease. The first stage involves the development of *erythema migrans,* a spreading annular erythematous lesion with central clearing occurring com-monly at the tick bite site 2-20 days after the bite. The second stage typically occurs within 6 months of the initial infection and is characterized by fever, fatigue, arthralgias, neuropathies (i.e., Bell's palsy), cardiac abnormalities (i.e., myocarditis presenting with conduction delay), and multiple annular lesions. Tertiary stage of Lyme disease occurs year after the infection and con-sists of chronic arthritis, subacute encephalopathy, and polyneuropathy.

Primary and secondary stages of the disease are treated with doxycy-cline. Tertiary stage is treated with IV ceftriaxone or penicillin.

Some sources refer to any facial nerve palsy as Bell's palsy **(a)**, whereas most consider Bell's palsy an idiopathic facial nerve paralysis. An easy way to look at it is that facial nerve paralysis may have an identifiable cause or may be idiopathic, in which case it is referred to as Bell's palsy. In either case, exclude Lyme disease in patients with facial nerve palsy by sending Lyme titer levels. Ramsay Hunt syndrome **(c)** is a facial nerve palsy sec-ondary to Varicella-Zoster virus (VZV). VZV causes chicken pox and may remain dormant in nerve ganglia for years. In addition to CN VII paralysis, the syndrome is characterized by severe ear pain, vertigo, hearing loss, and classic shingles in the ear. A brain tumor **(d)** may cause facial nerve com-pression centrally and may present with partial facial paralysis with forehead sparing. The forehead is bilaterally innervated, and the intact contralateral branch provides motor function. RMSF **(e)** is a tick-borne *R. rickettsii* infec-tion. The disease involves constitutional symptoms of high fever, myalgias, severe headache and a characteristic blanching erythematous macular rash which spreads from distal extremities to the trunk.

334. The answer is d. *(Rosen, pp 1714–1723.)* This patient is tachypneic, probably due to some underlying anxiety, which has resulted in paresthesias, carpal spasm, and tetany. This occurs as a result of an alkalemic environment that decreases ionized calcium levels. The treatment is reassurance, a rebreathing mask allowing for carbon dioxide retention and possibly sedation. The patient's metabolic profile is consistent with a *respiratory alkalosis (elevated pH, low CO_2).*

The blood gas indicates a pure alkalosis therefore an acidosis is not seen **(a, c)**. The bicarbonate level is normal and therefore it is not due to a metabolic disturbance **(b)**. Patients with hyperthyroidism may be tachycardic, hyperthermic with an elevated BP. Upon physical examination, these patients may also appear to be underweight, have bulging eyes (exopthalmos) and complain of palpitations, diarrhea, tremors, and generalized anxiety. Hyperthyroidism is not a direct cause of tetany.

Fever

Questions

335. A 43-year-old male intravenous (IV) drug user presents to the emergency department (ED) with 2 weeks of fever, back pain, and progressive weakness in his arms bilaterally. He denies any history of recent trauma. His blood pressure (BP) is 130/75 mm Hg, heart rate (HR) is 106 beats per minute, temperature is 103°F, and respiratory rate (RR) is 16 breaths per minute. On physical exam, he has tenderness to palpation in the mid-thoracic spine, and decreased strength in the upper extremities bilaterally with normal range of motion. Laboratory results reveal a white blood cell (WBC) count of 15,500/μL, hematocrit 40%, and platelets 225/μL. Which of the following is the most likely diagnosis?

a. Thoracic disk herniation
b. Ankylosing spondylitis
c. Spinal epidural abscess
d. Vertebral compression fracture
e. Spinal metastatic lesion

336. A 23-year-old man presents to the ED with left lower abdominal pain and left testicular pain that started 1–2 weeks ago and has gradually worsened. He denies nausea and vomiting. His HR is 98 beats per minute, BP 125/65 mm Hg, temperature 103°F, and RR is 18 breaths per minute. Physical exam reveals a tender left testicle with a firm nodularity on the posteriolateral aspect of the testicle. Pain is relieved slightly with elevation of the testicle and the cremasteric reflex in normal. Which of the following is the next best step?

a. Prescribe pain medications and penicillin for coverage of syphilis
b. Recommend bed rest and scrotal elevation with urology follow-up
c. Attempt to untwist the left testicle by rotating it in a clockwise direction and order an immediate scrotal ultrasound
d. Give ceftriaxone 250 mg intramuscularly (IM), plus a 10-day course of oral doxycycline
e. Confirm the diagnosis with transillumination of the testicle, and then consult urology for surgical drainage

337. A 40-year-old diabetic man presents to the ED with severe perineal pain and fever to 103°F. Physical exam demonstrates crepitus over the medial thigh and widespread discoloration with sharp demarcation over the scrotum. The scrotum is warm and markedly edematous. His pain appears out of proportion to the physical exam. Which of the following is the most likely diagnosis?

a. Epididymitis
b. Fournier's gangrene
c. Scrotal edema
d. Paraphimosis
e. Testicular torsion

338. A 55-year-old man with a history of alcoholism and osteoarthritis developed left knee pain several days after a fall from standing height. The patient was brought to the ED by ambulance after being found on a park bench stating he was unable to walk because of the pain. On physical exam, his left knee is warm, diffusely tender, and swollen with a large effusion. He has pain on passive range of motion. His BP is 150/85 mm Hg, HR is 105 beats per minute, temperature is 102.7°F, RR is 16 breaths per minute, and fingerstick glucose is 89 mg/dL. Which of the following is the most appropriate diagnostic test?

a. Knee radiographs
b. Magnetic resonance imaging (MRI)
c. Erythrocyte sedimentation rate (ESR) and C-reactive protein
d. Arthrocentesis
e. Bone scan

339. A 43-year-old woman presents to the ED with fever, diarrhea, sweating, weight loss despite an increased appetite, and palpitations. She is accompanied by her family, who state that she has been acting a little confused over the last several days and that her mood is very labile. Her vitals are HR of 155 beats per minute, BP of 140/65 mm Hg, RR of 18 breaths per minute, and temperature 102°F. On physical exam, she is diaphoretic and appears agitated. She is tachycardic and, on pulmonary exam, has rales at the bases bilaterally. She has a tremor and a diffuse, nontender, enlargement of her anterior neck. Her electrocardiogram (ECG) shows sinus tachycardia. Labs are significant for an elevated free T4 and a low thryotropin, TSH. You order a chest x-ray (CXR), start IV fluids, and place her on a monitor. You order a dose of propranolol, which slows her HR and makes her more comfortable. Which of the following is the next most appropriate step in management?

a. Begin thyroid replacement and admit her to the hospital
b. Begin thyroid replacement and discharge her with close outpatient follow-up

c. Begin iodine then propylthiouracil (PTU), and admit her to an intensive care unit (ICU)

c. Begin iodine then PTU, and discharge her with close outpatient follow-up

d. Begin PTU then iodine, and admit her to an ICU

340. A 35-year-old woman with systemic lupus erythematosus (SLE) is brought to the ED by her brother after he found her febrile and confused. Physical exam reveals fever, tachycardia, a waxing and waning mental status, petechiae over her oral mucosa, pallor, and mildly heme-positive stool. Her urinalysis is positive for blood, red cell casts, and proteinuria. Laboratory results reveal a blood urea nitrogen (BUN) of 40 mg/dL, creatinine of 2 mg/dL. Her bilirubin is elevated (unconjugated > conjugated) and her International Normalized Ratio (INR) is 0.98. Her complete blood count reveals WBC 12,000/μL; Hct 29%; and platelet count 17,000/μL with schistocytes on the peripheral smear. Which of the following is the most appropriate next step in management?

a. Admit to the ICU for plasmaphoresis and close monitoring for acute bleeds

b. Transfuse platelets then admit to the ICU

c. Begin corticosteroids, transfuse platelets, and call surgery for immediate splenectomy

d. Arrange for emergent dialysis then admit to the ICU

e. Perform a noncontrast head computed tomography (CT) followed by a lumbar puncture (LP) for analysis of cerebrospinal fluid

341. A 30-year-old woman presents to the ED with fever, headache, a "sunburn-like" rash, and confusion. A friend states that the patient has complained of nausea, vomiting, diarrhea, and a sore throat over the past few days. Her last menstrual period began 4 days ago. Vital signs are HR 110 beats per minute, BP 80/45 mm Hg, RR of 18 breaths per minute, and temperature of 103°F. On physical exam, you note an ill-appearing female with a diffuse blanching erythroderma. Her neck is supple without signs of meningeal irritation. You note a fine desquamation of her skin, especially over the hands and feet, and hyperemia of her oropharyngeal, conjunctival, and vaginal mucus membranes. Laboratory results reveal a creatine phosphokinase (CPK) of 5000, WBC 15,000/μL, platelets of 90,000/μL, BUN 40 mg/dL, Cr 2 mg/dL, and elevated liver enzymes. Which of the following is the most likely causative organism?

a. *Staphylococcus aureus*

b. *Rickettsia rickettsii*

c. *Streptococcus pyogenes*

d. *Neisseria meningitidis*

e. *Neisseria gonorrhoeae*

342. A 32-year-old diabetic man steps on a nail through his running shoe. Two weeks later, he presents to the ED with fever and right foot pain. On physical exam, his heel is mildly erythematous and diffusely tender to palpation, with overlying warmth and edema. There is a small amount of purulent drainage through the puncture hole in his heel. A plain radiograph of his foot demonstrates a slight lucency of the calcaneus. He has decreased range of motion, but you are able to passively dorsiflex and plantarflex his ankle without difficulty. His vital signs are temperature 101.4°F, HR 98 beats per minute, BP 130/75 mm Hg, and RR 16 breaths per minute. For adult patients with osteomyelitis, which of the following is the most common causative organism?

a. *Salmonella* sp.
b. *Pseudomonas aeruginosa*
c. *S. aureus*
d. Group B *Streptococci*
e. *Pasteurella multocida*

343. A 55-year-old man presents to the ED with fever, drooling, trismus, and a swollen neck. He reports a foul taste in his mouth since a tooth extraction 2 days ago. On physical exam, the patient appears anxious. He has bilateral submandibular swelling and elevation and protrusion of the tongue. He appears "bull-necked" with tense and markedly tender edema and brawny induration of the upper neck, and he is tender over the lower second and third molars. There is no cervical lymphadenopathy. His vital signs are a HR 105 beats per minute, BP 140/85 mm Hg, RR 26 breaths per minute, and temperature 102°F. Which of the following is the most appropriate next step in management?

a. Administer a dose of oral antibiotics and obtain a soft-tissue radiograph of the neck
b. Place the patient in a supine position, perform incision and drainage at the bedside, and start IV antibiotics
c. Begin steroids to decrease inflammation and obtain an ear, nose, and throat (ENT) consult
d. Discharge the patient with oral antibiotics and ENT follow-up
e. Secure his airway, start IV antibiotics, and obtain an emergent ENT consult

344. A 67-year-old woman presents to the ED with a painful facial rash that has been worsening over the past 2 days. On physical exam, she has a deeply erythematous, shiny area of warm and tender skin on her left face with a sharply-demarcated and indurated border. There is minimal edema. Vitals are HR 88 beats per minute, BP 125/70 mm Hg, RR 16 breaths per minute, and temperature 101°F. Which of the following is the most appropriate next step in management?

a. IV antibiotics and hospital admission
b. Oral cephalexin four times daily for 10 days
c. Oral acyclovir 800 mg five times daily for 7 days
d. Systemic steroids and immunosuppression
e. Dermatology consult and biopsy of the rash

345. A 3-year-old boy is brought to the ED by his mother with 5 days of rash, fever, and a tender lump on his neck. The mother states his pediatrician prescribed acetaminophen 2 days ago, but his fever has not resolved despite the medicine. On physical exam, the boy appears irritable. His lips appear dry, red, fissured, and crusted and his tongue is hyperemic with prominent lingual papillae. The conjunctivae are injected bilaterally without discharge. He has a polymorphous rash with confluent, erythematous patches, and plaques on the soles of his feet. His neck exam is notable for a 1.5 cm right anterior lymph node. Vitals are HR 160 beats per minute, RR 22 breaths per minute, and temperature 102°F. In additional to medical treatment, this boy will require which of the following?

a. Hemodialysis
b. LP
c. Lymph node biopsy
d. Echocardiogram
e. Testing for fluorescent treponemal antibody absorption (FTA-ABS)

346. A 22-year-old college student presents to the ED with a painful, swollen finger. He states that he was playing with a roommate's dog and was bitten 3 days earlier. On physical exam, vitals are HR 70 beats per minute, BP 115/65 mm Hg, RR 16 breaths per minute, and temperature 101.6°F. Bilaterally, the radial pulses remain equal, and the hands and fingers are intact to sensation. His right second finger is held in flexion, and is symmetrically swollen from the distal tip to the metacarpalphalangeal joint. Both your attempt to extend the digit passively and palpate the flexor tendon sheath produce great pain. Based on these findings you make your diagnosis and notify the hand surgeon immediately. What name is given to the criteria used to make the diagnosis?

a. Finkelstein
b. Trousseau
c. Tinel
d. Kanavel
e. Phalen

347. A 47-year-old man presents to Urgent Care complaining of a 2-day history of sore throat and subjective fever at home. He denies cough or vomiting. His BP is 130/75 mm Hg, HR is 85 beats per minute, temperature is 101°F, and his RR is 14 breaths per minute. He has tonsillar swelling but no exudates and bilateral enlarged and tender lymph nodes of the neck. The rapid streptococcal antigen test is negative. Which of the following is the next best step in management?

a. Administer penicillin and discharge the patient
b. Schedule a lymph node biopsy to rule out lymphoma
c. Observe for 6 hours
d. Perform a throat culture, symptomatic care, and treat if results are positive
e. Administer amantadine to patient and all contacts

348. A 28-year-old man who just finished a 7-day course of antibiotics for pharyngitis presents to the ED with progressive difficulty swallowing. His BP is 130/65 mm Hg, HR is 95 beats per minute, temperature is 100.1°F, RR is 16 breaths per minute, and O_2 saturation is 99%. On exam, the patient is in no acute distress but has a fluctuant mass on the right side of the soft palate with deviation of the uvula. Which of the following is the most appropriate next step in management?

a. Needle aspiration, antibiotics, and follow up in 24 hours
b. Pain control, observation for 6 hours
c. Admission for incision and drainage in the OR
d. Antibiotics and follow up in 24 hours
e. CT scan, antibiotics, and follow up in 24 hours

349. A 50-year-old man presents to the ED complaining of fever, sore throat, and neck pain for 24 hours. He states that 1 week ago he had two molars extracted from his mouth. His BP is 145/75 mm Hg, HR is 102 beats per minute, temperature is 101.2°F, and his RR is 16 breaths per minute. On exam you notice that the patient is drooling. There is erythema and swelling of his submandibular area that gives the appearance of a "bull neck." His tongue is swollen and elevated and the floor of his mouth is tender. There is no fluctuant mass in his mouth. Which of the following is the most likely diagnosis?

a. Acute mastoiditis
b. Peritonsillar abscess
c. Ludwig's angina (LA)
d. Acute necrotizing ulcerative gingivitis (ANUG)
e. *Streptococcus* pharyngitis

350. A 44-year-old man presents to the ED complaining of right foot pain. He states while playing basketball 2 weeks ago he stepped on a nail that punctured through his sneaker and cut his great toe. He went immediately to the ED and they took an x-ray, which was negative, and administered tetanus prophylaxis. On physical exam, his toe is swollen, erythematous, and tender to palpation. There is no obvious break in the skin or abscess present. His BP is 120/75 mm Hg, HR is 80 beats per minute, temperature is 100.4°F, and his RR is 16 breaths per minute. Which of the following organisms is the most likely pathogen?

a. *N. gonorrhoeae*
b. *Staphylococcus epidermidis*
c. *Sporothrix schenckii*
d. *P. aeruginosa*
e. *Salmonella* sp.

351. A 42-year-old diabetic man presents to the ED with 3 days of rapidly worsening scrotal and perineal pain. His HR is 115 beats per minute, BP is 135/90 mm Hg, RR is 18 breaths per minute, and temperature is 102.9 °F. Labs are notable for a WBC of $18,000/\mu$L. Physical exam demonstrates a necrotizing infection of the scrotum and perineal subcutaneous fascia. Which of the following is the most appropriate next step in management?

a. A 14-day course of levofloxacin and early urology follow-up
b. Oral metronidazole and cephalexin with early urology follow-up
c. Pain medications, daily warm soaks, and follow-up with an urologist
d. Aggressive fluid resuscitation, bedside incision and drainage, and urology consult
e. Surgical debridement, broad-spectrum IV antibiotics, and hospital admission

352. A 45-year-old woman presents to the ED complaining of 3 days of fever and worsening throat pain and painful odynophagia without cough or coryza. She sits on a chair, leaning forward with her mouth slightly open. She has a cup of saliva and a box of facial tissues at her side. Vitals are HR 120 beats per minute, BP 110/70 mm Hg, RR 22 breaths per minute, O_2 saturation 99% on room air, and temperature 102°F. Her voice is hoarse, but she is able to open her mouth fully. Her posterior oropharynx is moderately hyperemic, without exudates or tonsillar enlargement. Soft tissue lateral cervical radiograph shows marked edema of the prevertebral and retropharyngeal soft tissues and absence of the vallecular space. Which of the following is the most likely diagnosis?

a. Retropharyngeal abscess
b. Peritonsillar abscess
c. Epiglottitis
d. Pharyngitis
e. Laryngotracheitis

353. A 19-year-old woman presents with bilateral lower abdominal pain, fever, nausea, vomiting, and general malaise. Her last menstrual period was 5 days ago. Vitals are HR 98 beats per minute, BP 110/65 mm Hg, RR of 18 breaths per minute, and temperature of 102.7°F. Pelvic exam demonstrates exquisite cervical motion tenderness and right adnexal tenderness. Labs are notable for a WBC 15,000/μL, an ESR of 95 mm/h, and a negative urine β-hCG. Transvaginal ultrasound demonstrates a right complex mass with cystic and solid components. Which of the following is the most appropriate next step in management?

a. Ceftriaxone IM plus a 14-day course of oral doxycycline and follow-up in the gynecology clinic
b. Oral ofloxacin plus metronidazole and follow-up in the gynecology clinic
c. Analgesics for a ruptured ovarian cyst and follow-up in the gynecology clinic
d. Admission for IV antibiotics and possible laparoscopic drainage
e. Admission for emergent medical or surgical treatment of an ectopic pregnancy

354. A 42-year-old IV drug user presents to the ED with fever, chills, pleuritic chest pain, myalgias, and general malaise. Vitals are HR 110 beats per minute, BP 110/65 mm Hg, RR of 18 breaths per minute, and temperature of 103°F. Physical exam is notable for retinal hemorrhages, petechiae on the conjunctivae and mucus membranes, a faint systolic ejection murmur, and splenomegaly. Which of the following is the most likely diagnosis?

a. Sick sinus syndrome
b. Myocarditis
c. Pericarditis
d. Cardiac tamponade
e. Endocarditis

355. A 21-year-old male on the college swim team complains of right ear pain, pruritis, and discharge. On physical exam, his BP is 115/65 mm Hg, HR 75, and temperature 101°F. He withdraws when you retract the pinna of his ear. The external auditory canal is erythematosus and edematous and contains a purulent discharge. The tympanic membrane is erythematosus and bulging. Which of the following is the most common organism that causes his diagnosis?

a. *Streptococcus pneumoniae*
b. *P. aeruginosa*
c. Nontypeable *Haemophilus influenzae*
d. *Moraxella catarrhalis*
e. *Escherichia coli*

356. A 26-year-old woman presents to the ED with fever, malaise, and an evolving rash in the right axilla that she initially thought was from an insect bite that she received while hiking 1 week earlier. She complains of generalized fatigue, nausea, headache, and joint pain over the past several days. Her vitals are BP 120/75 mm Hg, HR 75 beats per minute, RR 16 breaths per minute, and temperature 101°F. On physical exam, she is awake and alert with a nonfocal neurological exam. Her neck is supple, but she is diffusely tender over the shoulder, knee, and hip joints bilaterally without any distinct effusions. Her abdomen is soft and nontender. She has a 9 cm erythematosus annular plaque with a central clearing under her right axilla. Which of the following is the next best step?

a. Consult dermatology for a biopsy of the rash
b. Perform a LP and begin treatment with IV ceftriaxone
c. Prescribe doxycycline 21 days and arrange follow-up with her primary care doctor
d. Prescribe hydrocortisone cream for the rash and acetaminophen for the headache and joint pain
e. Perform serologic testing for *Borrelia burgdorferi* and begin treatment only if positive

357. A 22-year-old man presents to the ED with a 3-day history of rash, fever, malaise, and mouth sores. He has been unable to eat due to mouth pain. He denies arthralgias, penile discharge, new medications, drug allergies, or prior similar episodes. Vital signs are BP 100/60 mm Hg, HR 110 beats per minute, RR 20 breaths per minute, and temperature 102°F. The patient appears alert but uncomfortable. He has multiple vesiculobullous lesions on his conjunctivae and mouth. Visual acuity is 20/20. Target lesions are found on his palms and soles. What is the most appropriate next step in management?

a. Discharge him with analgesics, antihistamines, and mouth rinses
b. Discharge him with acyclovir, analgesics, antihistamines, and mouth rinses
c. Discharge him after 1 L normal saline IV; prescribe analgesics, antihistamines, oral prednisone, and mouth rinses
d. Admit him and administer 1–2 L normal saline IV; oral prednisone, analgesics, antihistamines, and mouth rinses
e. Admit him and administer 1–2 L normal saline IV; analgesics, antihistamines, and mouth rinses

358. A 54-year-old man with a history of Hepatitis C, alcohol abuse, and cirrhotic ascites presents with increasing abdominal girth and abdominal pain. He complains of increasing difficulty breathing, especially when lying down, due to worsening ascites. On physical exam, the patient is cachectic and appears older than his stated age. He has a diffusely tender abdomen and tense ascites. The liver is palpable 4 cm below the costal margin. Vitals are BP 110/65 mm Hg, HR 110 beats per minute, RR 22 breaths per minute and temperature 102°F. Which of the following is the most common organism seen in spontaneous bacterial peritonitis?

a. *P. aeruginosa*
b. *Enterococcus*
c. *S. pneumoniae*
d. *Enterobacteriaceae*
e. Anaerobes

Fever

Answers

335. The answer is c. *(Rosen, pp 620–621.)* *Spinal abscesses* are most commonly found in *immunocompromised patients, IV drug users,* and the *elderly.* Signs and symptoms of epidural abscess usually develop over a week or two and include fever, localized pain, and progressive weakness. An elevated WBC count is also commonly seen. MRI is the most useful diagnostic test. *S. aureus* is the most common causative organism, followed by gram-negative bacilli and tuberculosis bacillus.

(a) Disk herniation is a common cause of chronic lower back pain, but is uncommon in the thoracic spine. L4-5 and L5-S1 are the most common sites affected. (b) Inflammatory conditions, including ankylosing spondylitis, may cause back pain. The key findings in this disease include gradual onset of morning stiffness improved with exercise in a patient less than age 40 years. On physical examination, these patients may have limited back flexion, reduced chest expansion, and sacroiliac joint tenderness, all of which are nonspecific. Fever and weakness would not be expected. (d) Back pain may result from vertebral compression fractures. These may be secondary to trauma or may be atraumatic in a patient with osteoporosis. Osteoporotic compression fractures usually involve patients over 70 years or patients with acquired bone weakness (e.g., prolonged steroid use). (e) Metastatic lesions invade the spinal bone marrow, leading to compression of the spinal cord. Most common primary tumors include breast, lung, thyroid, kidney, prostate (BLT with Kosher Pickles), as well as lymphoma and multiple myeloma. Maintain a high level of suspicion for any cancer patient who develops back pain; these patients must be investigated for spinal metastases.

336. The answer is d. *(Tintinalli, pp 617–618.)* *Epididymitis* is an inflammation of the epididymis, often caused by age-dependent bacterial infection. Sexually transmitted diseases (STDs), such as gonorrhea and *Chlamydia,* in patients younger than 35 years; and common urinary pathogens such as *E. coli* and *Klebsiella* are most common in patients older than 40 years. Unlike testicular torsion, the onset of pain is usually gradual. Scrotal elevation may transiently relieve pain (positive Prehn sign). Treatment includes bed rest, scrotal elevation or support when ambulating, avoidance of heavy lifting, and antibiotics for infection. **(a)** This patient may require pain medications but coverage with appropriate antibiotics will help relieve symptoms. While penicillin is appropriate therapy for primary syphilis, this patient has epididymitis. **(b)** While scrotal elevation may be helpful, definitive treatment for epididymitis requires appropriate antibiotic coverage. **(c)** Epididymitis must be differentiated from testicular torsion, a true emergency. Testicular torsion is a twisting of the testicle on its root, and often occurs during strenuous activity or as a result of trauma. It is acute in onset and pain is not typically relieved with scrotal elevation and the cremasteric reflex may be absent of the affected side. Manual detorsion may be attempted, but an immediate Doppler ultrasound must be obtained to look for blood flow to the testicle. **(e)** Hydrocele is a fluid accumulation in a persistent tunica vaginalis due to obstruction, which impedes lymphatic drainage of the testicle. On physical exam, transillumination may help confirm the diagnosis. Treatment includes reassurance, and possibly surgical follow-up for drainage.

337. The answer is b. (*Tintinalli, pp 614–615.*) *Fournier's gangrene* is a polymicrobial *necrotizing fasciitis* of the perineal subcutaneous tissue and male genitalia that originates from the skin, urethra, or rectum. It usually begins as a simple abscess or benign infection that quickly spreads, especially in an immunocompromised patient, often a diabetic male. If not promptly diagnosed, it can lead to end-artery thrombosis in the subcutaneous tissue and widespread necrosis. Treatment includes aggressive fluid resuscitation; broad-spectrum antibiotics to cover gram-positive, gram-negative, and anaerobic bacteria; wide surgical debridement; and possibly hyperbaric oxygen therapy. **(a)** Epididymitis is a bacterial infection of the epididymis, with a gradual onset of lower abdominal or testicular pain. The involvement in this case is far more extensive and the crepitus and widespread discoloration indicate a more virulent infection. **(c)** Scrotal edema can be idiopathic, but usually occurs secondary to an insect or human bite. Scrotal edema associated with penile edema may be seen in older men in conjunction with lower extremity edema in fluid overload states (e.g., congestive heart failure). **(d)** Paraphimosis is the inability to reduce the proximal foreskin over the glans penis (the foreskin becomes "stuck" behind the glans penis). It may lead to decreased arterial flow and eventual gangrene. **(e)** Testicular torsion is the twisting of a testicle on its root that usually occurs during strenuous activity or following trauma, but can occasionally occur during sleep. It is most common in infants and young adults.

338. The answer is d. *(Rosen, pp 1588–1591.) Septic arthritis* is an infection of a joint space, most commonly the knee, followed by the hip, shoulder, and wrist. Patient's present with a warm, tender, erythematous, swollen joint and pain with passive range of motion. Fever and chills are common. *Arthrocentesis* is diagnostic with joint fluid demonstrating a WBC count > 50,000/μL with >75% granulocytes. *S. aureus* remains the predominant pathogen for all age groups. In young adults gonococcal septic arthritis is common. Patients with septic arthritis should receive a first dose of antibiotics in the ED prior to admission. If a coincident cellulitis is present over the involved joint, arthrocentesis may need to be delayed.

(**a**) Plain radiographs should be obtained to identify any underlying osteomyelitis or joint disease, but are often negative. Preexisting arthritis (osteoarthritis or rheumatoid arthritis), immunocompromised states (alcoholism, diabetes, or cancer), and risky sexual behavior are risk factors for the development of septic arthritis. (**b**) MRI plays no role in the diagnosis of septic arthritis, but may be useful in other musculoskeletal injuries involving the knee. (**c**) The ESR and C-reactive protein are often elevated in septic arthritis, but neither is diagnostic. (**e**) A warm, swollen, painful knee is concerning for osteomyelitis, which may cause decreased active range of motion. However, passive range of motion should not be severely compromised. A bone scan will detect osteomyelitis within 48 hours that may not be immediately apparent on a plain radiograph.

339. The answer is e. *(Tintinalli, pp 1311–1313.) Thyroid storm* is a rare—but life-threatening—hypermetabolic state due to hyperthyroidism. Hyperthyroidism is 10 times more common in women than men. Graves' disease, is by far the most common etiology, accounting for 80% of cases of hyperthyroidism in the United States. The diagnosis of thyroid storm is made clinically as thyroid function tests are not always available to emergency physicians. The classic presentation of thyroid storm is fever, sinus, or supraventricular tachycardia out of proportion to fever, changes in mental status (confusion, delirium, or coma), and gastrointestinal symptoms. Patients often present with heat intolerance, palpitations, weight loss, sweating, tremor, nervousness, weakness, and fatigue. Sinus tachycardia, widened pulse pressure, and increased cardiac output resemble a state of increased adrenergic activity despite relatively normal levels of catecholamines. Patients must be admitted to a monitored environment for further evaluation and care. Treatment begins with the ABCs: stabilization, airway protection, oxygenation, IV fluids, and monitoring. β-Blockers (often propranolol) are used to treat the severe adrenergic symptoms, such as tachycardia and tremors. Propranolol has the added benefit of inhibiting the peripheral conversion of T_4 (thyroxine) to T_3 (triiodothyrinine), which is biologically more active than T_4. PTU and methimazole (MMI) are two medications that decrease the synthesis of additional thyroid hormone.

(a) and **(b)** Thyroid replacement is appropriate for patients with *hypo*thyroidism. This patient has *hyper*thyroidism and her condition will worsen with the addition of synthetic thyroid hormone. **(c)** and **(d)** Following PTU administration, treatment is directed toward decreasing the release of preformed thyroid hormone by administering iodine. Iodine must not be administered until the PTU has taken effect (1.5 hours). Otherwise, the addition of iodine will promote further hormone production. This patient must be monitored further and required hospital admission to a monitored setting.

340. The answer is a. (*Harrison, pp 689–690.*) This patient has *thrombotic thrombocytopenic purpura (TTP)*, caused by increased platelet destruction. In TTP, platelet-fibrin thrombi deposit in vessel and cause injury to red blood cells (RBCs) and platelets, resulting in microangiopathy hemolytic anemia and thrombocytopenia. Patients tend to be females who are 10–45 years of age. Risk factors include pregnancy, autoimmune disorders (e.g., SLE), infection, allogenic bone marrow transplantation, malignancy, and certain medications. The pentad can be remembered with the mnemonic FAT RN: Fever, hemolytic Anemia, Thrombocytopenia, Renal failure, and Neurologic change (waxing and waning mental status). Treatment includes daily *plasmaphoresis* until platelet count normalizes. RBCs may be transfused in patients symptomatic from anemia (e.g., tachycardia, hypoxia, orthostatic hypotension). All patients with TTP should be admitted to an ICU for close monitoring of acute bleeds.

(b) The therapy for TTP does *not* include platelet transfusion, as this could worsen the condition and increase mortality. **(c)** Corticosteroids and splenectomy are used in refractory cases, but plasmaphoresis is the mainstay of treatment of TTP. **(d)** Hemolytic uremic syndrome (HUS) is a condition, most common in children, thought to be on the same continuum as TTP. The diagnostic triad includes renal failure, microangiopathic hemolytic anemia, and thrombocytopenia. Fever and altered mental status are usually absent, although seizures may result from complications of renal failure. HUS is often associated with infection with *E. coli* or *Shigella dysenteriae* or ingestion of undercooked meats or unpasteurized foods. **(e)** Fever and altered mental status may indicate meningitis, but this patient has other signs and symptoms consistent with TTP. A LP is unnecessary and could be dangerous given the very low platelet count.

341. The answer is a. (*Tintinalli, pp 870–871, 913–918, and 1517–1519.*) This patient suffers from *toxic shock syndrome (TSS)*, a severe, life-threatening syndrome characterized by *high fever, diffuse macular erythroderma,* profound *hypotension, desquamation,* and multisystem involvement (including vomiting or diarrhea, severe myalgias, mucus membrane hyperemia, renal or hepatic dysfunction, decreased platelets, and disorientation). TSS can rapidly progress to multisystem dysfunction and shock. TSS was initially recognized as a disease of young, healthy, menstruating women, in which tampon use increased the risk 33 times. With increased awareness and changes in tampon composition, cases of TSS have declined over the past 20 years. *S. aureus* is the causative organism. An exotoxin produced by *S. aureus* is the presumed cause in menstrual-related TSS (MRTSS) and two endotoxins have been implicated in non-menstrual-related TSS (NMRTSS). TSS should be considered in any unexplained febrile illness associated with erythroderma, hypotension, and diffuse organ pathology. Patients with MRTSS usually present between the third and fifth day of menses. In severe cases, headache is the most common complaint. The rash is a diffuse, blanching erythroderma, often described as a painless "sunburn" that fades within 3 days and is followed by desquamation, especially of the palms and soles. For severe cases, treatment includes aggressive IV fluid resuscitation, IV oxacillin or cefazolin, and hospital admission in a monitored setting.

(b) Rocky Mountain spotted fever (RMSF) is caused by *R. rickettsii*, which is transmitted by ticks. The organism multiplies in endothelial cells lining small vessels, causing generalized vasculitis as well as headache, fever, confusion, rash, myalgias, and shock. The rash usually appears on day 2–3, initially on the wrists, ankles, palms, and soles, spreading rapidly to the extremities and trunk. Lesions begin as small, erythematous blanching macules that become maculopapular and petechial. The location and type of rash, along with the history distinguish RMSF from TSS. Serologic tests are confirmatory, but treatment with doxycycline or chloramphenicol should be started prior to confirmation. (c) Streptococcal scarlet fever is an acute febrile illness primarily affecting young children, caused by *S. pyogenes* (group A streptococci [GAS]). The "sandpaper" rash of scarlet fever differs from the macular sunburn rash of TSS. The treatment is penicillin or a macrolide in penicillin-allergic patients. While *S. aureus* is the causative organism of TSS, a less common, but more aggressive, TSS-like syndrome, streptococcal TSS (STSS), has recently emerged. The treatment is similar to TSS, with aggressive fluid management along with IV penicillin and clindamycin. These patients may progress to a necrotizing fasciitis or myositis, requiring surgical intervention. (**d**) Meningococcemia is an infectious vasculitis caused by disseminated *Neisseria meningitides,* a gram-negative diplococcus. Fever, headache, arthralgias, altered mental status, and abnormal vitals may also be found, along with neck stiffness. There is no indication of meningeal irritation in this patient. Furthermore, the rash of meningococcemia is distinctly different from that of TSS, involving petechial, hemorrhagic vesicles, macules, and papules with surrounding erythema, especially on the trunk and extremities. The treatment is IV ceftriaxone. (**e**) Disseminated gonococcemia, usually seen in young, sexually active females, is caused by *N. gonorrhoeae.* The rash of gonococcemia is pustular with an erythematous base, rather than petechial and hemorrhagic, as are the lesions of RMSF and meningococcemia. It can also be associated with fever and arthralgias. The treatment is IV ceftriaxone or oral ciprofloxacin.

342. The answer is c. (*Tintinalli, p 326. Rosen, pp 1928–1937.*) Osteomyelitis is an infection or inflammation of a bone with an incidence following plantar puncture wounds of 0.1–2%. For patients overall, *S. aureus* is the leading cause of osteomyelitis, followed by *Streptococcus* species. Pain, swelling, fever, redness, and drainage may all occur, but pain is the presenting complaint in most cases. Risk factors include trauma, surgery, soft tissue infections, and being immunocompromised (e.g., HIV, diabetes, IV drug user, sickle cell disease, alcoholism). Definitive diagnosis is made by bone scan which will demonstrate osteomyelitis within 72 hours of symptom onset. Radiographs may be normal early on, but will demonstrate periosteal elevation within 10 days. ESR is often elevated, but a normal or slightly elevated ESR does not rule out the diagnosis. The ESR is most valuable in following response to treatment, as the ESR should fall as the infection resolves. Blood cultures, which are positive in 50% of cases, should be used to guide antibiotic treatment. All patients with puncture wounds should receive tetanus prophylaxis.

(**a**) Patients with sickle cell disease and asplenism are at higher risk for *Salmonella* osteomyelitis, although *S. aureus* remains the most common cause. (**b**) *Pseudomonas* causes bone and joint infections primarily in three settings. Patients receiving implanted prosthetic devices during orthopedic surgery are at higher risk for osteomyelitis from *pseudomonas*. Puncture wounds to the foot also increase the risk of osteomyelitis from *Pseudomonas. Pseudomonas* does not appear to grow on puncture objects, but rather appears to grow on the footwear and may be inoculated into the wound. Thirdly, IV drug users may develop hematogenous osteomyelitis, often in the spine, from *Pseudomonas* bacteria. (**d**) For patients overall, *S. aureus* is the leading cause of osteomyelitis, followed by *Streptococcus*. In neonates, group B *Streptococcus* is a common infecting bacterium of bone and joint infections, and group A *Streptococcus* may be seen in children 3 months to 14 years. (**e**) Infection of the skin or bone following a cat bite is most likely due to *P. multocida*.

343. The answer is e. *(Rosen, pp 977–978.)* Ludwig's Angina (LA) is a potentially life-threatening *cellulitis* of the connective tissue of the *floor of the mouth and neck* that begins in the *submandibular space*. An infected or recently extracted tooth is present in most cases. Typically, it is a *polymicrobial infection* involving aerobic and anaerobic bacteria of the mouth. The most commonly isolated organisms include *Streptococci, Staphylococci,* and *Bacteroides* sp. The most common physical findings in LA are bilateral submandibular swelling and tongue protrusion or elevation. A tense edema and brawny induration of the neck above the hyoid may be present and is described as a "bull neck." Marked tenderness to palpation of the neck and subcutaneous emphysema may be noted. *Trismus* and *fever* are often present, but usually no palpable fluctuance or cervical lymphadenopathy. The involved teeth may be tender to palpation. Patients with LA should *never* be left alone as airway impairment can suddenly occur. Signs of impending airway compromise include stridor, tachypnea, dyspnea, drooling, and agitation. The upper airway may be distorted making endotracheal intubation difficult or impossible. Cricothyrotomy may also be difficult and increases the risk of spreading infection into the mediastinum. Fiberoptic nasotracheal intubation is preferred.

(**a**) Ludwig's angina is usually a clinical diagnosis. Soft-tissue radiographs of the neck may confirm the diagnosis by demonstrating edema of the affected area, airway narrowing, and gas collections. However, radiographs should not delay treatment or place the patient in an area where emergent airway management is difficult. (**b**) Prior to antibiotics, incision and drainage was the treatment of choice. Today, surgery is used only for those patients who fail to respond to antibiotic therapy or those with purulent collections. In these rare cases, surgery, including incision and drainage then excision of facial planes, would best be performed in an operating room (OR), not at the bedside. Patients with LA without respiratory compromise should be maintained in a sitting position. (**c**) While steroids have been used for peritonsillar abscesses to decrease inflammation, their value for LA is unclear. (**d**) Antibiotics must be started immediately. Appropriate regimens include high-dose penicillin with metronidazole, or cefoxitin used alone.

Clindamycin, ticarcillin-clavulanate, piperacillin-tazobactam, or ampicillin-sulbactam may also be used. Oral antibiotics are not adequate.

344. The answer is a. *(Tintinalli, p 1523.)* *Erysipelas* is an *acute superficial cellulitis* of the dermis, lymphatics, and subcutaneous tissue. It is characterized by a *sharply demarcated border* surrounding skin that is raised, deeply erythematous, indurated, and painful, and is associated with small breaks in the skin, nephrotic syndrome, and postoperative wounds. Erysipelas is more superficial than cellulitis and is more likely to occur in the young and in the elderly, but the distinction between the two is often subtle and therapeutically irrelevant. Treatment of erysipelas and facial cellulitis requires hospital admission and parenteral antibiotics. Treatment is aimed at the predominant organism, group A *Streptococcus*, but *Staphylococcus* and *Streptococcus* species are also found. An immediate ophthalmologic consult should be obtained if there is any orbital or periorbital involvement.
(b) While cellulitis may often be treated with oral antibiotics, treatment for erysipelas or facial cellulitis warrants parenteral antibiotics. (c) Erysipelas and facial cellulitis may be unilateral or bilateral. When unilateral, they must be distinguished from early herpes zoster infection, especially if vesicles are present. (d) Erysipelas with bilateral involvement may be confused with the malar rash of SLE. The malar or "butterfly" rash of SLE consists of erythema on the medial cheeks and across the bridge of the nose. Women of childbearing age comprise 90% of affected individuals, and clinical presentation generally includes multisystem involvement. (e) Erysipelas remains a clinical diagnosis. Skin biopsy is rarely necessary and often unhelpful.

345. The answer is d. *(Paller and Mancini, pp 566–571.)* This patient presents with the classic symptoms of *Kawasaki disease*, an acute febrile childhood disease and *one of the leading causes of acquired heart disease worldwide*. The diagnostic criteria include *fever for ≥5 days, plus* at least four of the following five clinical signs: *bilateral conjunctival injection, oral mucous membrane changes* (injected pharynx, injected or fissured lips, or strawberry tongue), *peripheral erythema or edema* or *periungal desquamation, polymorphous rash,* and *cervical lymphadenopathy* ≥1.5 cm. The cardiac sequelae, which may occur during the acute or latent stage of Kawasaki disease, represent its most serious complications. Patients may develop pericardial effusions and myocarditis, but the most significant complication is coronary artery aneurysm, which occurs in up to 5–10% of patients despite appropriate therapy. An *echocardiogram* should be performed as part of the diagnostic work-up and as part of the 2-month follow-up plan once the clinical diagnosis has been established.

(a) Electrolyte abnormalities and renal dysfunction are not generally present; therefore, hemodialysis should not be required. (b) While patients are febrile and may appear irritable or lethargic, if clinical diagnosis can be established based on multiple other signs and symptoms, a LP should not be required. If an LP is performed, CSF may demonstrate pleocytosis, but this finding is neither sensitive nor specific. (c) Unilateral cervical lymphadenopathy is the least common finding, occurring in only 50–75% of patients with Kawasaki disease. When present, it is usually quite apparent. Kawasaki disease is a clinical diagnosis and lymph node biopsy would not be expected to contribute to the diagnosis. (e) Secondary syphilis may present with fever, malaise, lymphadenopathy, and rash that begins on the trunk and spreads to the palms and soles. Specific treponemal antibody tests (fluorescent treponemal antibody absorption, or FTA-ABS) may be used to diagnose the disease. However, secondary syphilis, a STD, would be highly unusual in this 3-year-old without evidence of primary disease.

346. The answer is d. *(Tintinalli, p 1791.) Kanavel* criteria for *flexor tenosynovitis* include (1) **S**ymmetric swelling of the finger, (2) **T**enderness over the flexor tendon sheath, (3) **E**xtension (passive) of the digit is painful, and (4) **P**osture of the digit is flexed (**STEP**). A tenosynovitis is an infection of the flexor tendon sheath caused by penetrating trauma and dirty wounds (e.g., a dog bite). It is a surgical emergency. Infection spreads along the tendon sheath; therefore, failure to diagnose and treat a flexor tenosynovitis may lead to loss of function of the affected digit and eventually the entire hand. Treatment includes hand immobilization and elevation, immediate consultation with a hand surgeon, and IV antibiotics. Pain control and tetanus immunization should be provided, if not up-to-date.

(a) The Finkelstein test for DeQuervain's tenosynovitis is positive when, with the thumb cupped in a closed fist, ulnar deviation reproduces pain along the extensor pollicis and abductor pollicis. (b) Trousseau's sign for hypocalcemia is positive when a BP cuff inflated above the systolic BP for 3 minutes induces carpal spasm. (c) and (e) Compression of the median nerve may result in carpal tunnel syndrome, which presents with pain and paresthesias in the median nerve distribution. Tinel's sign is positive when tapping over the median nerve at the wrist produces pain and paresthesia, while the Phalen test is positive when one minute of forced palmar flexion produces pain and paresthesia over the median nerve distribution.

347. The answer is d. (*Centor, pp 239–246. Tannenbaum, pp 75–83.*) The patient has a modified *Centor score of 2* (history of fever, tender adenopathy, no cough, age > 45 years). The *Centor criteria*, seen below, is used for predicting *streptococcal pharyngitis* and whether or not to treat the patient with antibiotics.

Centor Criteria	Points
Presence of tonsillar exudates	+1
Tender anterior cervical adenopathy	+1
Fever by history	+1
Absence of cough	+1
Age <15 years	+1
Age >45	−1

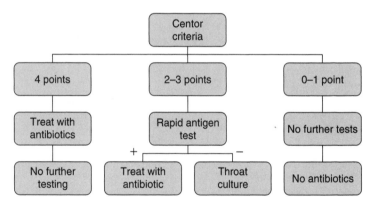

Since his rapid antigen test was negative, the patient should receive a *throat culture* and be treated only if the results are positive. In addition, he should be treated symptomatically with fluids, topical anesthetics, and acetaminophen or ibuprofen.

(a) According to the Centor criteria, the patient should not receive antibiotics. The negative predictive value for is approximately 80%. (b) There is no indication that this patient has lymphoma, his symptoms are only present for 2 days. (c) Observation is unnecessary in this patient. (e) Amantadine is used in the treatment of influenza, which typically presents with a high fever, myalgias, and headache. Cervical lymphadenopathy is rare.

348. The answer is a. *(Rosen, pp 975–977.)* The patient's presentation is typical for a *peritonsillar abscess.* Signs and symptoms include a sore throat, muffled voice, trismus, fluctuant mass, deviation of uvula, odynophagia, and drooling. Many patients recently have been treated for strep throat. The abscess is usually unilateral and in the superior pole of the tonsil. Airway patency must be assessed due to the obstructing potential of an abscess. Treatment includes either *needle aspiration* or *incision and draining* of the abscess in addition to *antibiotic treatment.* Some studies demonstrate the safety and cost-effectiveness of needle aspiration over incision and draining.

(b) The abscess will not resolve without an intervention. **(c)** Incision and drainage of the abscess may be performed in the OR depending on the size and degree of airway compromise. However, that is not necessary in this patient. **(d)** Drainage of the abscess is the most important factor in treating these patients. Antibiotics alone are not sufficient. **(e)** A CT scan may aid in the diagnosis of a peritonsillar abscess in patients with severe trismus.

349. The answer is c. *(Rosen, pp 977–978.)* *Ludwig's angina* is a potentially fatal disease that can progress to death within hours. It is a *progressive cellulitis* of the *floor of the mouth and neck* that begins in the submandibular space. A dental cause, such as an extraction, is present in approximately 90% of cases. The most common symptoms include dysphagia, neck pain, and swelling. Physical findings include bilateral submandibular swelling, tongue swelling, and protrusion. A tense edema and induration of the neck may occur that is described as a "bull neck." Management involves securing an airway and starting IV antibiotic therapy immediately. There is debate on whether these patients should be managed surgically with incision and drainage or medically with antibiotics.

(a) Acute mastoiditis usually presents with swelling of the mastoid, fever, and earache. **(b)** Peritonsillar abscess typically presents with a fluctuant soft palate mass. **(d)** ANUG is an infection of the gingival. **(e)** Pharyngitis is limited to the oropharynx and should not involve the tissues of the neck.

350. The answer is d. *(Rosen, pp 1928–1937.)* This is a typical scenario for *osteomyelitis.* Conventional radiography on the day of injury is insensitive to the detection of osteomyelitis and even 1 week after the injury x-ray diagnosis is limited. The most common pathogen in osteomyelitis is *S. aureus.* However, *Pseudomonas* is responsible for bone and joint infections in three settings. First, a puncture wound through a shoe. *Pseudomonas* does not grow on the puncture object, but rather is associated with the shoe itself and may be inoculated into bone as the sharp object passes through the colonized shoe into the wound. Second, prosthetic devices implanted for orthopedic surgery. Third is IV drug use.

(a) *N. gonorrhoeae* is the most common organism causing septic arthritis in individuals under 30 years old. (b) *S. epidermidis* is not a common organism to cause osteomyelitis. (c) *S. schenckii* is the causative agent of sporotrichosis or "rose handler's disease." (e) *Salmonella* is a cause of osteomyelitis in asplenic individuals such as those with sickle cell disease, due to their lack of ability to fend off encapsulated organisms. However, the most common causative organism in sickle cell patients is *S. aureus.*

351. The answer is e. (*Tintinalli, pp 614–615.*) The patient has *Fournier's gangrene,* a polymicrobial necrotizing fasciitis of the perineal subcutaneous fascial and male genitalia. Treatment is aggressive fluid resuscitation, surgical debridement, broad-spectrum antibiotics, and possibly hyperbaric oxygen therapy. These patients require hospital admission. If not promptly treated, the overall mortality is approximately 20%.

(a) and (b) These are polymicrobial infections and antibiotics must cover gram-negative, gram-positive, and anaerobic bacteria. These patients may require surgical debridement. IV antibiotic treatment and hospital admission are recommended as these patients have a relatively high mortality if not adequately and aggressively treated. (c) While these patients will require pain medications, fluid hydration, IV antibiotics, surgical debridement, and hospital admission are also recommended. (d) Urologic consultation may be necessary when a periurethral abscess is the inciting event, or when there is involvement of the urinary tract and supravesical urinary drainage is needed. However, widespread involvement of the fascia and genital structures makes a bedside incision and drainage inadequate. In addition, the treatment is incomplete without antibiotic coverage.

352. The answer is c. (*Tintinalli, pp 851 & 1494–1497.*) *Epiglottitis* is a life-threatening inflammatory condition, usually infectious, of the epiglottis and the aryepiglottic and periglottic folds. Since most children are immunized against *H. influenzae* type B (Hib), most cases of epiglottitis are now seen in adults, with an average age of 46 years. Signs and symptoms include a prodromal period of 1–2 days, high fever, dysphagia, odynophagia, drooling, and dyspnea. Stridor is primarily inspiratory and softer and lower-pitched than croup. The "thumbprint sign" seen on *lateral cervical radiograph* demonstrates a swollen epiglottis obliterating the vallecula.

(a) Retropharyngeal abscess can present with similar signs and symptoms as epiglottitis. Cervical lymphadenopathy is prominent and inflammation may be so severe that patients develop an inflammatory torticollis, causing the patient to rotate the head toward the affected side. Soft tissue cervical radiograph may demonstrate excess prevertebral swelling. Treatment is IV hydration and antibiotics, which should be started in the ED, and drainage in the OR. (b) Peritonsillar abscess would present with swollen erythematous tonsils and uvula deviation. It is most common during the second and third decades of life. Diagnosis is easily made by computed tomography (CT) scan or ultrasound, but aspiration of purulent material is sufficient for diagnosis. Treatment is incision and drainage or needle aspiration, followed by high-dose penicillin or clindamycin. (d) Pharyngitis is an infection of the pharynx and tonsils that occur in adults, but has a peak incidence in children aged 4–7 years. The etiology is most often viral. *S. pyogenes* (group A, beta-hemolytic strep) is the most common cause of bacterial pharyngitis (5–15%) in adults. Patients present with erythematous tonsils, tonsillar exudates, enlarged and tender anterior cervical lymph nodes. (e) Laryngotracheitis, or croup, is generally seen in children aged 6 months to 3 years and rarely seen after age 6 years.

353. The answer is d. (*Center for Disease Control, Treatment Guidelines 2006, Sexually Transmitted Diseases pp 58–63*) This patient has a *tubo-ovarian abscess (TOA),* a common and potentially fatal complication of *pelvic inflammatory disease (PID).* While PID can usually be treated with outpatient antibiotics, the Center for Disease Control lists several guidelines for inpatient admission including: surgical emergencies (e.g., appendicitis) cannot be excluded; pregnancy; failure of outpatient therapy; inability to tolerate oral intake; severe illness, nausea and vomiting, or high fever; and TOA. This patient has several of these factors and should therefore be admitted for further management. IV antibiotics are curative in 60–80% of cases and must be selected to cover *N. gonorrhoeae* and *Chlamydia trachomatis,* the most common pathogens responsible for PID, as well as *Bacteroides,* the most common cause of TOA. Surgical drainage or salpingectomy and oophorectomy may be required in resistant cases.

(a) and (b) Both of these regimens are appropriate for outpatient treatment of PID, but this patient requires IV antibiotics and an inpatient admission for optimal management. (**c**) The ultrasound is consistent with a TOA, not a ruptured ovarian cyst, and requires closer monitoring and IV antibiotics in an inpatient setting. (**e**) The β-hCG is negative, virtually ruling out an ectopic pregnancy.

354. The answer is e. (*Rosen, pp 1149–1152.*) Symptoms of *endocarditis* are nonspecific and vary widely, but the most common include fever (85%) and malaise (80%). In IV drug users, fever is present 98% of the time. Other symptoms include weakness, myalgias, dyspnea, chest pain, cough, headache, and anorexia. Neurologic signs and symptoms (e.g., confusion, personality changes, decreased level of consciousness, and focal motor deficits) are seen in 30–40% of patients. Vasculitic lesions, including petechiae, splinter hemorrhages, tender fingertip nodules (Osler's nodes), nontender palmar plaques (Janeway lesions) are seen in 35% of patients. Splenomegaly, new heart murmur, and retinal hemorrhages may also be detected on physical exam. Risk factors for infective endocarditis include rheumatic or congenital heart disease, calcific degenerative valve disease, prosthetic heart valve, mitral valve prolapse, a history of IV drug use, or a history of endocarditis. Although any valve can be affected, IV drug use is the most common cause of right-sided endocarditis. The recurrence rate in these patients is 41%, significantly higher than the rate of less than 20% in other patients.

(**a**) Also known as sinus node dysfunction or tachy-brady syndrome, sick sinus syndrome results from any combination of intermittent fast and slow heart rhythms associated with AV block and inadequate escape rhythm. The diagnosis is usually made with outpatient Holter monitoring. (**b**) Myocarditis results from inflammatory damage to the myocardium. The etiology may be infectious. Bacteria and enteroviruses, especially coxsackie B virus and adenovirus, predominate as causative agents. Worldwide, Chagas disease is the leading cause, especially in South America. Often myocarditis presents with flu-like complaints, including fever, fatigue, and myalgias. Tachycardia out of proportion to the temperature or clinical picture may be present. Vasculitis lesions, Janeway lesions, and retinal hemorrhages are not expected. (**c**) Pericarditis is caused by inflammation of the pericardial sac. The etiology is broad, including infection, trauma, metabolic diseases (e.g., uremia), medications, systemic autoimmune diseases, and most often the cause is idiopathic. (**d**) Cardiac tamponade is a large pericardial effusion that restricts ventricular filling and eventually stroke volume. The classic findings are hypotension, JVD, and muffled heart sounds (Beck's triad).

355. The answer is b. (*Tintinalli, pp 1466–1469.*) This patient suffers from *otitis externa (OE),* or "swimmer's ear." This is an infection of the external auditory canal (EAC), characterized by pain, pruritis, and tenderness of the external ear. Signs and symptoms include erythema and edema of the EAC, which may spread to the tragus and auricle, as well as fever, pruritis, clear or purulent otorrhea, and crusting of the EAC. The most common organisms responsible for OE are *P. aeruginosa* and *S. aureus,* although these organisms are often not isolated from suspect water samples. Treatment includes analgesia, cleansing of the EAC with hydrogen peroxide, topical antimicrobials, and sometimes steroids.

(a), (c), and (d) *S. pneumoniae,* nontypeable *H. influenzae,* and *M. catarrhalis* are the three most common causes of otitis media, an infection of the middle ear that is usually secondary to a viral URI in children aged 6 months to 3 years. (e) Newborns can get suppurative otitis media with *E. coli,* but it is not a common pathogen for otitis externa.

356. The answer is c. (*Marx, pp 2123–2128.*) Recommended treatment for early *Lyme disease* includes *doxycycline,* amoxicillin (for children younger than 8 years or for pregnant or lactating women), or cefuroxime. Erythromycin and azithromycin can be used, but are less effective. The same drugs can be used for the second stage of disease, but their course of therapy needs to be longer.

(a) This patient has Lyme disease, which is seen in the late spring and early summer. Up to a week or so after a bite from an infected tick, patients may develop a rash, erythema migrans (EM), at the site of the bite. The lesion is characterized by a bright red border and central clearing and quickly spreads outward. EM is the most characteristic clinical manifestation of Lyme disease, and is recognized in 90% or more of patients. Serologic testing may be positive weeks after inoculation, but a biopsy of the rash would neither be necessary nor informative. (b) If meningitis is suspected, a LP is an appropriate aspect of the work-up. In this case, however, the patient has a clear history and characteristic rash for Lyme disease without meningeal signs or focal neurological signs. A LP would not be warranted. (d) Untreated Lyme disease may progress to a second stage, involving neurologic and cardiac abnormalities, 4 weeks after the bite. (e) Lyme disease is largely a clinical diagnosis based on history and physical exam and serologic testing should be used discriminately to confirm the diagnosis. Serum immunofluorescent antibody assays are usually negative until approximately 6 weeks, when immunoglobulin M (IgM) peaks and indicates active disease. IgG antibodies are detected when the arthritis présents and peak at 12 months. Syphilis can cause false-positive titers, but the different clinical presentations should distinguish the diseases.

357. The answer is e. (*Tintinalli, p 1513.*) The patient has signs suggestive of *Erythema Multiforme (EM),* an acute inflammatory skin disease that ranges from a localized eruption (EM minor) to a severe multisystem illness (EM major) with extensive vesiculobullous lesions and erosion of the mucous membranes known as *Stevens-Johnson syndrome (SJS).* It affects all age groups with the highest incidence in males 20–40 years of age. SJS has significant morbidity and a mortality rate of approximately 10%. Death is usually due to infection and dehydration. As in this case, patients with severe disease should be admitted. Therapy consists of IV fluids, oral prednisone, analgesics, antihistamines, mouth rinses, and skin care. While no causative factor can be found in 50% of cases, known triggers include infection, especially *Mycoplasma* and herpes simplex virus, drugs, especially anticonvulsants and antibiotics, and malignancies.

(a), (b), and (c) Because of the high morbidity and mortality, patients with EM, especially the more severe form, SJS, should be admitted to the hospital. Outpatient therapy of EM minor with topical steroids is possible. Patients with extensive disease, systemic toxicity, or mucous membrane involvement require hospitalization, optimally in an intensive care unit or a burn unit. (e) Systemic steroids are used to provide symptomatic relief, although they show no proven benefit in altering the duration and outcome of SJS.

358. The answer is d. (*Tintinalli, p 570.*) *Spontaneous bacterial peritonitis (SBP)* is the most common complication of cirrhotic ascites and should be suspected in all patients with a history of cirrhosis who present with fever, abdominal pain or tenderness, worsening ascites, or encephalopathy. *Paracentesis* should be performed to confirm the diagnosis. Ascitic fluid should be tested for glucose, total protein, lactate dehydrogenase, Gram's stain, and WBC count. Culture results are often negative but yield may be improved by placing 10 mL of fluid in a blood culture bottle. Total WBC count >1000/μL or neutrophil count >250/μL is diagnostic for SBP. Gram negative *Enterobacteriaceae* (*E. coli, Klebsiella,* etc.) account for 63% of all cases. Empiric treatment for suspected SBP includes third-generation cephalosporins, ticarcillin-clavulanic acid, piperacillin-tazobactam, or ampicillin-sulbactam.

(a), (b), (c), and (e) Other causes of SBP include *S. pneumoniae* (15%), enterococci (6–10%), and anaerobes (1%).

Poisoning and Overdose

Questions

359. After being fired from his job, a 35-year-old man attempts suicide by drinking from a bottle labeled "Insecticide." Three hours later, emergency medical service (EMS) brings him in to the emergency department (ED) and you notice he is extremely diaphoretic, drooling, and vomiting. He is awake but confused. His vital signs are blood pressure (BP) 170/90 mm Hg, heart rate (HR) 100, respiratory rate (RR) 22, temperature 98.6°F, and O_2 saturation 95% on room air. Physical exam demonstrates pinpoint pupils and crackles on lung exam. What is the treatment to reverse this patient's poisoning?

a. Naloxone
b. N-acetylcysteine (NAC)
c. Atropine and pralidoxime (2-PAM)
d. Flumazenil
e. Bicarbonate and Kayexalate

360. A 19-year-old man is brought to the ED by EMS after he was found lying on the floor at a dance club. EMS states that the patient seemed unconscious at the dance club but as soon as they transferred him onto the gurney he became combative. Upon arrival in the ED, his BP is 120/65 mm Hg, HR is 75 beats per minute, temperature is 98.9°F, RR is 12 breaths per minute, and O_2 saturation is 98% on room air. On physical exam, his pupils are mid-sized, equal, and reactive to light. His skin is warm and dry. Lung, cardiac, and abdominal exam are unremarkable. As you walk away from the bedside, you here the monitor alarm signaling zero respirations and the O_2 saturation starts to drop. You perform a sternal rub and the patient sits up in bed and starts yelling at you. As you leave him for the second time, you hear the monitor alarm again signal zero respirations. You administer naloxone, but there is no change in his condition. Which of the following is most likely the substance ingested by this patient?

a. γ-Hydroxybutyrate (GHB)
b. Diazepam
c. Cocaine
d. Phencyclidine (PCP)
e. Heroin

361. A 43-year-old woman presents to the ED with a 3-week history of intermittent headache, nausea, and fatigue. She was seen at her private doctor's office 1 week ago along with her husband and children, who also have similar symptoms. They were diagnosed with a viral syndrome and told to increase their fluid intake. She states that the symptoms began approximately the same time it started to get cold outside. The symptoms are worse in the morning and improve while she is at work. Her BP is 123/75 mm Hg, HR is 83 beats per minute, temperature is 98.9°F, and O_2 saturation is 98% on room air. Physical exam is unremarkable. You suspect her first diagnosis was incorrect. Which of the following is the most appropriate next step to confirm your suspicion?

a. Order a mono spot test
b. Perform a nasal pharyngeal swab to test for influenza
c. Consult psychiatry to evaluate for malingering
d. Order a carboxyhemoglobin (COHb) level
e. Perform a lumbar puncture

362. An 18-year-old woman is brought to the ED by her mother. The patient is diaphoretic and vomiting. Her mom states that she thinks her daughter tried to commit suicide. The patient admits to ingesting a few handfuls of extra-strength Tylenol approximately 3 hours ago. Her temperature is 99.1°F, BP is 105/70 mm Hg, HR is 92 beats per minute, RR is 17 breaths per minute, and O_2 saturation is 99% on room air. On exam, her head and neck are unremarkable. Cardiovascular and pulmonary exam are within normal limits. She is mildly tender in her right upper quadrant but there is no rebound or guarding. Bowel sounds are normoactive. She is alert and oriented and has no focal deficits on neurologic exam. You administer 50 g of activated charcoal with sorbitol. At this point, she appears well and has no complaints. Her 4 hour serum acetaminophen (APAP) concentration returns at 350 μg/mL. You plot the level on the nomogram seen on the next page. Which of the following is the most appropriate next step in management?

a. Discharge home with instructions to return if symptoms return
b. Observe for 6 hours and if the patient still has no complaints discharge her home
c. Admit to the hospital for serial abdominal exams
d. Admit to the psychiatry unit and keep on suicide watch
e. Begin NAC and admit to the hospital

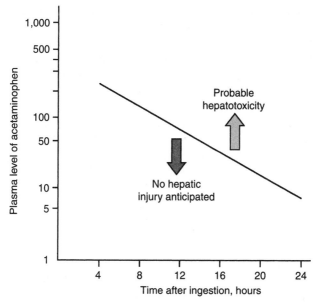

(Reproduced, with permission, from Brunton LL et al. Goodman and Gilman's The Pharmacological Basis Therapeutics. *New York, NY: McGraw-Hill, 2006: 694.)*

363. A 47-year-old man is brought to the ED by EMS after being found wandering in the street mumbling. His BP is 150/75 mm Hg, HR is 110 beats per minute, temperature is 100.5°F, RR is 16 breaths per minute, O_2 saturation is 99% on room air, and fingerstick glucose is 98 mg/dL. On exam, the patient is confused with mumbling speech. His pupils are dilated and face is flushed. His mucous membranes and skin are dry. Which of the following toxic syndromes is this patient exhibiting?

a. Sympathomimetic syndrome
b. Anticholinergic syndrome
c. Cholinergic syndrome
d. Opioid syndrome
e. Ethanol syndrome

364. A 25-year-old man is carried into the ED by two of his friends who state that he is not breathing. The patient has a history of heroin abuse. His vital signs are BP 115/70 mm Hg, HR 99 beats per minute, temperature 98.9°F, RR 3 breaths per minute and O_2 saturation 87% on room air. You notice fresh needle marks and miotic pupils. You begin bag-valve-mask ventilation and his O_2 saturation increases to 99%. Which of the following is the most appropriate next step in management?

a. Continue bag-mask-ventilation until he breathes on his own
b. Administration of naloxone
c. Administration of flumazenil
d. Place a nasogastric tube and administer activated charcoal
e. Place a nasogastric tube and administer syrup of ipecac

365. A 42-year-old man who is actively seizing is brought to the ED by EMS after a massive ingestion of an unknown substance. The man is known to have a history of acquired immunodeficiency syndrome (AIDS). An intravenous (IV) line is established and anticonvulsant therapy administered. After high doses of diazepam, phenobarbital, and phenytoin, it is determined that the seizures are refractory to standard anticonvulsant therapy. Which of the following substances did this patient most likely ingest?

a. Cocaine
b. Diphenhydramine
c. Tricyclic antidepressant
d. Camphor
e. Isoniazid (INH)

366. A 60-year-old woman with a history of diabetes is brought into the ED by EMS workers who state that the patient was found on a bus lethargic and diaphoretic. Her fingerstick at the scene was 35 mg/dL. EMS workers quickly administered dextrose through an IV line and the patient became alert and responsive and remained this way throughout her trip to the ED. However, in the ED you notice that the patient is again diaphoretic and is mumbling her speech. Her fingerstick glucose is 47 mg/dL. You administer dextrose and she perks right up. Which of the following diabetes medications commonly causes hypoglycemia for which the patient is likely to require hospital admission?

a. Regular insulin
b. Metformin

c. Glyburide
d. Troglitazone
e. Acarbose

367. A 23-year-old woman presents to the ED complaining of abdominal pain, nausea, and vomiting. She has a history of depression but is not currently taking any antidepressant medications. Upon further questioning, the patient states that she ingested a bottle of pills in her medicine cabinet approximately 3 hours ago. Her BP is 115/65 mm Hg, HR is 101 beats per minute, temperature is 100.1°F, RR is 29 breaths per minute, and O_2 saturation is 100% on room air. Physical exam is unremarkable except for mild diffuse abdominal tenderness. Laboratory results reveal white blood cell (WBC) count 10,300/μL, hematocrit 46%, platelets 275/μL, aspartate transaminase (AST) 70 U/L, alanine transaminase (ALT) 85 U/L, alkaline phosphatase 75 U/L, sodium 143 mEq/L, potassium 3.7 mEq/L, chloride 98 mEq/L, bicarbonate 8 mEq/L, blood urea nitrogen (BUN) 22 mg/dL, creatinine 0.9 mg/dL, and glucose 85 mg/dL. Arterial blood gas values on room air are pH 7.51, PCO_2 11 mm Hg, and PO_2 134 mm Hg. Which of the following substances did this patient most likely ingest?

a. Diphenhydramine (Benadryl)
b. Ibuprofen
c. APAP
d. Aspirin
e. Pseudoephedrine

368. A 35-year-old agitated man presents to the ED in police custody. He denies any past medical history and takes no medication. He admits to using some drugs today. His BP is 195/90 mm Hg, HR is 121 beats per minute, temperature is 100.1°F, RR is 18 breaths per minute, and O_2 saturation is 99% on room air. On exam, he is diaphoretic, pupils are 8 mm in diameter, and has 3+ patella reflexes bilaterally. Electrocardiogram (ECG) reveals sinus tachycardia with a rate of 123. Which of the following toxic syndromes is this patient exhibiting?

a. Anticholinergic
b. Cholinergic
c. Sympathomimetic
d. Opioid
e. Serotonin

369. A 31-year-old woman with a known psychiatric history presents to the ED after ingesting an unknown quantity of pills from her medication vial. In the ED, she complains of nausea, abdominal cramping, and feels unsteady on her feet. On physical exam you observe that she is tremulous, ataxic, and exhibits dystonia. Which of the following substances is *not* adsorbed by activated charcoal?

a. Digoxin
b. Diphenhydramine
c. Amitriptyline
d. Lithium
e. APAP

370. A 27-year-old man presents to the ED extremely agitated complaining of mild chest pain and dyspnea. He states that he was snorting cocaine all afternoon. You place him on a monitor and get his vital signs. His BP is 215/130 mm Hg, HR is 112 beats per minute, temperature is 100.1°F, RR is 17 breaths per minute, and O_2 saturation is 98% on room air. An ECG reveals sinus tachycardia at a rate of 116. Which of the following is the most appropriate medication to administer?

a. Haloperidol
b. Labetolol
c. Esmolol
d. Diltiazem
e. Diazepam

371. A 30-year-old man is brought to the ED by police officers. The patient is agitated, vomiting, and complaining of body aches. He states that he is withdrawing from his medication. His vital signs are BP 160/85 mm Hg, RR 20 breaths per minute, HR 107 beats per minute, and temperature 99.7°F. On exam he is diaphoretic, has rhinorrhea, piloerection, and hyperactive bowel sounds. Which of the following substances is this patient most likely withdrawing from?

a. Ethanol
b. Cocaine
c. Nicotine
d. Methadone
e. Clonidine

372. A 25-year-old man is brought into the ED by two police officers because of suspected drug use. The patient is extremely agitated and is fighting the police officers. It takes three hospital staff members and the two police officers to keep him on the stretcher. His vital signs are: BP 150/80 mm Hg, HR 107 beats per minute, temperature 99.7°F, RR 18 breaths per minute, and O_2 saturation 99% on room air. Physical exam is unremarkable except for cool, diaphoretic skin, persistent vertical and horizontal nystagmus, and occasional myoclonic jerks. Which of the following is the most likely diagnosis?

a. Cocaine intoxication
b. Cocaine withdrawal
c. Amphetamine intoxication
d. PCP intoxication
e. Opiate withdrawal

373. An undomiciled 49-year-old man presents to the ED with altered mental status. His BP is 149/75 mm Hg, HR is 93 beats per minute, temperature is 97.5°F, RR is 18 breaths per minute, and O_2 saturation is 99% on room air. Physical exam reveals an unkempt man with the odor of "alcohol" on his breath. His head is atraumatic, pupils are 4 mm, equal, and reactive. The neck is supple. Cardiovascular, pulmonary, and abdominal exam is unremarkable. There is no extremity edema and his pulses are 2+ and symmetric. Neurologically, he withdraws all four extremities to deep stimuli. ECG is sinus rhythm.

Laboratory results reveal:

sodium 141 mEq/L	arterial blood pH 7.26
potassium 3.5 mEq/L	lactate 1.7 mEq/L
chloride 101 mEq/L	ethanol level undetectable
bicarbonate 14 mEq/L	measured serum osmolarity 352 mOsm/L
BUN 15 mg/dL	calculated serum osmolarity
creatinine 0.7 mg/dL	292 mOsm/kg.
glucose 89 mg/dL	urinalysis: no blood, ketones, or protein

Which of the following statements below best describes the laboratory findings?

a. Anion gap metabolic acidosis and osmol gap
b. Anion gap metabolic acidosis without osmol gap
c. Nonanion gap metabolic acidosis and osmol gap
d. Nonanion gap metabolic acidosis without osmol gap
e. Metabolic alkalosis

374. A 26-year-old woman, who was found lying on the floor of her apartment next to an unlabeled empty pill bottle, is brought into the ED. Her HR is 117 beats per minute, BP is 95/65 mm Hg, RR is 14 breaths per minute, and O_2 saturation is 97% on 2 L nasal cannula. She is obtunded. Her pupils are 3 mm and reactive. Her oropharynx is dry and there is no gag reflex to pharyngeal stimulation. Her neck is supple. The heart is tachycardic without murmurs, the lungs are clear to auscultation, and the abdomen is soft. There is normal rectal tone and brown stool that is heme negative. Her skin is cool and moist with no signs of needle tracks. Neurologically, she is unresponsive, but withdraws all extremities to deep palpation. Finger stick blood glucose is 85 mg/dL. Her ECG reveals sinus tachycardia at 119 with a QRS complex of 120 msec and a terminal R wave in lead aVR. Which of the following is the most appropriate next step in management?

a. Orotracheal intubation, administer activated charcoal through orogastric tube, and IV narcan
b. Orotracheal intubation, administer activated charcoal through orogastric tube, and IV sodium bicarbonate
c. Orotracheal intubation, administer activated charcoal through orogastric tube, and IV NAC
d. Orotracheal intubation, administer syrup of ipecac through orogastric tube, and IV sodium bicarbonate
e. Induce vomiting prior to intubation to lower the risk of aspiration, then administer IV sodium bicarbonate

375. A 37-year-old woman is brought into the ED by her friend who states that the patient swallowed approximately 50 capsules of 325 mg APAP 6 hours ago in an attempted suicide. The patient states she feels nauseated and vomits while you take her history. Her BP is 100/75 mm Hg, HR is 97 beats per minute, temperature is 98.9°F, RR is 18 breaths per minute and O_2 saturation is 99% on room air. Examination is unremarkable except for mild epigastric tenderness. Which of the following is the correct antidote for APAP overdose?

a. NAC
b. Physostigmine
c. Flumazenil
d. Naloxone
e. Digibind

376. A 31-year-old man is brought to the ED by EMS who state that the man was found lying on the floor of his garage. He is arousable in the ED, speaks with slurred speech, and vomits. His BP is 140/85 mm Hg, HR is 94 beats per minute, temperature is 98.8°F, RR is 17 breaths per minute, and O_2 saturation is 99% on room air. You place an IV line, draw blood, and start a liter of normal saline running through the line. Laboratory results reveal serum sodium 139 mEq/L, potassium 3.5 mEq/L, chloride 101 mEq/L, bicarbonate 14 mEq/L, BUN 15 mg/dL, creatinine 1 mg/dL, glucose 105 mg/dL, arterial blood pH 7.27, COHb 4%, and lactate 2.8 mEq/L. Urinalysis shows: 1+ protein, trace ketones, WBC 4/hpf, red blood cell (RBC) 2–3/hpf, and multiple envelope-shaped and needle-shaped crystals. Which of the following conditions would best explain his metabolic acidosis?

a. Carbon monoxide (CO) poisoning
b. Ethylene glycol poisoning
c. Diabetic ketoacidosis
d. Lactic acidosis
e. Uremia

377. A 35-year-old man who is employed as a forklift operator was found sitting outside of a warehouse. He came stumbling out complaining of dizziness and headaches. Coworkers in an adjoining warehouse also complained of headache and nausea. After collapsing outside, he regained consciousness immediately but appeared confused. In the ED, his BP is 100/54 mm Hg, HR is 103 beats per minute, temperature is 100°F, and RR is 23 breaths per minute. Physical exam is unremarkable. Laboratory results reveal WBC 10,500/μL, hematocrit 45%, platelets 110/μL, sodium 137 mEq/L, potassium 4 mEq/L, chloride 103 mEq/L, bicarbonate 21 mEq/L, BUN 8 mg/dL, creatinine 0.5 mg/dL, and glucose 89 mg/dL. Arterial blood gas results are pH 7.32, PCO_2 32 mm Hg, PO_2 124 mm Hg, and COHb 18%. Which of the following is the most likely diagnosis?

a. Methemoglobinemia
b. Hypoglycemic syncope
c. Hydrocarbon poisoning
d. Opioid overdose
e. CO poisoning

378. A 51-year-old man presents to the ED complaining of nausea and abdominal pain after drinking some "bitter stuff." He is one of the "regulars" who is usually there with ethanol intoxication. His temperature is 97.9°F, BP is 130/65 mm Hg, HR is 90 beats per minute, RR is 16 breaths per minute, and O_2 saturation is 97% on room air. Physical exam is unremarkable except for slurred speech and the smell of acetone on the patient's breath. Laboratory results reveal serum sodium 138 mEq/L, potassium 3.5 mEq/L, chloride 105 mEq/L, bicarbonate 23 mEq/L, BUN 10 mg/dL, creatinine 1.7 mg/dL, glucose 85 mg/dL, arterial blood pH 7.37, and lactate 1.4 mEq/L. Urinalysis shows moderate ketones. Which of the following is the most likely diagnosis?

a. Diabetic ketoacidosis (DKA)
b. Ethanol intoxication
c. Methanol intoxication
d. Isopropyl alcohol intoxication
e. Ethylene glycol intoxication

379. A 55-year-old man presents to the ED 6 hours after ingesting two bottles of his baby aspirin. He complains of nausea, vomiting, dizziness, and tinnitus. His temperature is 100.3°F, BP is 140/80 mm Hg, HR is 105 beats per minute, RR is 31 breaths per minute, and O_2 saturation is 99% on room air. Arterial blood gas on room air reveals a pH of 7.52, PCO_2 10 mm Hg, and PO_2 129 mm Hg. The blood salicylate level returns at 45 mg/dL. Which of the following is the most appropriate next step in management?

a. Administer activated charcoal, begin IV hydration, and alkalinize the urine with sodium bicarbonate
b. Administer activated charcoal and intubate the patient for respiratory failure
c. Administer activated charcoal then NAC
d. Arrange for immediate hemodialysis
e. Observe the patient overnight to allow the body to metabolize the salicylates

380. A 40-year-old man with a known history of ethanol abuse states that 2 hours ago he ingested two bottles of extra-strength Tylenol. The patient has no medical complaints except for some nausea. At 4 hours post ingestion you send blood to the laboratory to measure the serum APAP concentration. The level returns and falls above the treatment line when you plot it on the APAP nomogram. You administer activated charcoal and decide to start IV NAC. Which of the following is a known adverse effect of IV NAC administration?

a. Hepatic failure
b. Anaphylactoid reaction
c. Hypertensive crisis
d. Confusion
e. Change in urine color

381. A 19-year-old woman presents to the ED with abdominal pain, nausea, vomiting, diarrhea, and hematemesis after ingesting an unknown substance in a suicide attempt. Which of the following antidotes are correctly paired?

a. Organophosphate—Physostigmine
b. Iron overdose—Deferoxamine
c. Aspirin overdose—NAC
d. Benzodiazepine overdose—Narcan
e. Anticholinergic overdose—Fomepizole

382. A 34-year-old woman presents to the ED after ingesting an unknown quantity of her antidepressant pills. EMS workers found an empty bottle of amitriptyline on her apartment floor. She is awake but appears delirious. Her BP is 130/65 mm Hg, HR is 101 beats per minute, temperature is 99.1°F, RR is 16 breaths per minute, and O_2 saturation is 100% on room air. On exam, her pupils are 7 mm and reactive. Her face is flushed and mucous membranes are dry. Her lungs are clear and heart is without murmurs. The abdomen is soft, nontender, and with decreased bowel sounds. She is moving all four extremities. ECG reveals sinus rhythm at a rate of 99 and QRS just under 100 msec. In a tricyclic antidepressant overdose, which of the following is responsible for her mydriasis, dry mucous membranes, and delirium?

a. Sodium channel blockade
b. Muscarinic receptor blockade
c. Inhibition of serotonin and norepinephrine reuptake
d. Histamine receptor blockade
e. α-Receptor blockade

383. You receive a notification from EMS that they are brining in a 17-year-old male who was found unconscious by a police officer. The police officer at the scene states that he snuck up on a group of kids that he thought were using drugs. Two of them got away and one just fell to the floor seconds after standing up. On the ground at the scene are multiple lighters and plastic bags. The emergency medicine technician (EMT) states that the patient was in ventricular fibrillation. He was shocked in the field and is now in a sinus rhythm. The EMT also administered IV dextrose, thiamine, and narcan without any change in mental status. Which if the following substance was the patient most likely abusing?

a. Butane
b. Ethanol
c. Heroin
d. Cocaine
e. PCP

384. A 61-year-old man with a history of depression and hypertension is brought to the ED by EMS for altered mental status. The patient's wife states that he stopped taking his fluoxetine 1 month ago and now only takes metoprolol for his hypertension. The patient's BP is 75/40 mm Hg, HR is 39 beats per minute, RR is 14 breaths per minute, O_2 saturation is 99% on 100% O_2, and fingerstick glucose is 81 mg/dL. The patient is awake and moaning, responding only to deep stimuli. You suspect an overdose of metoprolol. You endotracheally intubate the patient for airway control. Which of the following is the most appropriate next step in management?

a. Syrup of ipecac, normal saline bolus, epinephrine
b. Cardioversion with 200 J then administer epinephrine
c. Cardioversion with 200 J then administer atropine
d. Normal saline bolus, atropine, and activated charcoal
e. Normal saline bolus, atropine, glucagon, and activated charcoal

385. A 22-year-old woman presents to the ED by ambulance from a dance club. The paramedics report that the patient was agitated in the club and had a generalized seizure. Her BP is 165/100 mm Hg, HR is 119 beats per minute, temperature is 100.9°F, RR is 17 breaths per minute, O_2 saturation is 98% on room air, and fingerstick glucose is 92 mg/dL. On exam, the patient is hyperactive and appears to be hallucinating. Her pupils are dilated to 6 mm bilaterally and reactive. Her neck is supple. Examination of the heart is unremarkable except for tachycardia. Her lungs are clear and abdomen is soft and nontender. The patient moves all four extremities. Laboratory results are as follows:

sodium 109 mEq/L   WBC 12,000/mm^3
potassium 3.5 mEq/L   Hct 49%
chloride 83 mEq/L   platelets 350/μL
bicarbonate 20 mEq/L
BUN 10 mg/dL
creatinine 1 mg/dL
glucose 103 mg/dL

Which of the following substances did this patient most likely consume?

a. Cocaine
b. Heroin
c. 3,4-Methylenedioxymethamphetamine (MDMA)
d. Ketamine (special K)
e. PCP

386. An asymptomatic young adult was brought to the ED by a police officer after his home was raided. The patient swallowed five small packets of an unknown substance before being arrested. His BP is 125/75 mm Hg, HR is 85 beats per minute, temperature is 98.7°F, and RR is 16 breaths per minute. Physical exam is unremarkable. An abdominal radiograph confirms intraluminal small bowel densities. Which of the following is the most appropriate treatment?

a. Magnesium citrate
b. Gastric lavage
c. Activated charcoal and polyethylene glycol
d. Syrup of ipecac
e. NAC

387. A 33-year-old woman presents to the ED with a painful sprained ankle. She has a past medical history of depression for which she is taking phenelzine, a monoamine oxidase inhibitor. After you ACE wrap her ankle, she asks you to prescribe her some pain medication. Which of the following mediation is contraindicated in patients taking a monoamine oxidase inhibitor?

a. Ibuprofen
b. APAP
c. Meperidine
d. Oxycodone
e. Hydrocodone

388. A 27-year-old woman presents to the ED 6 hours after the onset of body aches, abdominal cramping, and diarrhea. She is currently visiting relatives and normally lives in another state. She regularly takes six to eight tablets daily of hydrocodone for chronic low back pain, sumatriptan for migraines, and amitriptyline and paroxetine for bulimia nervosa. Her BP is 130/80 mm Hg, HR is 100 beats per minute, temperature is 98.6°F, RR is 16 breaths per minute, and O_2 saturation is 99% on room air. Examination shows diaphoresis, dilated pupils, and piloerection. Neurologically she is moving all four extremities and you do not note tremors. She is alert and cooperative but seems restless. She denies hallucinations or suicidal ideations. She becomes very angry when you ask her for the phone numbers of her regular physicians. Which of the following is the most likely explanation of her symptoms?

a. Anticholinergic overdose
b. Tricyclic antidepressant intoxication
c. Ethanol withdrawal
d. Serotonin syndrome
e. Opiate withdrawal

Poisoning and Overdose

Answers

359. The answer is c. (*Rosen, pp 2187–2190.*) The patient drank *insecticide,* which is primarily composed of *organophosphate compounds* (i.e., Malathion). These compounds *inhibit acetylcholinesterase,* the enzyme responsible for the breakdown of acetylcholine. The patient is having a "cholinergic crisis." Over stimulation of muscarinic and nicotinic receptors leads to his symptoms, commonly remembered by the mnemonics **SLUDGE** (Salivation, Lacrimation, Urination, Defecation, Gastrointestinal [GI] upset, Emesis) or **DUMBBELS** (Defecation, Urination, Miosis, Bronchospasm, Bronchorrhea, Emesis, Lacrimation, Salivation). The treatment for organophosphate toxicity is *atropine* and *pralidoxime (2-PAM).* Atropine is an anticholinergic, therefore it competitively inhibits the excess acetylcholine. Pralidoxime works to regenerate acetylcholinesterase, therefore also limiting the amount of acetylcholine.

(**a**) Naloxone is used to reverse opiate (i.e., heroin) overdoses. (**b**) NAC is used in APAP (Tylenol) overdoses. (**d**) Flumazenil reverses benzodiazepines (i.e., diazepam). (**e**) Bicarbonate and kayexalate are commonly used in hyperkalemia.

360. The answer is a. (*Rosen, pp 2214–2215.*) *GHB* is a natural neurotransmitter that induces sleep. GHB has been sold as a muscle builder (release of growth hormone), a diet aid, and a sleep aid. Patients with GHB overdose generally have a decreased level of consciousness. In contrast to other sedative/hypnotic overdoses, the level of consciousness tends to fluctuate quickly between agitation and depression. A distinctive feature of GHB intoxication is *respiratory depression with apnea, interrupted by periods of agitation and combativeness,* especially following attempts at intubation.

(**b**) Diazepam, a benzodiazepine, also depresses mental and respiratory function but typically patients remain sedate. (**c**) Cocaine is a stimulant that increases HR, BP, and usually causes the pupils to dilate. (**d**) PCP intoxication may cause bizarre behavior, lethargy, agitation, confusion, or violence. (**e**) Heroin intoxication can cause respiratory depression. Patients usually present with miotic pupils.

361. The answer is d. (*Goldfrank, pp 1478–1486.*) The most useful diagnostic test obtainable in a suspected *CO poisoning* is a *COHb level*. Normal levels range from 0 to 5%, as CO is a natural by-product of the metabolism of porphyrins. COHb levels average 6% in one-pack-per-day smokers. CO poisoning should be suspected when multiple patients, usually in the same family, present with flu-like symptoms, and were exposed to products of combustion (home heaters/generators). This most commonly occurs in the winter months. The mainstay of treatment is the delivery of O_2. Hyperbaric O_2 is usually used for patients with COHb levels greater than 25%.

(**a**) A mono spot test detects the Epstein-Barr virus, the causative agent of mono. (**b**) CO poisoning is often confused for a viral syndrome. Patients with influenza usually present to the ED with high fever. (**c**) Malingering is the intentional production of false or exaggerated symptoms motivated by external incentives. (**e**) A lumbar puncture is used to diagnose meningitis, which may present with headache, nausea, and fatigue.

362. The answer is e. (*Rosen, pp 2069–2074.*) APAP is one of the most common analgesic-antipyretic medications and causes more hospitalizations after overdose than of any other pharmaceutical agent. Risk of hepatotoxicity is best established by plotting the APAP concentration on the APAP nomogram. APAP concentration must be measured between 4 and 24 hours after ingestion and then plotted on the nomogram. Patients with APAP concentrations on or above the treatment line should be treated. This patient has a 4-hour serum APAP concentration of 350 μg/mL. According to the nomogram, at 4 hours any concentration above 200 μg/mL should be treated. Therefore, the *patient should be started on NAC* and *admitted to the hospital*. During her admission, she should be evaluated by a psychiatrist regarding her attempted suicide.

The patient is at risk for APAP toxicity and meets criteria for treatment with NAC. Without treatment with NAC, she is at risk of developing liver failure and possible death. The patient is in phase 1 of an APAP poisoning. This phase usually lasts 0.5–24 hours. Patients are usually asymptomatic or exhibit findings such as nausea, vomiting, anorexia, malaise, and diaphoresis.

363. The answer is b. (*Rosen, pp 2064–2066.*) The term *toxidrome* refers to *a constellation of physical findings* that can provide important clues in a toxic ingestion. This is particularly useful in patients that cannot provide an adequate history. The *anticholinergic syndrome* typically presents with delirium, mumbling speech, tachycardia, elevated temperature, flushed face, dry mucous membranes and skin, dilated pupils, and hypoactive bowel sounds. The anticholinergic syndrome can be remembered by the phrase "blind as a bat (mydriasis), red as a beet (flushed skin), hot as a hare (hyperthermia secondary to lack of sweating), dry as a bone (dry mucous membranes)."

(a) The sympathomimetic syndrome is usually seen after ingestion of cocaine, amphetamines, or decongestants. It typically presents with delirium, paranoia, tachycardia, hypertension, hyperpyrexia, diaphoresis, mydriasis, seizures, and hyperactive bowel sounds. Sympathomimetic and anticholinergic syndromes are frequently difficult to distinguish. The main difference is that sympathomimetics usually cause diaphoresis whereas anticholinergics cause dry skin. (c) The cholinergic syndrome is commonly remembered by the mnemonics SLUDGE (Salivation, Lacrimation, Urination, Defecation, GI upset, Emesis) or DUMBBELS (Defecation, Urination, Miosis, Bronchospasm, Bronchorrhea, Emesis, Lacrimation, Salivation). (d and e) Opioids and ethanol are part of the sedative-hypnotic syndrome. It typically presents with sedation, miosis, respiratory depression, hypotension, bradycardia, hypothermia, and decreased bowel sounds.

364. The answer is b. (*Goldfrank, pp 480–496.*) The patient presents to the ED with central nervous system (CNS) and respiratory depression and miotic pupils. Along with his history of heroin abuse and fresh needle marks, this is most likely a *heroin overdose*. Opioid toxicity is associated with the toxidrome of CNS depression, respiratory depression, and miosis. Attention is always first directed at *airway management* in emergency medicine. The first action for this patient is to provide O_2 via bag-valve-mask. Because his respiratory depression is most likely secondary to opioid overdose, an *opioid antagonist* should be administered. *Naloxone* is the antidote most frequently used to reverse opioid toxicity. The goal of naloxone therapy is not necessarily complete arousal; rather, to reinstitute adequate spontaneous respiration, attempting to avoid inducing acute opioid withdrawal.

(a) Theoretically, one can continue bag-valve-mask ventilation until the affects of the heroin wears off, however this is not practical. If the patient overdosed on a long acting opioid, respiratory depression can last greater than 24 hours. (c) Flumazenil is the antidote for acute benzodiazepine overdose. (d) Activated charcoal should not be administered in patients with CNS depression who are not intubated due to the risk of emesis and aspiration. (e) Cathartics such as syrup of ipecac are contraindicated in patients with CNS depression. In addition, it has no use in overdoses by the IV route.

365. The answer is e. (Goldfrank, pp 656–660.) An overdose of any of these agents can lead to seizures. However, INH is notorious for causing seizures that are refractory to standard therapy. Marked acidosis and respiratory compromise may also be present. Pyridoxine (vitamin B₆) is the treatment of choice for INH overdose. INH is used for the treatment of tuberculosis, which is seen with a greater incidence in patients with AIDS. All of the other substances listed as answer choices should respond to standard therapy with benzodiazepines.

366. The answer is c. (Goldfrank, pp 593–603.) Glyburide is a commonly prescribed sulfonylurea. Sulfonylureas are oral agents that stimulate the beta cells of the pancreas to produce insulin. Many of the sulfonylureas have relatively long durations of action. Glyburide can act up to 24 hours after ingestion. Hypoglycemia secondary to sulfonylureas generally requires hospital admission to monitor for recurrent hypoglycemia.

(a) Excess insulin is the most common cause of hypoglycemia in patients who present to the ED. Often, the hypoglycemia results from the nonintentional overdose of a short or intermediate-acting insulin. After correcting the initial hypoglycemia, a meal and observation is usually enough for patients to be discharged. (b) Metformin, a biguanide, acts by increasing peripheral sensitivity to insulin and suppressing gluconeogenesis. Metformin should not produce hypoglycemia. (d) Troglitazone, a thiazolidinediones, also reduces insulin resistance, and decreases endogenous glucose production. Troglitazone should not produce hypoglycemia. (e) Acarbose is an α-glucosidase inhibitor that acts to decrease GI absorption of carbohydrates. It does not cause hypoglycemia.

367. The answer is d. (Goldfrank, pp 507–516.) The patient most likely ingested aspirin. Patients with an acute salicylate overdose may present with nausea, vomiting, tinnitus, fever, diaphoresis, and confusion. Salicylates are capable of producing several types of acid-base disturbances. Acute respiratory alkalosis, without hypoxia, is due to salicylate stimulation of the respiratory center in the brainstem. If the patient is hypoxic, salicylate-induced noncardiogenic pulmonary edema should be considered. Within 12–24 hours after ingestion, the acid-base status in an untreated patient shifts towards an anion gap metabolic acidosis due to interference with the Kreb's cycle, uncoupling oxidative-phosphorylation, and increased fatty-acid metabolism. A mixed respiratory alkalosis and metabolic acidosis is typically seen in adults.

(a) Diphenhydramine is a common decongestant that has antihistaminergic and anticholinergic properties. Overdoses may present as an anticholinergic toxidrome including altered mental status, mydriasis, flushed skin, hyperthermia, and dry mucous membranes. The antihistaminergic properties may cause sedation. (b) Ibuprofen overdose includes GI symptoms (nausea, vomiting, epigastric pain) and mild CNS depression. (c) APAP overdose usually lacks clinical signs or symptoms in the first 24 hours. Patients may have nonspecific GI complaints. (e) Pseudoephedrine is a commonly used decongestant. An overdose may present with CNS stimulation, hypertension, tachycardia, and dysrhythmias.

368. The answer is c. (*Rosen, pp 2064–2066.*) The *sympathomimetic syndrome* usually is seen after acute abuse of cocaine, amphetamines, or decongestants. Patients are usually *hypertensive* and *tachycardic* and exhibit *mydriatic pupils.* In massive overdoses, cardiovascular collapse can result in shock and wide-complex dysrhythmias. CNS effects include seizures. Sympathomimetic syndrome is sometimes difficult to distinguish from anticholinergic syndrome. The difference is that patients usually present with dry mucous membranes with an anticholinergic overdose, whereas patients are diaphoretic with sympathomimetics.

(a) The anticholinergic syndrome typically presents with delirium, mumbling speech, tachycardia, elevated temperature, flushed face, dry mucous membranes and skin, dilated pupils, and hypoactive bowel sounds. (b) The cholinergic syndrome is commonly remembered by the mnemonics SLUDGE (Salivation, Lacrimation, Urination, Defecation, GI upset, Emesis) or DUMBBELS (Defecation, Urination, Miosis, Bronchospasm, Bronchorrhea, Emesis, Lacrimation, Salivation). (d) Opioids are part of the sedative-hypnotic syndrome. It typically presents with sedation, miosis, respiratory depression, hypotension, bradycardia, hypothermia, and decreased bowel sounds. (e) Serotonin syndrome is characterized by altered mental status, fever, agitation, tremor, myoclonus, hyperreflexia, ataxia, diaphoresis, shivering, and sometimes diarrhea. It is difficult to distinguish from cocaine overdose and diagnosis relies on the medication history.

369. The answer is d. (*Rosen, pp 2066–2067.*) A major change has occurred in the approach of GI decontamination over the past decade. Previous recommendations indicated that the stomach should be emptied by either syrup of ipecac or gastric lavage. Activated charcoal (AC) alone has demonstrated similar or superior results and now is the recommended GI decontaminant. The complications of gastric emptying procedures, primarily aspiration, are largely avoided when only AC is used. Most ingested drugs and chemicals are adsorbed to activated charcoal. The few agents that do not adsorb to charcoal include *ions* (e.g., mineral acids and alkalis, lithium, borates, bromides), *hydrocarbons (HCs), metals* (e.g., iron), and *ethanol*.

The patient in question ingested *lithium* that is used to treat her bipolar disorder. A lithium level should be drawn and management decided based on those results. Potential treatments include whole-bowel irrigation and dialysis.

370. The answer is e. *(Goldfrank, pp 1004–1014. Rosen, pp 2119–2124.)* *Benzodiazepines (i.e., diazepam)* should be used as the first-line agent for nearly all cocaine toxicities. Many effects of cocaine are thought to be mediated through CNS stimulation by the release of or inhibiting the reuptake of catecholamines. The affects that acute cocaine intoxication have on the heart includes coronary vasoconstriction with increasing myocardial O_2 demand. The goal of lowering the BP in this patient is to reverse the vasoconstriction by norepinephrine at peripheral α-adrenergic receptors. Benzodiazepines restore the CNS inhibitory tone on the peripheral nervous system. The use of β-adrenergic antagonists should be avoided with cocaine because of paradoxical hypertension and coronary artery vasoconstriction due to unopposed α-adrenergic receptor stimulation.

(a) Although haloperidol can be used for sedation, its anticholinergic effects can limit cooling by impeding diaphoresis and may increase morbidity. **(b and c)** It is best to avoid β-adrenergic antagonists in the setting of cocaine intoxication. Their use leads to unopposed α-adrenergic stimulation that results in vasoconstriction and hypertension. Although labetolol is an α- and β-adrenergic receptor blocker, it has substantially more β-adrenergic antagonism than α-adrenergic antagonist effects. **(d)** The data regarding the efficacy of calcium channel blockers (CCBs) for the treatment of cocaine toxicity are contradictory. Therefore, their role in patients with cocaine intoxication remains unclear.

371. The answer is d. *(Goldfrank, pp 41059–41069.)* Opioid *withdrawal* initially presents with drug craving, yawning, rhinorrhea, piloerection and progresses to nausea, vomiting, diarrhea, hyperactive bowel, diaphoresis, myalgias, arthralgias, anxiety, fear, and mild tachycardia. *Methadone withdrawal* starts approximately 24 hours after the last dose and persists for 3–7 days. Heroin withdrawal begins about 6 hours after the last dose and usually fully manifests at 24 hours. Opioid withdrawal is not life-threatening as long as adequate hydration and nutritional support is maintained.

(a) Ethanol withdrawal is a life-threatening condition that develops 6–24 hours after the reduction of ethanol intake. It is characterized by autonomic hyperactivity including nausea, anorexia, coarse tremor, tachycardia, hypertension, hyperreflexia, sleep disturbances, hallucinations, and seizure. (b) When cocaine use is stopped or when a binge ends, a crash follows almost immediately. This is accompanied by a strong craving for more cocaine, fatigue, lack of pleasure, anxiety, irritability, sleepiness, and sometimes agitation or extreme suspicion. (c) Nicotine withdrawal manifests largely as cigarette craving and subjective dysphoric symptoms. There are some symptoms of irritability and restlessness. (e) Discontinuation of clonidine leads to headache, flushing, sweating, hallucinations, anxiety, and reflex tachycardia.

372. The answer is d. (*Goldfrank, pp 11034–11041. Rosen, pp 2145–2148.*) *PCP intoxication* is characterized by a wide spectrum of findings. Behavior may be bizarre, agitated, confused, or violent. The hallmark of PCP toxicity is the *recurring delusion of superhuman strength and invulnerability* resulting from both the anesthetic and dissociative properties of the drug. Patients have broken police handcuffs, fracturing bones in doing so. The major cause of death or injury from PCP is behavioral toxicity leading to suicide and provoked homicide. Typical neurologic signs include *nystagmus* (horizontal, vertical or rotary), ataxia, and altered gait. Pupils are usually midsized and reactive, but can be mydriatic or miotic. Bizarre posturing, grimacing, and writhing may be seen. Management is conservative. To prevent self-injury, the patient must be safely restrained. Antipsychotics or benzodiazepines are frequently administered for chemical sedation. PCP intoxication usually ranges from 8 to 16 hours, but can last longer in chronic users.

(a and c) Cocaine and amphetamines are sympathomimetics that can be confused with PCP intoxication. However, the hallmark to PCP intoxication that is not usually observed in sympathomimetic intoxication is the recurring delusion of superhuman strength and nystagmus. (b) When cocaine use is stopped or when a binge ends, a crash follows almost immediately. This is accompanied by a strong craving for more cocaine, fatigue, lack of pleasure, anxiety, irritability, sleepiness, and sometimes agitation or extreme suspicion. (e) Opioid withdrawal initially presents with drug craving, yawning, rhinorrhea, piloerection and progresses to nausea, vomiting, diarrhea, hyperactive bowel, diaphoresis, myalgias, arthralgias, anxiety, fear, and mild tachycardia.

373. The answer is a. (*Goldfrank, pp 980–988.*) An *anion gap* is the difference between unmeasured anions (e.g., proteins, organic acids) and unmeasured cations (e.g., potassium, calcium, magnesium). The anion gap can be calculated from the formula:

$$\text{Anion gap} = [Na^+] - [HCO_3 + Cl^-]$$

The normal anion gap is approximately 6–10 mEq/L. The cause of increased anion gap is frequently remembered by the mnemonic **MUD PILES**:

M: methanol, metformin   **P**: paraldehyde
U: uremia   **I**: iron, INH
D: diabetic ketoacidosis   **L**: lactate
     E: ethylene glycol, ethanol
     S: salicylate

Our patient's anion gap is $(141) - (101 + 14) = 26$

The *measured serum osmolarity* performed by the laboratory is measured by a depression in the freezing point or an elevation in the boiling point of the solution. If there is an increase in low–molecular weight molecules, such as acetone, methanol, ethanol, mannitol, isopropyl alcohol, or ethylene glycol, the osmolarity increases more than what is calculated from the regular serum molecules.

The formula to *calculate serum osmolarity* is:

$$\text{Serum Osm (mOsm/Kg)} = 2[Na^+] + \text{glucose}/18 + \text{BUN}/1.8 + \text{EtOH}/4.6$$

The difference between the actual measured osmolarity and the calculated osmolarity is the osmol *gap (measured − calculated)*.

Our patient's osmol gap is $(352) - (292) = 60$. When the osmol gap is greater than 50 mOsm/L, it should be considered nearly diagnostic of *toxic alcohol* ingestion. However, a normal or even negative osmol gap does not exclude the presence of *toxic alcohols*.

The patient's clinical presentation of altered mental status, anion gap metabolic acidosis, and osmol gap is consistent with a *toxic alcohol* ingestion. In this case, the ingested substance was methanol.

374. The answer is b. (*Goldfrank, pp 847–860. Rosen, pp 2087–2093.*) For young patients with altered mental status, toxic ingestion should be high on the differential. This clinical scenario is most consistent with toxic ingestion of a *tricyclic antidepressant (TCA)*. Treatment of all toxic ingestions should begin with assessment of airway, breathing, and circulation. Due to this patient's mental status and loss of gag reflex, *orotracheal intubation* is indicated for airway protection. Subsequently, *activated charcoal* can be administered. Due to the anticholinergic effects of TCAs, absorption is prolonged and GI motility is delayed leading to greater toxicity. Therefore, an additional dose of charcoal should be administered several hours later. In an obtunded patient, it is important to first secure an airway prior to administering charcoal to prevent aspiration in the event of vomiting.

Acute cardiovascular toxicity is responsible for most of the mortalities from TCA overdose. The characteristic features are conduction delays, dysrhythmias, and hypotension. The sodium blocking activity of TCAs leads to a widened QRS and rightward axis. It is believed that there is an increased chance of cardiac dysrhythmias if the QRS is greater than 100 msec. It is recommended that you treat this condition with IV *sodium bicarbonate* until the QRS narrows to 100 msec or the serum pH increases to 7.55. In addition, the patient is hypotensive and should receive a fluid bolus of normal saline and be placed in Trendelenberg position. If the hypotension does not resolve after these maneuvers and administration of bicarbonate, the patient should receive norepinephrine. TCA overdose may progress rapidly and is frequently unpredictable. It is common for a patient to present to the ED awake and alert and then develop life-threatening cardiovascular and CNS toxicity within a couple of hours.

(a) Narcan is the antidote for opioid toxicity; this patient requires sodium bicarbonate for a TCA overdose. (c) NAC is the antidote for APAP overdose. (d) Syrup of ipecac cannot be administered to a patient who is intubated. It must be given to patients with a normal mental status with nothing impeding their oropharynx. (e) Inducing vomiting is contraindicated given the potential for precipitous neurologic and hemodynamic deterioration.

375. The answer is a. (*Goldfrank, pp 480–496.*) NAC is the cornerstone of therapy for the potentially lethal APAP overdose. NAC acts as a glutathione precursor to reduce NAPQI (N-acetyl-p-benzoquinoneimine), the toxic metabolite of APAP. It can be administered orally or intravenously. NAC is most effective if administered within 8 hours of the ingestion, however, it may still be of benefit if given more than 24 hours after an acute APAP overdose.

(b) Physostigmine is used for an anticholinergic overdose. (c) Flumazenil is a benzodiazepine antagonist used occasional in a benzodiazepine overdose. Its use can precipitate benzodiazepine withdrawal and seizures in chronic benzodiazepine users. **(d)** Naloxone is a μ receptor antagonist and is used in opioid overdoses. **(e)** Digibind is the antidote for digitalis glycoside poisoning.

376. The answer is b. *(Rosen, pp 2129–2133.) Ethylene glycol* is a colorless, odorless, slightly sweet-tasting liquid that is found in antifreeze. Ingestions of antifreeze are either accidental, suicidal, or in substitute of ethanol. Ethylene glycol is metabolized to glycolic acid, which results in a profound *anion gap metabolic acidosis* (Na) − ([Cl] + [HCO₃]); (139 − [101 + 14]) = 24. Glycolic acid is subsequently metabolized to oxalic acid, which combines with calcium to form calcium oxalate crystals, which then precipitate in renal tubules, brain, and other tissues. The finding of *crystalluria* is considered the *hallmark of ethylene glycol ingestion,* however, its absence does not rule out the diagnosis. Another useful test in the ED involves examining freshly voided urine for fluorescence with a Wood's lamp. Sodium fluorescein is added to antifreeze to aid in the detection of radiator leaks. Ingestion of ethylene glycol is associated with neurologic, cardiopulmonary, and renal abnormalities.

(a) CO poisoning can cause a metabolic acidosis. However, this patient's CO level is within normal limits. **(c)** Diabetic ketoacidosis can cause a metabolic acidosis. Patients usually have a history of diabetes, elevated blood glucose (>200 mg/dL), and ketones in their urine. **(d)** Lactic acidosis can cause a metabolic acidosis. This patient's lactate is within normal limits. **(e)** The patient has a normal creatinine level.

377. The answer is e. *(Goldfrank, pp 1478–1486.) CO poisoning* is the leading cause of poisoning morbidity and mortality in the United States. People are exposed to CO through fires, vehicle exhaust, home generators, and the metabolism of methylene chloride. Workers also become symptomatic from use of propane-powered equipment indoors such as forklifts and ice skating resurfacers. Often, other people in the area have similar complaints. The earliest symptoms are nonspecific and readily confused with other illnesses such as viral syndromes. Mild symptoms include headache, nausea, and dizziness. Severe symptoms include chest pain, palpitations, and seizures. Diagnosis is made by detecting elevated CO in the blood. Normal levels range from 0 to 5%, while smokers may be as high as 10%. Treatment includes immediate O₂ therapy. Hyperbaric O₂ is the treatment of choice for patients with significant CO exposures.

(a) Methemoglobinemia occurs from exposures to nitrates, certain anesthetics, and various medications. Patients typically present cyanotic with a normal PO$_2$ that does not respond to supplemental O$_2$. **(b)** Hypoglycemia can cause syncope. However, this patient's blood glucose was normal. **(c)** Hydrocarbon poisoning (e.g., kerosene, gasoline, nail polish remover) typically occurs from an intentional exposure. The pulmonary system is most commonly affected. **(d)** Opioid overdose causes sedation and respiratory depression.

378. The answer is d. *(Rosen, pp 2133–2135.)* *Isopropyl alcohol* is one of the *toxic alcohols* (ethylene glycol, methanol, and isopropyl alcohol). It is a clear, colorless liquid with a *bitter taste.* It is commonly used as a *rubbing alcohol* and as a solvent in hair-care products, skin lotion, and home aerosols. Moreover, it is often ingested as an inexpensive and convenient substitute for ethanol. Clinically, GI and CNS complaints predominate. Its GI irritant properties cause patients to complain of abdominal pain, nausea, and vomiting. Pupillary size varies but miosis is commonly observed. Large ingestions can result in coma. Hypotension, although rare, signifies severe poisoning. Characteristically, metabolic acidosis, unlike the other *toxic alcohols,* is not present. This is because isopropyl alcohol is metabolized to *acetone,* a ketone, not an acid. It is also the cause for the presence of urinary ketones and the odor on the patient's breath. Isopropyl alcohol intoxication is often remembered by "ketosis without acidosis." Another unique finding is the presence of "pseudo renal failure" or isolated false elevation of creatinine with a normal BUN. This results from interference of acetone and acetoacetate by the colorimetric method of creatinine determination.

(a) If the patient had a history of diabetes with an elevated blood sugar and ketones present in the urine, then DKA would be highly suspected. **(b)** Differentiating between ethanol and isopropyl alcohol ingestion can be very difficult. However, the patient's clinical presentation of drinking a bitter liquid, abdominal pain, nausea, vomiting, odor of acetone and ketosis without acidosis is most consistent with isopropyl alcohol intoxication. **(c and e)** Methanol and ethylene glycol intoxication are typically associated with an anion gap metabolic acidosis.

379. The answer is a. *(Rosen, pp 2076–2078.)* The treatment of *salicylate toxicity* has three objectives: prevent further salicylate absorption, correct fluid deficits and acid-base abnormalities, and reduce tissue salicylate concentrations by increasing excretion. *Activated charcoal* should be administered as soon as possible to reduce salicylate absorption. Dehydration occurs early in salicylate intoxication and should be treated with

IV hydration. *Urine alkalization* should be considered in patients with salicylate levels greater than 35 mg/dL. Because salicylic acid is a weak acid, it is ionized in an alkaline environment and gets "trapped," limiting the amount that crosses the blood-brain barrier and increasing urinary excretion.

(b) Endotracheal intubation may be necessary in respiratory failure; however, in a salicylate poisoned patient, it is important to maintain hyperventilation and an alkalotic environment in order to keep salicylic acid ionized to limit it from crossing the blood-brain barrier. It is difficult to maintain an appropriate level of hypocarbia and hyperventilation through assisted ventilation. **(c)** NAC is the antidote for APAP poisoning. It is important, however, to obtain an APAP level in patients with an aspirin overdose because the two may occur together. **(d)** Hemodialysis for aspirin overdose should be considered in patients with severe salicylism associated with serum salicylate levels greater than 100 mg/dL, coma, renal, or liver failure, and pulmonary edema. Also with severe acid-base disturbances or the failure to respond to more conservative treatments such as activated charcoal and alkalization. **(e)** Observation without intervention is not recommended with an aspirin overdose as there is a risk of death.

380. The answer is b. *(Rosen, pp 2069–2074.)* IV NAC has been responsible for *anaphylactoid reactions, including rash, bronchospasm, hypotension, and death.* These complications are dose and concentration dependent and are prevented by slow administration of dilute NAC. Some other side effects include GI disorders, tachycardia, and chest tightness.

(a) NAC is used in the treatment of hepatic failure secondary to APAP overdose. **(c and d)** IV NAC is not known to cause these side effects. **(e)** Amitriptyline, indomethacin, doxorubicin, pyridium, and rifampin are some medications known to cause urine to change color.

381. The answer is b. *(Rosen, pp 2151–2152.)* *Deferoxamine* is a specific chelator of *ferric iron (Fe^{3+})*. It binds with iron to form a water-soluble compound, ferrioxamine, which can be excreted by the kidneys. Deferoxamine has a half-life of 1 hour, so continuous infusion is the preferred method of administration.

The patient's clinical presentation is consistent with *acute iron poisoning.* Initial presentation reflects the corrosive effects of iron on the gut and includes nausea, vomiting, diarrhea, and sometimes GI bleeding. Patients with severe overdose may present with shock or coma.

(a) The treatment for organophosphate toxicity is atropine and pralidoxime. Physostigmine is an antidote for the anticholinergic syndrome.

(c) Aspirin overdose is treated with decontamination, urine alkalinization, and sometimes dialysis. NAC is the antidote for APAP overdose. (d) Acute benzodiazepine overdose is treated with flumazenil. Narcan is the antidote for opioid overdose. (e) Anticholinergic overdose can be treated with physostigmine. Fomepizole is the treatment for toxic alcohol ingestion (i.e., ethylene glycol).

382. The answer is b. (*Rosen, pp 2087–2093.*) Overdose of *TCA* results in toxicity by a number of different mechanisms. The *anticholinergic properties* of TCAs results in the toxidrome "blind as a bat (mydriasis), red as a beet (flushed skin), hot as a hare (hyperthermia secondary to lack of sweating), dry as a bone (dry mucous membranes)." This is secondary to *muscarinic receptor blockade.* The cardinal signs of TCA overdose include ventricular dysrhythmias, hypotension, and decreased mental status. *Sodium bicarbonate* is a potentially life-saving intervention in TCA overdose because an alkaline pH combined with a sodium load increases conductance through cardiac fast sodium channels and prevents ventricular dysrhythmias as evidenced by narrowing of the QRS complex on an ECG.

(a) The most worrisome effect is sodium channel blockade causing conduction delays and dysrhythmias as evidenced by QRS widening, QT prolongation, and wide-complex tachycardias. (c) Inhibition of serotonin and norepinephrine reuptake results in catecholamine depletion and contributes to hypotension. (d) Histamine receptor blockade is associated with sedation. (e) α receptor blockade causes vasodilation and hypotension leading to a decrease in systemic vascular resistance and widened pulse pressure.

383. The answer is a. (*Rosen, pp 2159–2162.*) HCs are a diverse group of organic compounds that contain hydrogen and carbon. Some common products containing HCs are household polishes, glues, paint remover, and industrial solvents. Acute HC toxicity usually affects three main target organs: the lungs, the CNS, and the heart. The lungs are most commonly affected by aspiration of ingested HCs. Pulmonary toxicity is associated with cough, crackles, bronchospasm, pulmonary edema, and pneumonitis on chest radiograph. Certain HCs (e.g., toluene, benzene, gasoline, butane, chlorinated HCs) can have sedative/opioid-like effect and cause euphoria, disinhibition, confusion, and obtundation. HCs can also cause *sudden cardiac death,* particularly after sudden physical activity after intentional inhalation. It is thought that the HCs produce *myocardial sensitization* of endogenous and exogenous catecholamine, which precipitates ventricular dysrhythmias and myocardial dysfunction. One scenario is the solvent-abusing person.

EMS workers often describe an individual who has used inhaled solvents, performed some type of physical activity, then suddenly collapsed.

In the scenario above, the patient inhaling *butane* was approached by a police officer and tried to run away. This sudden exertion most likely led to a cardiac dysrhythmia. Paraphernalia is often found at the scene, including plastic bags used for "bagging" (pouring HCs in a bag, then deeply inhaling) or a HC-soaked cloth used for "huffing" (inhaling through a saturated cloth). Other paraphernalia include gasoline containers, multiple butane lighters, and spray paint cans.

384. The answer is e. (*Goldfrank, pp 741–753. Rosen, pp 2108–2110.*) *β-Adrenergic receptor blockers* (i.e., Metoprolol) are commonly prescribed medications for hypertension. *β*-Adrenergic antagonism overdose is often benign, with about 33% of patients remaining asymptomatic. This is partially explained by the fact that *β*-adrenergic antagonism is often well tolerated in healthy persons who do not rely on sympathetic stimulation to maintain cardiac output. Conversely, those with cardiac abnormalities may rely on sympathetic stimulation to maintain HR or cardiac output. The *hallmark of β-adrenergic receptor toxicity* is *bradycardia with hypotension*. Patients may also exhibit conduction and rhythm abnormalities. Onset of toxicity usually occurs within 4 hours of ingestion. If a patient remains asymptomatic after 4 hours there is a low risk for subsequent morbidity unless a delayed-release preparation is involved.

Management begins with addressing the ABCs. Airway and ventilation should be maintained with endotracheal intubation if necessary. The initial treatment of hypotension and bradycardia consists of *fluid resuscitation* and *atropine*. Patients should receive GI decontamination with *activated charcoal* and whole-bowel irrigation should be considered in patients who have ingested sustained-release preparations. Patients with significant toxicity (HR <40, BP <80, congestive heart failure (CHF), altered mental status) should also receive *glucagon,* which does not rely on *β*-receptors for its actions and has both inotropic and chronotropic effects. It also helps counteract the hypoglycemia induced by *β*-blocker overdose.

(a) Syrup of ipecac is contraindicated in any patient with depressed or potentially depressed consciousness. **(b and c)** Cardioversion is contraindicated in sinus rhythm. It is reserved for "shockable" rhythms such as ventricular fibrillation and pulseless ventricular tachycardia. Epinephrine may be used if administration of fluids, atropine, and glucagon fails to treat the patient. **(d)** This selection may be attempted with a patient who was not hypotensive. However, if atropine and fluids do not treat the hypotension then glucagon is required.

385. The answer is c. (*Goldfrank, pp 1020–1028.*) MDMA is currently one of the most widely abused *amphetamines* by college students and teenagers. It is commonly known as "ecstasy," "E," "XTC," and "M&M." MDMA is an entactogen, a substance capable of producing euphoria, inner peace, and a desire to socialize. Negative effects include ataxia, restlessness, confusion, poor concentration, and memory problems. MDMA, although classified as an amphetamine, is also a potent stimulus for the release of serotonin. MDMA can also cause significant *hyponatremia*. The increase in serotonin results in the excessive release of vasopressin (antidiuretic hormone [ADH]). Moreover, large free-water intake (increased thirst) combined with sodium loss from physical exertion (dancing) certainly contributes to the development of hyponatremia. This hyponatremia is mot likely responsible for the patient's seizure.

(**a**) Cocaine use can cause agitation and seizures but should not cause significant hyponatremia. (**b**) Heroin intoxication usually causes people to be more sedate rather than agitated. It should not cause seizures or hyponatremia. (**d and e**) Ketamine and PCP can cause agitation and hallucinations; however, significant hyponatremia is not usually present.

386. The answer is c. (*Goldfrank, pp 1013–1014.*) Patients being arrested whom swallow illegal drugs to conceal the evidence are referred to as "body stuffers." They commonly tend to ingest any and all the drugs they possess, potentially resulting in a polypharmaceutic overdose. Body stuffers are usually seen in the ED before symptoms have developed. *Activated charcoal* should be administered immediately and *whole-bowel irrigation* may be indicated. Sometimes there is radiographic evidence of the swallowed substances as seen in crack vials or staples on the packaging materials. Whole-bowel irrigation uses a *polyethylene glycol electrolyte solution (i.e., GoLYTELY)*, which is not absorbed and flushes drugs or chemicals through the GI tract. This procedure seems to be most useful when radiopaque tablets or chemicals, swallowed packets of street drugs, or sustained-released drugs have been ingested.

(**a**) Magnesium citrate is a cathartic whose action begins 4–6 hours after ingestion. It is contraindicated in patients with renal failure. (**b**) The packets are observed in the small bowel, too distal for effective gastric lavage. (**d**) Syrup of ipecac is also ineffective for the packets in the small bowel. (**e**) NAC is the antidote for APAP toxicity.

387. The answer is c. (*Goldfrank, p 889.*) Any patient taking a monoamine oxidase inhibitor (MAOI) is at risk for developing the *serotonin syndrome* if the individual coingests a selective serotonin reuptake inhibitor or another drug that raises CNS serotonin levels. Some medications that can cause this interaction include indirect-acting and mixed-acting sympathomimetics (cocaine, amphetamine), antidepressants (TCA, SSRI), *meperidine (Demerol)*, and dextromethorphan, which is found in many nonprescription antitussives. In contrast, morphine and its derivatives lack the serotonin-potentiating effects. Serotonin syndrome is characterized by altered mental status, hyperthermia, neuromuscular dysfunction, and autonomic dysfunction. Symptoms may also include shivering, trismus, akathisia, coma, and seizures.

(a, b, d, and e) Ibuprofen, APAP, oxycodone, and hydrocodone are all safe to use in patients taking MAOIs.

388. The answer is e. *(Rosen, pp 2180–2185.)* Hydrocodone is an opioid used for pain relief. *Opioid withdrawal* occurs in tolerant individuals when opioid exposure is discontinued or an antagonist is administered. Its effects are secondary to *increased sympathetic discharge* that is responsible for the clinical signs and symptoms. Although these can be significant, they are typically not life-threatening. Withdrawal is associated with CNS excitation, tachypnea, and mydriasis. Pulse and BP may be elevated. The patient may preset with nausea, vomiting, diarrhea, abdominal cramps, myalgias, and insomnia. Examination often reveals piloerection, yawning, lacrimation, rhinorrhea, and diaphoresis. Neurologic manifestations include restlessness, agitation, and anxiety, but cognition and mental status are unaffected. Dysphoria and drug craving are usually prominent.

(a and b) Amitriptyline is a TCA that has anticholinergic properties. Overdose of TCAs results in toxicity by a number of different mechanisms. The anticholinergic properties of TCAs results in the toxidrome "blind as a bat (mydriasis), red as a beet (flushed skin), hot as a hare (hyperthermia secondary to lack of sweating), dry as a bone (dry mucous membranes)." The cardinal signs of TCA overdose include ventricular dysrhythmias, hypotension, and decreased mental status. (c) Early alcohol withdrawal may occur 6 hours after cessation or decrease of alcohol consumption. It is characterized by autonomic hyperactivity: nausea, anorexia, coarse tremor, tachycardia, hyperreflexia, hypertension, fever, decreased seizure threshold, hallucinations, and delirium. (d) Serotonin syndrome occurs when a serotonin reuptake inhibitor is combined with another drug that potentiates serotonin. The opioid meperidine (Demerol), but not hydrocodone, is known to potentiate serotonin. It presents with abdominal pain, diarrhea, diaphoresis, hyperpyrexia, tachycardia, hypertension, myoclonus, irritability, agitation, seizures, and delirium.

Environmental Exposures

Questions

389. A 58-year-old man presents to the emergency department (ED) with reported blister formation over both feet that initially began 2 days ago. He denies any past medical history, medications, or allergies. His social history is significant for alcohol dependence and recently becoming undomiciled. He denies any sick contacts or recent travel. Upon physical examination, these lesions are fluid-filled and his feet are grossly cyanotic and tender to the touch. His foot is shown below. What is the most likely diagnosis in this patient?

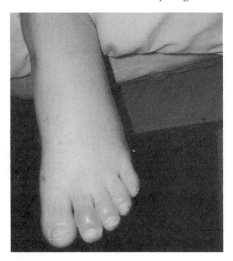

(Reproduced, with permission, from Knoop KJ, Stack LB, Storrow AB. Atlas of Emergency Medicine. New York, NY: McGraw-Hill, 2002: 517.)

a. Chilbains
b. Frostbite
c. Trench foot
d. Thermal burn
e. Herpes

390. A 43-year-old insulin-dependent diabetic woman presents with an intensely pruritic rash across her back for the last several days. She reports a recent trip to the Caribbean with her family last week, none of whom has similar symptoms. She denies any insect bites, new detergents, soaps, or clothes and has otherwise been at her baseline of health with no constitutional symptoms. The patient is on insulin glargine for her diabetes and reports a hemoglobin A1C of <7 mg/dL. Upon physical examination, the patient has small vesicular lesions on an erythematous base with no visible purulence. The rash does not follow a dermatome distribution and is clustered across her back. Which of the following is the most appropriate treatment choice for this patient?

a. Calamine lotion
b. Acyclovir
c. Chlorhexadine lotion
d. Benadryl
e. Parenteral antibiotics

391. A 32-year-old otherwise healthy man develops dizziness, nausea, and confusion after running a race. Emergency medical services are available on-site and the patient is given intravenous (IV) resuscitation with crystalloids. He is oriented to person and year, but not place. He appears generally confused and it is difficult to obtain contact information from him. The patient is brought to the ED whereupon his symptoms generally resolve, except for diffuse muscle fatigue. Labs are drawn at this time, which are essentially normal, except for minimally elevated hepatic transaminases. Given this patient's symptoms and laboratory evaluation, what is the most likely diagnosis?

a. Heat syncope
b. Heat edema
c. Rhabdomyolysis
d. Heat stroke
e. Heat exhaustion

392. A 2-year-old girl is brought in to the ED by her father who reports that he found the child crying in the next room holding her right index finger. An unprotected electrical wall socket was nearby. Upon presentation, the child is easily consolable but holds her right index finger in the air. Visual inspection reveals localized erythema at the distal tip but good capillary refill, 2+ radial, and ulnar pulses and full range of motion of that hand and extremity. The child's chest auscultation reveals a normal S1 and S2 with clear and equal breath sounds bilaterally. There are no other signs of trauma. What diagnostic test should be performed next in the complete evaluation of this child?

a. Urinalysis
b. Basic metabolic panel
c. Chest x-ray
d. Electrocardiogram (ECG)
e. Arterial Doppler

393. A 27-year-old Greek woman, upon arriving at the airport of her native country, develops left upper quadrant (LUQ) abdominal pain that is sharp and severe in nature. She is brought to the ED by local officials who report that she syncopized. Upon arrival, she is awake and alert and states that she has no medical history except for an abnormal blood trait. She denies any prior hospitalizations and states that her last menstrual period was 2 weeks ago. Upon physical examination, her abdomen is soft with significant LUQ pain upon palpation and deep inspiration. A subsequent pelvic exam reveals no tenderness or abnormalities. Which of the following is the most likely underlying cause for this patient's pain?

a. Left ovarian torsion
b. Appendicitis
c. G6PD-deficiency
d. Sickle cell trait
e. Ectopic pregnancy

394. An 18-year-old man presents to the ED with right leg pain and swelling after swimming at a local beach. He reports swimming in the ocean, whereupon he felt a sharp sting in his right leg. Upon physical examination, there is no gross deformity of the right lower extremity and there is a palpable dorsalis pedis and posterior tibial pulse. There is tenderness to palpation over the lateral calf with many punctuate, erythematous lesions as seen below. Which of the following is the most appropriate treatment of choice for this patient?

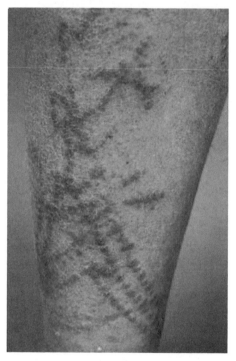

(Reproduced, with permission, from Wolf K, Johnson RA, Suurmond D. Color Atlas and Synopsis of Clinical Dermatology. New York, NY: McGraw-Hill, 2005: 869.)

a. Fresh water
b. Vegetable oil
c. Vinegar
d. Toothpaste
e. Household window cleaner

395. A 49-year-old man presents to the ED with pain, erythema, and swelling to his left forearm after a chemical spill sustained at work. He irrigated the area with water and applied a cold packet before arriving but states that the burning sensation in his arm is now worse. The patient works in a glass factory and reports using a rust-removing agent. What tissue-saving treatment must be administered emergently?

a. Limb tourniquet
b. Calcium gluconate
c. Alkalinization of urine
d. Silver silvadene ointment
e. Surgical debridement

396. A 23-year-old construction worker is brought by ambulance to the ED with bilateral knee pain. He reports mixing cement the day before and kneeling in the process. The patient states that his jeans were soaked through most of the day but did not attempt to wash the cement off. Upon physical examination, you see marked tissue necrosis of both knees extending to the bone in some places. Which chemical was this patient most likely exposed to?

a. Hydrocarbon
b. Phenol
c. Ammonia
d. Formic acid
e. Lime

397. A 40-year-old veterinary assistant presents to the ED with puncture wounds over her right upper extremity and neck. She reports being bitten multiple times by a cat in her care, also stating that the cat's immunizations were up to date. The injury was sustained 2 days ago with minimal initial symptoms. However, today the patient noticed redness and pain in that area. She denies any fever, chills, nausea, vomiting, or any other constitutional symptoms. Her initial vitals include an oral temperature of 99.7°F, a heart rate (HR) of 90 beats per minute, blood pressure (BP) of 125/75 mm Hg, respiratory rate (RR) of 14 breaths per minute and an O_2 saturation of 99% on room air. Multiple punctate wounds may be seen over her right lateral neck extending down to her deltoid with surrounding erythema and edema. Which antibiotic coverage for the specific organism involved in this type of injury would be most appropriate?

a. A first-generation cephalosporin/*Staphylococcus aureus*
b. Amoxicillin/Clavulanate (Augmentin)/*Pasteurella multocida*
c. Clindamycin/Streptococcus species
d. Vancomycin/Methicillin resistant *S. aureus*
e. Bacitracin ointment/*S. aureus*

398. A 16-year-old girl presents to the ED with a history of spilling hot soup over her left arm earlier in the day. She states that she immediately put her hand under cold water and applied ice. Upon physical examination, the involved area covers the dorsum of her hand and extends up to the middle of her forearm with no circumferential or digital involvement. She can freely flex and extend all joints of that upper extremity. In addition, two large fluid-filled bullae are noted in the area of the forearm. What is the burn degree and relative area of involvement in this patient?

a. First-degree/9%
b. Second-degree/9%
c. Second-degree/2.25%
d. Third-degree/9%
e. Third-degree/4.5%

399. A 60-year-old male cook reports spilling hot oil over his left thigh while attempting to pull a pan off of the stove. He presents to the ED with erythema extending over his left thigh without any blister formation or circumferential involvement. The patient reports that he was wearing thick pants at the time of the accident which he removed quickly and promptly irrigated the area with water. There are no other signs of injury. What is the burn degree and relative area of involvement in this patient?

a. First-degree/9%
b. First-degree/4.5%
c. Second-degree/2.25%
d. Second-degree/9%
e. Third-degree/4.5%

400. A 29-year-old male mountain-climber presents to the ED with nausea, vomiting, and dizziness. Upon review of systems, he denies fever, cough, abdominal pain, or dysuria but does report anorexia and some ankle swelling. What diuretic is the drug of choice in this patient?

a. Furosemide
b. Hydrochlorothiazide
c. Bumetanide
d. Fosinopril
e. Acetazolamide

401. A 25-year-old female scuba diver presents to the ED with multiple areas of periarticular joint pain and red, itchy skin. Her initial vitals include an oral temperature of 98°F, BP of 110/65 mm Hg, a HR of 88 beats per minute, a RR of 14 breaths per minute and an O_2 saturation of 97% on room air. Upon physical examination, the patient has pain upon palpation of bilateral knees and ankles with full range of motion in these joints. Areas of erythema that do not follow a specific dermatomal pattern cover most of the lower extremities, torso, and back with areas of excoriation where patient reports scratching. There are no other lesions. Which of the following is the most likely diagnosis?

a. Sexually transmitted disease
b. Decompression sickness
c. Descent barotrauma
d. Ascent barotrauma
e. Nitrogen narcosis

402. A 19-year-old rookie Navy Seal presents to the ED with a history of syncopizing upon ascent from a dive. The length and depth of the dive was within decompression regulation. He currently complains of feeling light-headed with a moderate frontal headache. Vital signs include a HR of 86 beats per minute, a BP of 130/65 mm Hg, a RR of 16 breaths per minute with an O_2 saturation of 93% on room air. Upon physical examination, he appears somewhat confused and is oriented only to person and place. He has no focal neurological deficits. What underlying event is the cause for this patient's symptoms?

a. Pulmonary embolism
b. Cardiac ischemia
c. Transient ischemic attack
d. Dysbaric air embolism
e. Decompression sickness

403. A farmer in Texas presents to the ED with right leg numbness, local-ized edema, and tremors. He reports being out in the field when the symp-toms began. He denies contact with insecticides and reports being at his baseline of health prior to the event. His initial vitals include a HR of 105 beats per minute, a BP of 175/90 mm Hg, and a RR of 22 breaths per minute with an O_2 saturation of 97% on room air. Which of the following is the most appropriate initial treatment of choice in this patient?

a. Antivenin
b. Tetanus prophylaxis
c. Antibiotic prophylaxis
d. Sedation
e. Atropine

404. A 3-year-old boy is brought in by his parents after sustaining a bee sting. The patient is crying and points to his left arm when asked where the pain is. Upon physical examination, you see a single puncture wound with surrounding erythema and swelling. The patient is in no respiratory distress and is phonating well. Chest auscultation reveals clear breath sounds bilaterally with no wheezing. The oropharynx is patent without any tonsillar or uvular displacement. Which of the following is the most appropriate next step in management?

a. Subcutaneous epinephrine 0.01 mL/kg
b. IV epinephrine 0.01 mL/kg
c. Steroids
d. Observation
e. Antihistamines

405. An 8-year-old boy is brought into the ED by a babysitter who reports that the child was bitten by a stray dog at the park. The child complains of right forearm pain, where he was bitten. Upon physical examination, you note a superficial macerated laceration on the dorsal surface of the distal forearm with no active bleeding. The child is able to freely flex and extend all joints in the right upper extremity. In addition to localized wound care, antibiotics, and tetanus prophylaxis, what other expeditious measures should be taken in the care of this child?

a. Reporting the incident to local authorities
b. Rabies immunization
c. Tight suturing of the laceration
d. Antihistamines
e. Irrigation with betadine solution

406. A 35-year-old man presents to the ED with right hand swelling, pain, and erythema that began 3 days ago. He denies any trauma, sick contacts, insect bites, or recent travel. The patient's vitals are significant for an oral temperature of 101°F. Upon physical examination, you note an area of erythema surrounding multiple punctate lacerations over the right third and fourth metacarpalphalangeal joints with localized tenderness. The patient is neurovascularly intact with limited flexion due to the swelling and pain. Given this, what is the most appropriate disposition for this patient?

a. Suture and close follow-up with a hand surgeon
b. Suture and prescription for oral antibiotics
c. Wound irrigation and prescription for oral antibiotics
d. Wound irrigation and tetanus prophylaxis
e. Admission for IV antibiotics

407. A 31-year-old man presents to the ED with left calf pain. He reports general malaise, nausea, and myalgias since a recent trip to Arkansas. His initial vitals include an oral temperature of 99°F, HR of 76 beats per minute, BP of 128/70 mm Hg, RR of 16 breaths per minute and an O_2 saturation of 98% on room air. Upon physical examination, there are diffuse petechiae of the left lower extremity from the anterior distal tibia to the mid-thigh. Closer examination reveals a small necrotic lesion at the level of the lateral mid-calf with surrounding edema as seen below. The patient's calf is tender to the touch and upon dorsiflexion. Which of the following is the most likely cause of this patient's clinical symptoms?

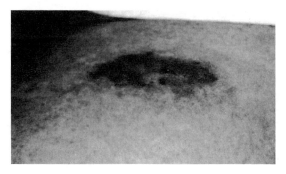

(Reproduced, with permission, from Knoop KJ, Stack LB, Storrow AB. Atlas of Emergency Medicine. *New York, NY: McGraw-Hill, 2002: 531.)*

a. Deep venous thrombosis
b. Scorpion sting
c. Brown recluse spider bite
d. Folliculitis
e. Thrombocytopenia

408. A 50-year-old man presents to the ED with bloody otorrhea. He denies any history of trauma but reports ear fullness and pain since a recent vacation where he went scuba diving. His physical examination is significant for serosanguinous fluid draining from his left ear without direct visualization of the tympanic membrane. Which of the following is the most likely cause for this patient's symptoms?

a. Otitis externa
b. Descent barotrauma
c. Ascent barotrauma
d. Descent and ascent barotrauma
e. Decompression sickness

409. A 23-year-old avid high altitude skier presents to the ED with intense pain, tearing and bilateral ocular foreign body sensation. He denies any trauma, past medical problems or contact lens use. His physical examination is significant for bilateral decreased visual acuity, injected conjunctiva, and diffuse punctuate corneal lesions with a discrete inferior border. His pupils are equal, round, and reactive to light. Given this patient's history and physical examination, which of the following is the most likely diagnosis?

a. Corneal abrasion
b. Iritis
c. Ultraviolet keratitis
d. Corneal foreign body
e. Corneal laceration

410. A 44-year-old woman returns from a mountain excursion with headache symptoms, nausea, and vomiting that are improving. Her initial vital signs in the ED are a HR of 93 beats per minute, BP of 120/60 mm Hg, RR of 18 breaths per minute and an O_2 saturation of 96% on 2 L nasal cannula. Her chest examination is clear to auscultation with no palpable overlying crepitus and there are no signs of peripheral edema. Which of the following medications is indicated in this patient?

a. Acetazolamide
b. Dexamethasone
c. Nifedipine
d. Furosemide
e. Morphine

411. A 39-year-old woman presents to the ED in agony from diffuse abdominal pain, stating that the ambulance ride to the hospital worsened her symptoms. The patient reports that her pain was initially dull, gradually becoming sharper over the course of the day. Her symptoms began after cleaning out her barn a few hours prior to presentation. Upon physical examination of her abdomen, the patient involuntarily guards and is tender in all four quadrants. There is no flank tenderness and a urine dip is negative for blood, ketones, or leukocytes. What is the diagnosis in this patient?

a. Acute appendicitis
b. Acute pyelonephritis

c. New-onset diabetes with ketoacidosis
d. Black widow spider bite
e. Anaphylaxis

412. A 20-year-old college student presents to the ED with a cutaneous lesion as depicted below. He is brought in by friends who report being out in an open field during stormy weather when the injury occurred. The patient denies any recent travel or sick contacts. He also denies any symptoms except for some generalized confusion. Which aspect of the physical examination of this patient is initially most pertinent to the nature of this type of injury?

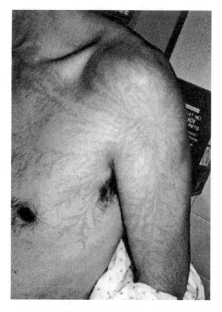

(Reproduced, with permission, from Tintinalli J, Kelen G, and Stapczynski J. Emergency Medicine A Comprehensive Study Guide. New York, NY: McGraw-Hill, 2004: 1238.)

a. Testing of cranial nerves
b. Otoscopic evaluation of tympanic membranes
c. Evaluation of gait cadence
d. Testing of cerebellar deficits
e. Palpating the cervical spine for tenderness

413. A 32-year-old man presents to the ED with a chief complaint of "I got stung by something." He reports that he is an underwater photographer who was specifically photographing starfish when he was stung on his right leg. He reports pulling something out of his leg, but is still experiencing pain. He denies parestheisas, difficulty breathing, weakness, or pruritis. Upon physical examination, there is a circular 1 cm area of erythema on the patient's right lateral lower leg with no palpable subcutaneous foreign body. What is the initial treatment of choice in this patient?

a. Washing the area with vinegar
b. Washing the area with water
c. Tetanus prophylaxis
d. Topical antibiotics
e. Antivenin

414. A 14-year-old boy presents to the ED with diffuse facial pain, pruritis, erythema and dizziness after reportedly falling on to an anthill. His initial vital signs include HR of 102 beats per minute, BP of 118/75 mm Hg, RR of 18 breaths per minute with an O_2 saturation of 98% on room air. What is the initial appropriate assessment in this clinical scenario?

a. Give tetanus prophylaxis
b. Begin local wound care
c. Assess airway, breathing, and circulation
d. Start IV fluid administration
e. Give oral antihistamines

415. A 4-year-old girl is brought in to the ED by her parents who report that she was found next to an open can of gasoline in the garage. Some of the gasoline had spilled on the child's clothing but they are sure that the child did not ingest any of the solution given that she was left alone for a very short period of time. They brought her directly to the ED without any intervention prior to arrival. The child appears to be in no apparent distress and is playing with toys. What exposure has this child sustained and what is the contained substance?

a. Lye/NaOH
b. Phenol/carbolic acid
c. Hydrocarbon/Tar
d. Hydrofluoric acid (HF)
e. Acetic acid

416. An undomiciled man of unknown age presents to the ED unresponsive. His ECG is shown below. What is the most appropriate next step in treatment?

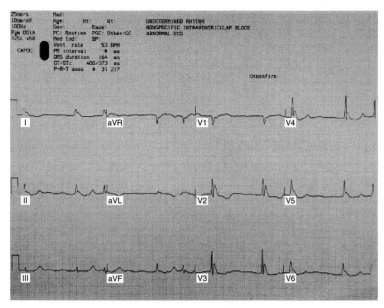

(Reproduced, with permission, from Knoop KJ, Stack LB, Storrow AB. Atlas of Emergency Medicine. *New York, NY: McGraw-Hill, 2002: 516.)*

a. Defibrillation
b. Cardiac pacing
c. Advanced cardiac life support
d. Advanced cardiac life support and rewarming
e. Cardiopulmonary bypass

417. A 16-year-old man presents to the ED in agony with a Gila Monster still attached to his arm after being bitten. He reports that he is the animal's main handler, with no prior biting incidents. He reports localized pain but denies weakness, nausea, or feeling lightheaded. The animal bite occurred about 45 minutes ago. After the animal is carefully removed, what should be done next in the care of this patient?

a. Check for any remaining embedded teeth and begin wound care
b. Administer antivenin
c. Give tetanus prophylaxis
d. Administer broad-spectrum antibiotics
e. Apply suction device

418. A 24-year-old woman presents to the ED with a human bite that was sustained 5 days ago. The patient reports that she did not seek immediate medical care because of the benign-appearing nature of the bite, which has since dramatically worsened with erythema, swelling, and pain. She reports intermittently taking some of her friends' oral antibiotics. You counsel the patient about the seriousness of her condition, emphasizing the high infection rates associated with these injuries. Which of the following pathogens is most likely responsible for this patient's symptoms?

a. *P. multocida*
b. *Capnocytophaga canimorsus*
c. Herpes virus
d. *Streptococcus pneumoniae*
e. *Eikenella corrodens*

419. An anxious college student presents to the ED at 2 AM stating that he was woken up by a bat in his apartment. He heard something flying around his bedroom and when he turned the lights on, he saw a bat fly into his closet. He is unsure if he was bit by the bat but noticed bat droppings in his bed. Which is the most appropriate management for the patient?

a. Reassure him that there is nothing to do and discharge him
b. Immunoprophylax with human rabies immune globulin and human diploid cell vaccine
c. Administer ciprofloxacin 500 mg
d. Admit him to the hospital for 24 hours of observation
e. Immunoprophylax with human diploid cell vaccine

Environmental Exposures

Answers

389. The answer is b. (*Rosen, pp 1972–1978.*) Frostbite usually occurs when temperatures fall below 0°C. There are essentially three phases to the freezing injury cascade. Phase 1 (Prefreeze) includes initial skin cooling, increased blood viscosity, and microvascular leakage which causes localized edema formation. Phase 2 (Freeze-Thaw) is when extracellular crystal formation begins thereby causing intracellular shrinkage and essentially collapse of the cellular network. Finally, Phase 3 (vascular stasis/progressive ischemia) involves further coagulation, interstitial leakage, and cell death thus resulting in blister formation, cyanosis, and ultimately mummification of the tissue. The bullae formed may also have a hemorrhagic appearance. It is important to note that wind and moisture may increase the freezing rate. Management includes rapid rewarming with water at a temperature of 37–40°C with care in preventing refreezing. Friction massage, which furthers tissue loss, should be avoided. Rewarming is a painful procedure that requires parenteral analgesia. Patients may also have a degree of dehydration and benefit from crystalloid administration.

(**a**) Chilblains, also known as pernio, is a condition commonly seen in the homeless population due to chronic dry-cold exposure and mostly affects the face, hands, and pretibial areas. Trench foot (**c**), also known as immersion injury, is common in this population however, it usually presents as a loss of sensation with pallor and mottling. (**d**) Thermal burns may present with bullae formation but do not elicit cyanosis. (**e**) Herpes is also unlikely given the distribution and lack of contacts with similar lesions.

390. The answer is c. (*Rosen, p 2002.*) This patient is suffering from *miliaria rubra*, more commonly known as *prickly heat or heat rash*. This is an acute inflammatory disorder of the skin that occurs in tropical climates, also lending the term "lichen tropicus." It occurs because of sweat gland blockage and staphylococcal infection. The acute phase is noted by vesicular lesions that are caused by obstruction of the sweat glands, which subsequently rupture. The rash is confined to *clothed areas* and may progress to a profunda stage, in which the obstruction delves deeper into the skin and produces larger vesicles that may become infected. These, however, are not pruritic and may resemble a chronic dermatitis. The antibacterial treatment of choice is **Chlorhexadine**, which is to be used in the acute phase. Salicylic acid may also be used to assist in desquamation, but should not be used on large areas because of possible salicylate intoxication.

(**a and d**) Although Calamine lotion and Benadryl may assist in symptomatic relief, they do not offer treatment. (**b**) Acyclovir is to treat herpes infection. (**e**) Treatment is especially important in this patient with insulin-dependent diabetes mellitus (IDDM) to prevent further infectious complications that necessitate parenteral antibiotics.

391. The answer is e. (*Rosen, pp 1997–2008.*) The diagnosis of *heat exhaustion* is initially made upon clinical presentation. Patients may have general malaise, fatigue, frontal headache, impaired judgment, diaphoresis, nausea, and show signs of dehydration with tachycardia and orthostatic hypotension. Heat exhaustion may progress to heat stroke and lies along a spectrum in which intermediate cases may often be difficult to delineate, however the treatment is essentially the same. It is important to bring the patient to a cool location and start fluid replacement slowly as to prevent cerebral edema, especially in younger patients. To help distinguish between heat exhaustion and heat stroke, hepatic transaminases are helpful. Elevations to several thousand units may be seen in heat exhaustion or healthy runners after a marathon, whereas in heat stroke the levels are elevated to tens of thousands.

(**a**) Heat syncope results from the dilatation of cutaneous vessels to assist in the delivery of heat to the skin's surface, thereby pooling the blood to the periphery and causing syncope. Elderly patients and those who stand for long periods are especially prone to this. (**b**) Heat edema occurs in patients who are not acclimated to warmer temperatures and thereby develop swollen feet and ankles. This is not a central process and altered mental states do not occur. (**c**) Rhabdomyolysis may result in any case where there is muscle breakdown due to dehydration, stress, or exogenous factors however, it alone does not explain this patient's symptoms. (**d**) Neurologic dysfunction, including seizures and coma, are a hallmark of heat stroke, which result when treatment is not initiated and thermoregulatory responses fail. These patients often have dry, hot skin with core temperatures above 105°F.

392. The answer is d. (*Rosen, pp 2010–2019.*) This child sustained a *low-voltage (<1000 volts) electrical injury* from an unprotected wall socket. All patients sustaining such an injury warrant an *ECG* and *cardiac monitoring* in the ED. In the United States, household wiring has 120 volts of alternating current with a frequency (number of switches from positive to negative) of 60 Hz. Alternating current causes continuous muscle contraction and stimulation that may cause ventricular fibrillation. Direct current usually just causes a single muscle spasm and is the less dangerous of the two, depending upon the voltage. The current is equal to the voltage over the resistance (Ohm's Law). This child sustained a superficial thermal burn and most likely did not become part of the circuit given that there were not any clear entry or exit wounds as seen in direct contact injuries. Disposition of this patient should include localized wound care, close follow-up, and instructions to return if there are any worsening symptoms. In older patients, it is important to check that tetanus is up-to-date.

(a and b) Although a urinalysis to screen for myoglobin and a basic metabolic panel to check renal function might be performed, it is not necessary given the nature of this child's injury. (c and e) A chest x-ray and arterial Doppler will not prove efficacious given the clinical exam.

393. The answer is d. (*Rosen, pp 2046–2048.*) The acute abdomen in a childbearing female is often a difficult diagnostic dilemma for the emergency medicine physician. In this clinical scenario, it is important to note the details that lend clues as to the underlying diagnosis that was provoked by the environmental factors. This patient experienced a *high-altitude aircraft* flight that provided a stress. The patient tells you of a *blood trait* that she is aware of but has not caused any prior complications or hospitalizations. *Sickle cell trait,* commonly seen in individuals of African descent, may also be seen in individuals of Mediterranean descent. Although many people with sickle-cell trait remain asymptomatic, splenic ischemia or infarction has been seen especially in this subgroup. Treatment includes oxygen, IV fluid administration, rest, and analgesia in order to relieve the vaso-occlusive crisis. Surgery may be warranted if further splenic necrosis, coagulapathy, or hemodynamic instability occurs.

(a) Given the patient's pelvic examination, torsion is also less likely but can be further evaluated with a Doppler ultrasound. (b) Appendicitis should always be considered in any patient with an acute abdomen and needs further evaluation here. (c) G6PD-deficiency has been seen in patients of Mediterranean descent who might attend wine and cheese parties or take sulfa-containing medications but is not provoked by changes in altitude. (e) The patient's LMP was 2 weeks ago and a pregnancy can be ruled out with a simple urine test, thereby making an ectopic pregnancy less likely.

394. The answer is c. (*Rosen, pp 797–799.*) This patient sustained an injury from a *venomous marine animal*. Approximately 50,000 such incidents occur yearly. Marine animals may be divided into two classes: *stingers and nematocysts*. Stingers include sea urchins, stingrays, catfish, cone shells, and starfish. Radiographs may be useful in delineating the calciferous material deposited in the skin for removal. Nematocysts are much more prevalent and account for the majority of envenomations and most likely account for this patient's distress. This class includes jellyfish, fire corals, Portuguese man-o-war, and anemones. These creatures have spring-loaded venomous glands that discharge upon mechanical or chemical stimulation. The number of nematocysts on a tentacle can number in the thousands. These stinging cells can remain activated after weeks of the animal being beached. The venom contains various peptides and enzymes that may cause progression of symptoms including nausea, muscle cramps, dyspnea, angioedema, and anaphylaxis. The preferred treatment is *vinegar,* which deactivates the nematocyst. In cases where medical attention cannot be sought in a timely manner, urine has been shown to be just as efficacious. An attempt may be made to shave off nematocysts after proper analgesia. Patient should be given tetanus prophylaxis and antihistamines as needed.

(a) Fresh water activates the nematocyst and should be avoided. (b, d, and e) Vegetable oil, toothpaste, and household window cleaners should also be avoided as they might cause further irritation and pain.

395. The answer is b. (*Rosen, pp 2117–2118.*) Chemical burns are a common occupational hazard and can be caused by a variety of solvents containing acidic or alkali mixtures. Initially, it is important to remove the patient from the offending chemical and irrigate with copious amounts of water to dilute the agent. It is important to assess the affected area, size, and depth of the burn, as some patients will need transfer to a burn center. This patient was chemically burned by a rust-removing agent, which commonly holds HF. Other solvents include high-octane gas and germicides. *Pain out of proportion to sustained injury* is usually seen in these cases. As HF is a relatively weak acid, its extreme electronegativity however makes it very dangerous. Fluoride avidly binds to available cations, such as calcium and magnesium, thereby causing cell death. Profound *hypocalcemia* has been demonstrated in HF exposure. ECG monitoring and administration of exogenous cations such as topical *calcium gluconate gel,* can act as chelating agents to the fluoride ions. IV or intradermal calcium gluconate may also be used. Calcium chloride should be avoided given its ability to cause tissue necrosis upon extravasation.

(a) Placing a tourniquet upon the limb may cause ischemia and further cell death. (c) Alkalinization of urine would not be of benefit in this type of exposure. (d) Silver silvadene may be applied later on for wound care. (e) The extent of this injury at this time does not warrant surgical debridement, however, close wound care monitoring should be instilled to recognize cases when tissue necrosis progresses.

396. The answer is e. *(Rosen, pp 816–818.)* This patient was exposed to *lime,* which is present in *cement.* When water interacts with dry cement, hydrolysis occurs forming an alkali with a pH of 10–12. *Alkali burns* form a *liquefaction necrosis,* causing quick dissolution of involved tissue. Acid burns form a coagulation necrosis, which is somewhat slower in nature. The best treatment is *intense irrigation* upon initial contact, a ritual performed by the more experienced individuals who work with lime. This patient will need further debridement and wound care because of his exposure.

(a) Hydrocarbons are present in mainly gasoline and paint thinners. (b) Phenol is found in dyes, deodorants, disinfectants, and agriculture solvents, which causes cell denaturing upon contact. Ammonia (c) is present in many household cleaners, as a cooling agent in refrigerator units and as a fertilizer due to its high nitrogen content and may act differently depending in what form it is in. For example, it may freeze skin on contact or affect breathing due to its vapors. Formic acid (d) is a caustic organic acid used in many industries that causes a coagulation necrosis. Treatment for exposure to all of these chemicals includes copious irrigation and observation for systemic side effects.

397. The answer is b. *(Rosen, pp 775–776.)* *Cat bites* involve *puncture wounds* often extending down through skin into tendons and bones due to the nature of the animals' sharp teeth. The reported incidence of infection from these bites may be as high as 30–50%, with many patients presenting only after an infection has incurred. It is important to note that cat bites have a higher infection rate compared to dog bites, given the typical puncture wound that inoculates bacteria down the track deep into tissue and becomes enclosed. *P. multocida* is a strong gram-negative, facultative anaerobic rod found in the oral cavity of the majority of healthy cats and may cause severe systemic infection, especially in the immunocompromised. Patients need to be followed closely as these infections may seed deep into joints and tissue requiring debridement.

(a) First-generation cephalosporins have proven to be only minimally effective. The organism is resistant to (d) vancomycin and (c) clindamycin.

(e) Antibiotic topicals such as bacitracin would be inappropriate given the high virulence of this organism.

398. The answer is c. (*Rosen, pp 801–812.*) This patient sustained a *second-degree burn involving 2.25% of her body surface area (BSA),* according to the rule of nines. The rule of nines aids in estimating the area of involvement as seen below. In the adult, each anterior or posterior surface of the upper extremity and head are equal to 4.5%. Each surface of the lower extremity is equal to 9%. Each surface of the chest and torso is equal to 18%. Perineal areas account for 1% of BSA. Children and infants have increased total BSA relative to their weight, thereby requiring different fluid requirements and area estimation. More percentage is dedicated to the head given their larger head-to-body ratios (7% in children and 9% in infants). The *treatment for this patient involves silver silvadene dressings and close follow-up.* Prophylactic antibiotics are not warranted in these cases, given the chance of increased future resistance rates. For areas of greater involvement and inhalation burns, fluid resuscitation may become necessary to account for losses. This is done using the *Parkland Formula:* 4 mL/kg/%TBSA, one-half to be given

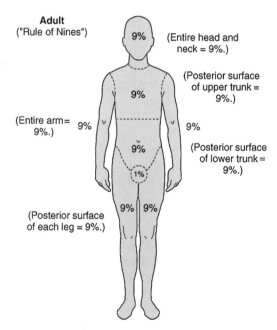

(*Reproduced, with permission, from Tierney LM, McPhee SJ, Papadakis MA.* Current Medical Diagnosis & Treatment. *New York, NY: McGraw-Hill, 2006.*)

over first 8 hours and the remaining half to be given over the next 16 hours. Ringer's lactate is the fluid of choice. It is also important to protect against hypothermia and provide adequate analgesia. Depending on the extent and area of the burn, some patients may need transfer to a burn facility where further escharotomy and debridement may be performed.

First-degree burns (a) are characterized primarily by erythema, having the appearance of a simple sunburn. It involves the epidermis only and usually heals without scar formation. Second-degree burns (b, c) are superficial partial thickness burns involving the epidermis and part of the dermis resulting in painful erythema and blister formation. Follicles and glands may or may not be involved. These blisters are best left intact. Third-degree burns (d, e) are full thickness burns involving the epidermis, dermis, and subcutaneous fat that results in pale, charred skin. Surgical debridement and grafting is necessary in these cases. Fourth-degree burns extend through the skin, fat, muscle, and bone and are often limb and life-threatening.

399. The answer is b. (*Rosen, pp 801–812.*) Please see explanation in previous question.

400. The answer is e. (*Rosen, pp 2035–2048.*) This patient is an otherwise healthy male with no reason to have congestive heart failure (CHF), renal failure, hepatic failure, or cardiomyopathy. Instead, he is an avid *mountain-climber*, which should hint at *acute mountain sickness (AMS)* in this clinical scenario. Early on, symptoms may mimic an acute viral syndrome with nausea, vomiting, headache, and anorexia. However, these symptoms progress to include *peripheral edema, oliguria, retinal hemorrhages, and finally high-altitude pulmonary or cerebral edema.* The initial treatment for all of these conditions across the spectrum of AMS, include *gradual descent.* A descent of 1500–3000 ft reverses high-altitude sickness in most cases. Supplemental *oxygen* is indicated in all cases. Diuretics, such as *acetazolamide* have been proven effective not only for treatment but for prophylaxis. Symptomatic treatment for vomiting and headache may also be indicated. Hyperbaric oxygen therapy is indicated in severe cases. Risk factors for AMS include, but are not limited to, rapid ascent, chronic obstructive pulmonary disease (COPD), sickle-cell disease, cold exposure, heavy exertion, and sleeping at higher altitudes.

Furosemide (a) and Hydrochlorothiazide (b) are indicated in CHF and hypertension. Bumetanide (c) is a more potent loop diuretic, also not indicated. Fosinopril (d) is an angiotensin-converting enzyme (ACE)-inhibitor.

401. The correct answer is b. (*Rosen, pp 2020–2033.*) This patient is suffering from *decompression sickness,* more commonly known as "the bends." This term refers to a spectrum of states whereupon bubbles of nitrogen gas collect in the blood and tissues. To help illustrate, picture a bottle of soda being opened, allowing the bubbles to rapidly come out of the solution to the top. Clinically, the degree of collection is a result of the depth and length of the dive. Other risk factors include inherent fatigue, heavy exertion, dehydration, and flying after a dive. A patent foramen ovale may also prove to be dangerous in causing gas bubbles to embolize to the arterial system. Decompression sickness can progress from its initial musculoskeletal involvement to include the cardiovascular, respiratory, and central nervous systems. Divers should ascend in a slow, gradual manner to avoid to collection of nitrogen gas in these tissues. Transport to the nearest *hyperbaric chamber* is the treatment of choice. IV fluid hydration and supplemental oxygen may also be warranted.

A sexually transmitted disease (**a**) is unlikely. Descent barotrauma (**c**) include sinus, ear, and skin squeeze. Divers who hold their breath upon descent may also develop lung squeeze. Ascent barotrauma (**d**) involves similar conditions in addition to pneumomediastinum and pneumothorax. Nitrogen narcosis (**e**), also known as "rapture of the deep," is an interesting phenomenon in which prolonged dives produce a euphoric effect upon the diver due to the collection of nitrogen gas in the tissues. This may prove dangerous in the face of an emergency, given a false sense of security and impaired motor skills.

402. The answer is d. (*Rosen, p 2025.*) Being a rookie diver, this patient ascended to the surface too quickly. As in decompression sickness, nitrogen gas bubbles form and subsequently travel to the arterial system through the pulmonary veins into the cardiac chambers. *Arterial gas embolism* may also occur in patients with an underlying patent foramen ovale. Symptoms are usually sudden and dramatic. Divers, who may have been thought to drown, actually passed out during ascent due to an underlying embolism. Treatment includes hyperbaric oxygen therapy and the avoidance of air transport.

Although cardiac ischemia (**b**) may occur because of this, it is not the precipitating event. Pulmonary embolism (**a**) in otherwise healthy individuals with no risk factors is low probability as the inciting event. Transient ischemic attacks (**c**) may present in a variety of ways, but given this clinical scenario, a serious diving-related cause must be investigated first.

403. The answer is a. (*Rosen, pp 786–792.*) This patient suffered a *venomous snakebite*. Pit vipers, such as rattlesnakes, copperheads, and water moccasins, are the most prevalent and are present in all states except Alaska, Maine, and Hawaii. Coral snakes are the second most prevalent and are present mainly in the southern states. *Red on yellow, kill a fellow; Red on black, venom lack* is a commonly used phrase to help remember which snakes are dangerous. Venomous snakes can also be recognized by their triangular-shaped heads, elliptical pupils, fangs, and the presence of a pit between the eye and nostril—characteristics that may not noticed by the victim initially. Therefore, there is a snakebite grading system, which requires antivenin with progressive symptoms of edema, coagulopathy, and neurological manifestations. The amount of antivenin is dependent on the severity of these symptoms. Venom itself has a number of substances including proteolytic enzymes and polypeptides, which promote coagulation, neuromuscular blockage, cell lysis, and death. Anaphylaxis may also occur. Airway, breathing, and circulation (ABCs) must always be initially assessed.

Tetanus prophylaxis (**b**) should be given at some point in treatment, but it is not the initial treatment of choice. Antibiotic prophylaxis (**c**) is not clinically indicated in these cases. Sedation (**d**) with benzodiazepines may be used in other venomous bites, such as scorpions, due to the extreme pain and neurological manifestations but is not clinically indicated here. Atropine (**e**) and pralidoxine are used in cases of organophosphate exposure.

404. The answer is d. (*Rosen, pp 793–794.*) History-taking should include prior bee stings in this child, as each successive sting increases the possibility of anaphylaxis given sensitization. The ABCs must be initially addressed. Stings most commonly present with localized burning, erythema, and edema at the sting site lasting for about 24 hours. The patient is asymptomatic and only warrants *observation* at this time. Toxicity and anaphylaxis are evident soon after the sting and include vomiting, diarrhea, fever, and neurological manifestations such as seizures and altered mental status. This child most likely sustained a sting from a honeybee or bumblebee, given the single puncture wound. Aphids contain retroserrate-barbed stingers, which are removed upon stinging, thereby eviscerating and killing the insect. Vespids, such as wasps, hornets, and yellow jackets, do not contain this mechanism and may sting many times. "Killer bees," as popularized by the film industry, contain the same amount of venom as other species. The difference is that they are more aggressive, not more toxic.

Our patient's condition at this time does not warrant epinephrine (**a and b**) in any form. Steroids (**c**) and antihistamines (**e**) are usually given in patients with systemic signs. β_2-agonists (i.e., Albuterol) may also be given for respiratory symptoms.

405. The answer is b. (*Rosen, pp 774–780, 1839–1840.*) Given that the bite was sustained by an *unknown stray dog* that may be difficult to locate, *rabies immunization* should given promptly. If the dog could be found, quarantining the animal for 10 days for observation may be a valid option and could save the patient from the rigorous postexposure prophylaxis schedule. It is important to note the powerful effects of *water and soap irrigation* in these cases, as it has been proven as the most effective means of lowering the virulence of the organism and should be initiated quickly. For immunizing against the rabies virus, it is important to give the *immunoglobulin* in addition to the *cell vaccine.* As much of the initial dose should be infiltrated around the wound site and then be given intramuscularly. Pregnancy is not a contraindication to giving the vaccine. All patients should be monitored for an antibody response. In the United States, the predominant threat to humans is *bats,* which most commonly carry the virus. This should be considered in individuals who are cave spelunkers and present with hydrophobia and neurological symptoms. Small rodents (squirrels, rats, chipmunks) and lagomorphs are herbivores and do not carry the virus.

(**a**) Reporting the incident to local health officials is also warranted, but may be done later. Suturing the sustained lacerations in these types of injuries is controversial, but should never be tight (**c**). Head and neck lacerations may be sutured for cosmetic reasons. Given the adequate blood supply to these areas, infection rates are low. Antihistamines (**d**) are not usually indicated in cases of dog bites. Irrigation of the wound with betadine solution (**e**) should never be performed as it causes further maceration of the skin edges and tissue necrosis.

406. The answer is e. (*Rosen, pp 780–783.*) This patient most likely sustained a *closed-fist injury,* which have high infection rates and evidence of poor wound healing. Wounds sustained by punches to the jaw and human bites, also known as "fight bites," are classically over the *metacarpal joints.* Penetration deep into the joint space and infection is common given the positioning of the hand during the injury, human oral flora, and delay in seeking treatment. Infected wounds are *polymicrobial* and specifically include *E. corrodens,* a facultative anaerobic gram-negative rod harbored in human dental plaque. It acts synergistically with aerobic organisms to increase the morbidity of these injuries. The joint spaces must be examined under full range of motion to detect any tendon lacerations or presence of foreign bodies. Hand radiographs should also be obtained to examine for any bony involvement. *IV antibiotics* and *admission* is the appropriate disposition. The antibiotics of choice are *penicillin and second-generation cephalosporins* with broader coverage in the immunocompromised. The wounds should be left open with a sterile dressing, splinted in the position of function (hand-holding-glass position) and elevated. Human bites have resulted in the transmission of hepatitis B, hepatitis C, syphilis, and herpes. Although HIV is present in human saliva, it is in relatively small amounts and considered a low risk of transmission. Appropriate antivirals and testing should be considered in these patients.

(**a and b**) You should never suture these lacerations. (**c and d**) Wound irrigation and tetanus prophylaxis is warranted in conjunction with *IV antibiotics.*

407. The answer is c. (*Rosen, pp 795–796.*) This patient's *necrotic lesion* and travel to the *south-central states* is classic for a *brown recluse spider bite.* These injuries may present with systemic symptoms of fever, chills, myalgias, hemolysis, petechiae and eventually seizure, renal failure, and death. The brown recluse spider can be distinguished by its *violin-shaped cephalothorax.* Its venom contains hemolytic enzymes and substances that cause vasoconstriction. Initial lesions may appear targetoid, as blood supply to the central area is diminished and becomes necrotic. Lesions have been shown to cause significant scarring and infection. Initial treatment should include the ABCs, wound care, analgesia, and tetanus prophylaxis. Patients may be observed in the ED for a period of 6 hours to see if envenomation occurred. Antibiotics may become warranted if infection ensues. Loxosceles reclusa antivenin is manufactured in Brazil, but is not currently available in the United States.

Although these bites may cause a coagulapathy, a DVT (**a**) and thrombocytopenia (**e**) are not the underlying causes but rather a manifestation of envenomation. Scorpion stings (**b**) are not so subtle. Patients feel immediate localized pain followed by neurological symptoms that may include salivation, fasciculations, and blurred vision. Folliculitis (**d**) may have the appearance of petechiae given the erythema surrounding each hair follicle, but it does not usually present with necrotic lesions.

408. The answer is d. (*Rosen, pp 2020–2033.*) Both *ascent and descent barotrauma* may cause *ear squeeze.* Symptoms of middle ear squeeze, or barotitis media, includes ear fullness or pain, nausea, vertigo, and hemotympanum. External ear squeeze can be caused by occlusion of the external ear canal with cerumen and causes a bloody otorrhea and petechiae in the canal. Inner ear squeeze is rare and is associated with rapid descent. Patients may present with hearing loss. Reverse ear squeeze is mainly seen with ascent barotrauma and may result with tympanic membrane rupture and bloody otorrhea. It is important to keep in mind that this injury may occur with either descent or ascent barotraumas, which also each have their own specific comorbidities.

Otitis externa (**a**) is associated with excruciating external ear pain, erythema, and mucopurulent discharge. Decompression sickness (**e**) is due to undissolved nitrogen bubbles in the blood, which form upon ascent and do not affect open air spaces such as the sinuses.

409. The answer is c. (*Rosen, p 911.*) This patient has *ultraviolet keratitis*, also known as *snow blindness*. This is essentially a radiation burn when an individual comes in close contact with an *ultraviolet-ray-containing light source*. It may be caused by sun lamps, tanning booths, or high-altitude environments. Patients usually present about 6–10 hours postexposure complaining of eye pain, blepharospasm, tearing, photophobia, and foreign body sensation. Physical examination reveals an injected eye with decreased visual acuity. Corneal examination reveals punctuate lesions that are clearly demarcated by a protective covering from the ultraviolet rays, such as the inferior conjunctiva. Treatment consists of a short-acting cycloplegic agent for pain management and broad-spectrum ophthalmologic antibiotics. Treatment is guided to assist in the quick, natural healing capacity of the cornea, in which the patient should feel better in a couple of days.

Although a corneal abrasion (**a**) is probable given the patients' symptoms, his history and lack of trauma or contact lens use suggests otherwise. Regardless, the treatment for both is the same. Iritis (**b**) usually is an injury of blunt trauma, resulting in ciliary spasm. Patients complain of photophobia and eye pain. Physical examination reveals ciliary flush, cells and flare in the anterior chamber and a small, poorly dilating pupil. Corneal foreign bodies (**d**) and corneal lacerations (**e**) are usually traumatic injuries in which the patient can recall a specific event. Corneal foreign bodies can be visualized upon physical examination using fluorescent dye and may present with an abrasion or ulceration. Small corneal lacerations may be difficult to diagnose. A positive Seidel test in which fluorescent dye streams from a corneal wound, indicates leaking aqueous humor, can be diagnostic. This is an ophthalmologic emergency that may warrant surgical repair.

410. The answer is a. *(Rosen, pp 2035–2048.)* This patient is recovering from AMS with no signs of CHF or pulmonary edema. The first-line treatment is descent and oxygen supplementation, which is already accomplished in this patient. Other treatment considerations include hyperbaric oxygen therapy, which improves hypoxemia for all altitude illnesses. As for medication regimens, *acetazolamide* is indicated even in patients with a history of altitude illness as prophylaxis. It works to decrease the formation of bicarbonate by inhibiting carbonic anhydrase. This diuretic action counters the fluid retention in acute mountain illness. It also decreases bicarbonate absorption in the kidney, causing a metabolic acidosis, which stimulates hyperventilation. This compensatory mechanism is turned off when the pH is close to the physiologic range of 7.4. It's this hyperventilation that counters the altitude-induced hypoxemia, thereby relieving symptoms.

Dexamethasone **(b)** works to decrease vasogenic edema and decrease intracranial pressure. It is generally used as adjunctive therapy in high-altitude cerebral edema. Nifedipine **(c)** works by decreasing pulmonary artery pressure in high-altitude pulmonary edema as does the diuresis resulting from **(d)** furosemide. Morphine **(e)** is thought to reduce pulmonary blood flow and decrease hydrostatic forces in pulmonary edema.

411. The answer is d. *(Rosen, pp 794–795.)* The key to the answer in this question is in the history-taking of environmental exposure. The patient states that her symptoms began after *cleaning out her barn*, a perfect place for *Black widow spiders* to live. This patient has *pseudo-peritoneal symptoms* due to the painful muscle spasm inflicted by the envenomation. Individuals may not feel the initial bite, especially if they are working. Spasms may resolve spontaneously or progress to hypertension and cardiovascular failure. Initial first aid includes applying an ice packet to the area. Pain control and muscle relaxants in addition to tetanus prophylaxis and wound care are the usual methods of treatment, after assessing the ABCs. Antivenin is available in the United States for severe reactions and has only been used at the extremes of age. Prior to this, all patients must be tested for horse serum sensitivity, which suspends the antivenin. Black widow spiders might be confused with other spiders given that the signature hourglass bright-red marking is present on the underside of the abdomen. This is contrary to the way the insect is depicted in the public media where the marking is clearly visible. Only females have the ability to envenomate humans and usually become aggressive when they are protecting their eggs.

Although acute appendicitis **(a)**, pyelonephritis **(b)**, and new-onset diabetes **(c)** presenting with ketoacidosis are high on the differential for this patient, a simple urine dip lessens the likelihood of these. Anaphylaxis **(e)** to things in her barn is even more unlikely given the nature of her symptoms.

412. The answer is b. *(Rosen, pp 2010–2019.)* This patient sustained a *direct lightning injury,* as evidenced by the typical *fern-like pattern* exhibited. These injuries may inflict fractures, cardiovascular collapse, burns, blunt abdominal injuries, and neurological damage. *Tympanic membrane ruptures* are a common associated injury due to the outflow tract of the lightning strike and it is important to check for blood in the ear canals of these patients. It is important to quickly assess the ABCs of these patients and establish an airway. Immobilization of the cervical spine is often indicated as well as close ECG monitoring. Patients should be admitted for observation after obtaining a complete blood count, creatinine kinase with MB fraction, basic metabolic panel, and appropriate radiographs of involved areas. Although 50–300 people die because of lightning strikes each year in the United States, most injuries sustained are not lethal.

413. The answer is b. *(Rosen, pp 797–799.)* The main difference in treatment between a *stinger* and a nematocyst is that irrigation involves *water* for the stinger and vinegar for the nematocyst. Water is contraindicated in nematocyst exposures because it can actually activate the venom. Stingers include stingrays, starfish, sea urchins, scorpion fish, catfish, lion fish, and cone shells. As a whole, they are less common than nematocyst envenomations which include the Portuguese man-of-war, corals, anemones (tentacled creatures that attach themselves to coral shells), sea wasps (box jellyfish), and most commonly jellyfish (bell-shaped invertebrates).

Tetanus prophylaxis **(c)** may be done later in the assessment of this patient. Topical antibiotics **(d)** and antivenin **(e)** are not indicated. If the stinger is still present, local exploration and removal is warranted.

414. The answer is c. *(Rosen, pp 793–794.)* *Fire ants* have proven to be a real threat to humans. Ninety-five percent of clinical cases result from the *Solenopsis invicta* species, another member of the *Hymenoptera,* which was imported from Brazil in the 1930s. This ant is found in many of the southern states given that it cannot survive long winters and is slowly replacing the less dangerous species native to North America. It is small and light-reddish to dark brown and its venom is 99% alkaloid, which is unique to the animal kingdom. This causes hemolysis, membrane depolarization, local tissue destruction, and activation of the complement pathway all of which could be especially dangerous in this patient with facial injuries. The sting usually produces a pustule within 24 hours. Local burning, erythema, and pruritis are common. About 10% of cases have progressive, systemic symptoms including nausea, vomiting, dizziness, respiratory distress, and further hypersensitivity. Therefore, assessment of this patient's airway and circulation are imperative. Continuous monitoring is indicated to detect hemodynamic instability.

Local wound care (**b**) may be performed after the patient is deemed stable. Beginning IV fluids (**d**) may be done if the patient becomes hemodynamically unstable but is not initially warranted. Tetanus prophylaxis (**a**) may be administered after the initial assessment. IV antihistamines, not oral (**e**), may be given as indicated. It is unclear as to whether this patient's symptoms of dizziness are due to trauma or initial systemic effects of the envenomation and therefore continuous monitoring is warranted.

415. The answer is c. (*Rosen, pp 816–818.*) This patient was exposed to *gasoline,* which is a *hydrocarbon.* Thermal burns mainly occur as a result of the *tar* that is found within this specific hydrocarbon. It is important to dilute the gasoline with water. Neosporin (polysorbate) may be used to take particles of tar off of skin. It is important to avoid using other solutions such as acetone to remove it, as these will cause the tar to further stick to the skin. Given that direct skin contact did not occur in this patient, gentle irrigation and a brief observation to look for local irritation is warranted in this child.

Lye/NaOH (**a**) is a strong alkali present in agricultural products and cement which can lead to liquefaction necrosis. Treatment is aggressive irrigation and local wound care. Phenol/carbolic acid (**b**) is found in dyes, deodorants, and disinfectants that causes a local coagulation necrosis and protein denaturation. Dilution with water is warranted in these exposures and isopropyl alcohol has been thought to decrease local absorption and necrosis. HF acid (**d**) penetrates tissues like alkali burns and releases fluoride, which immobilizes intracellular calcium and magnesium. Treatment is irrigation with water and detoxification with calcium gluconate. Acetic acid (**e**) is a weak acid with little systemic effects.

416. The answer is d. (*Rosen, pp 1972–1978.*) In all critically ill patients, it is important to remove clothing, obtain a rectal temperature and initiate continuous monitoring, including an ECG, while assessing the airway, breathing, and circulatory status of the patient. The clinician must initiate *advanced cardiac life support* and *rewarm* the patient once a rectal temperature has confirmed *hypothermia.* A tympanic temperature is not accurate below 94°F. It is important to remember that severely hypothermic patients who appear dead have a good chance of a normal neurological outcome with continued resuscitation and rewarming. Remember that a *patient is not dead until they're warm and dead!* Those at extremes of age, users of sedative-hypnotics, undomiciled individuals, and those with chronic illness, altered mental status, or sepsis are at most risk for hypothermia. Rewarming should begin with removing all wet clothing and placing warm blankets over the patient with progressive attempts made to rewarm the patient; mechanical warming blanket, warm IV fluids, gastric lavage/peritoneal warming, and lastly cardiopulmonary bypass.

Defibrillation (a) and cardiac pacing (b) are not currently indicated in this patient. Osborne (J) waves are indicative of a junctional rhythm, as seen in this patient, and are consistent with hypothermia. Prolongation of any interval, bradycardia, asystole, atrial fibrillation/flutter, and ventricular tachycardias may also be seen.

417. The answer is a. (*Rosen, pp 788–793.*) Only two venomous lizards are found in the world, both of which whose natural habitat is in the southwestern United States and Mexico. These animals are usually not aggressive, despite the Gila Monster's name, and bites are usually a result of direct handling as in this case. Both the Gila Monster and the Mexican-beaded lizard are easily identified by their thick bodies, beaded scales with either white and black or pink and black configuration. Envenomation from these bites occurs from the glands along the lower jaw and introduced into the victim through grooved teeth, which the animal uses to continuously chew after it has bitten down. These teeth may become embedded in the victim, thereby distributing more venom.

Antivenin (b) is not available for these bites, as they are rarely fatal. Broad-spectrum antibiotics (d) and tetanus prophylaxis (c) should be administered at a later interval. Applying a suction device (e) as in snakebites is not warranted. The patient should be observed for at least 6 hours for systemic effects.

418. The answer is e. (*Rosen, pp 780–783.*) *E. corrodens* is unique to human oral flora. *P. multocida* (a) is found in cats. *C. canimorsus* (b) is found in canine species. Herpes (c) may be transmitted with monkey bites. *Streptococcus viridans* not *S. pneumoniae* (d) is present in oral flora and a possible pathogen in the evolution of this patient's symptoms.

419. The answer is b. (*Rosen, pp 1834–1841.*) The patient should receive *full immunoprophylaxis* for the *rabies virus.* The CDC recommends postexposure prophylaxis when a bat is found indoors in the same room as a person who might be unaware that a bite or direct contact had occurred and rabies cannot be ruled out by testing the bat. Full prophylaxis in the United States includes passive immunization with human rabies immune globulin and active immunization with human diploid cell vaccine. Immune globulin is administered in and around a bite wound if visualized. Human diploid cell vaccine is administered at a distant site from the immunoglobulin, usually in the deltoid, to avoid cross reactivity. Human diploid cell vaccine is subsequently administered on days 3, 7, 14, and 28.

(a) The patient should not be sent home without full immunoprophylaxis. Ciprofloxacin (b) has no role in this patient or in rabies treatment. Rabies is caused by a virus. Admitting the patient for observation (c) is incorrect because rabies virus incubation ranges from 30 to 90 days with some reporting up to 7 years. The patient should receive immunoprophylaxis and be sent home. (e) The patient should receive both active and passive immunoprophylaxis unless they already received it in the past. In that case, they only receive the vaccine.

Vaginal Bleeding

Questions

420. A 23-year-old woman presents to the emergency department (ED) with irregular menstrual bleeding. She denies any abdominal pain, dizziness, or palpitations. The patient reports that her last menstrual period was 2 weeks ago with normal flow and duration. Which of the following ancillary tests is critical in defining the differential diagnosis for this patient?

a. Type and screen
b. Coagulation panel
c. β-hCG
d. Complete blood count
e. No ancillary tests are needed

421. A 30-year-old G_2P_{2002} presents to the ED with acute onset of lower abdominal pain associated with vaginal bleeding that began 2 hours prior to arrival. She denies any prior medical history but does report having a tubal ligation after the birth of her second child. Her vitals are significant for a heart rate (HR) of 120 beats per minute and a blood pressure (BP) of 90/60 mm Hg. On physical examination, the patient has right adnexal tenderness with blood in the posterior vaginal vault. Her cervical os is closed. Given this patient's history and physical examination, which of the following is the most likely diagnosis?

a. Appendicitis
b. Pelvic inflammatory disease (PID)
c. Placenta previa
d. Ectopic pregnancy
e. Abruptio placentae

422. A 28-year-old woman presents with severe abdominal pain with distention and vaginal bleeding. She reports being pregnant with a due date in approximately 4 weeks. Her pain came on suddenly, shortly before arrival to the ED. Upon further history-taking, the patient reports recent cocaine use. What condition needs to be considered in this patient?

a. Uterine rupture
b. Normal contractions
c. Placenta accreta
d. Vasa previa
e. Ruptured ovarian cyst

423. A 24-year-old G_2P_{0010} in her second trimester presents to the ED with vaginal spotting for the past day. She denies any abdominal pain and is otherwise in her usual state of health. Her vital signs are a HR of 76 beats per minute, BP of 120/65 mm Hg, respiratory rate (RR) of 16 breaths per minute, and temperature 98.9°F. Which of the following conditions does this patient most likely have?

a. Ectopic pregnancy
b. Placenta previa
c. Abruptio placentae
d. Uterine rupture
e. Ovarian torsion

424. A 7-year-old girl presents to the ED with vaginal bleeding, noticed by her mother as she was bathing the child. Birth history is unremarkable and the child is otherwise well with no past medical history. The mother reports that this has never happened before and cannot report any change in the child's behavior. What is the most probable diagnosis in this child?

a. Anovulatory bleeding
b. Cervical dysplasia
c. Cervical polyp
d. Cervicitis
e. Sexual abuse

425. A 24-year-old G_3P_{1112} presents to the ED with vaginal bleeding and clots. Her vital signs include a HR of 110 beats per minute, BP of 130/70 mm Hg, RR of 14 breaths per minute with an O_2 saturation of 99% on room air. She is afebrile and in mild distress. Recent medical history is significant for vaginal delivery 2 days ago with prolonged labor. Pelvic examination is significant for a large, boggy uterus and a normal vaginal wall. What is the most likely diagnosis in this patient?

a. Genital tract trauma
b. Endometritis
c. Uterine atony
d. Ectopic pregnancy
e. Uterine artery rupture

426. A 40-year-old G_1P_{0101} presents to the ED with suprapubic pain and general malaise for the last 3 days without improvement. Her vitals are significant for a HR of 115 beats per minute, BP of 100/60 mm Hg, and a temperature of 101°F. Upon physical examination, her abdomen is soft with significant suprapubic tenderness to light palpation but no rebound or guarding. Her pelvic examination reveals a scant amount of dark red vaginal blood and yellow discharge. Her past medical history is significant for an emergent cesarean section 2 weeks ago without any other gynecological history. What is the most likely diagnosis in this patient?

a. Uterine atony
b. Retained products of conception
c. Uterine inversion
d. Endometritis
e. Tubo-ovarian torsion

427. A 17-year-old girl presents to the ED with vaginal bleeding, nausea, and vomiting. Her vitals include a HR of 80 beats per minute, BP of 190/100 mm Hg, and a temperature of 99°F. She reports her last menstrual period was 7 weeks ago. Her physical examination is significant for a fundal height at the umbilicus. After obtaining a positive β-hCG, sonographic evaluation reveals the following image shown below. What is the most likely underlying condition for this patient's symptoms?

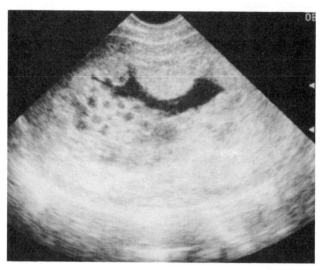

(Reproduced, with permission, from Knoop KJ, Stack LB, Storrow AB. **Atlas of Emergency Medicine.** *New York, NY: McGraw-Hill, 2002: 272.) (Courtesy of Robin Marshall, MD))*

a. Ectopic pregnancy
b. Hydatidiform mole
c. Ovarian torsion
d. Abruptio placentae
e. Hyperemesis gravidarum

428. A 25-year-old G_1P_0 presents to the ED with vaginal bleeding. She recently discovered that she was pregnant and has yet to be medically evaluated. Prior to presentation, the patient was in her usual state of good health with no history of trauma or any other symptoms. She reports using two absorbent pads an hour for the bleeding and does not notice passing fetal tissue. On physical examination, her cervical os is open. Which of the following is the most appropriate diagnosis?

a. Threatened abortion
b. Complete abortion
c. Inevitable abortion
d. Incomplete abortion
e. Missed abortion

429. A 27-year-old G_2P_{1001} presents to the ED with vaginal spotting. She reports occasional abdominal cramping associated with the bleeding, without fetal product passage, approximately 6 hours prior to presentation. She is currently in her first trimester and reports that her previous pregnancy was uncomplicated. She has been compliant with her prenatal vitamins and does not report any other medications or drug use. Her vitals are within normal limits and her physical examination is significant for a closed cervical os. Which of the following is the most likely diagnosis?

a. Placenta previa
b. Inevitable abortion
c. Complete abortion
d. Septic abortion
e. Threatened abortion

430. A 28-year-old woman presents to the ED with heavy menstrual flow for the last 2 days with clots. She reports using about 2 pads every hour. The patient states that she has occasional metromenorrhagia in the past and has been treated with oral contraceptives. She reports symptoms of feeling lightheaded but denies any syncope, palpitations, chest pain, abdominal pain, or weakness. Her initial vital signs include a HR of 96 beats per minute, BP of 135/70 mm Hg, RR of 14 breaths per minute with an O_2 saturation of 99% on room air. Upon physical examination, the patient is obese and you note a pronounced hairline. Which of the following conditions is most consistent with this patient's presentation?

a. Pregnancy
b. Polycystic ovaries
c. Ectopic pregnancy
d. Follicular cyst rupture
e. Corpus luteum cyst rupture

431. A 22-year-old woman presents to the ED with diffuse pelvic pain and vaginal bleeding. She reports that it is about the same time that she normally has her menses. She also reports some pain with defecation, dyspareunia, and points of dysmenorrhea in the past. The patient states that she has felt this way before, but that the pain has now worsened and is intolerable. Her physical examination reveals a soft abdomen with normal bowel sounds without rebound tenderness. The patient does not guard and there is no costovertebral tenderness. Her pelvic examination is significant for blood in the posterior vaginal vault, a closed os and no palpable masses or cervical motion tenderness. Given this patient's history and physical examination, which of the following is the most likely diagnosis?

a. Ureteral colic
b. Pregnancy
c. Ruptured ectopic pregnancy
d. Endometriosis
e. Appendicitis

432. A 51-year-old woman presents to the ED with heavy vaginal bleeding. She reports that she has bleeding for 12 consecutive days. She also reports missing a period 3 months ago, with an ensuing menses that she states was quite heavy. She denies having any hot flashes, vaginal dryness, night sweats, or changes in weight. The patient further denies any abdominal or back pain, syncope, palpitations but states that recently she often feels lightheaded and can't perform her normal activities of daily living. Her initial vital signs include a HR of 110 beats per minute, BP of 140/88 mm Hg, RR of 18 breaths per minute with an O_2 saturation of 98% on room air. Upon physical examination, she appears pale with a nontender abdomen and warm skin. Her pelvic examination reveals blood clots in the vaginal vault with a closed os, an enlarged uterus, and no adnexal tenderness. An ultrasound is performed which does not show any abnormalities. Which of the following diagnostic tests is most appropriate for this patient?

a. Endometrial biopsy
b. Hormonal therapy trial
c. Laparoscopic examination
d. Dilation and curettage
e. Hysterectomy and salpingectomy

433. A 29-year-old G_1P_{0010} presents to the ED with sharp, right-sided flank pain of acute onset associated with nausea. The pain began approximately 1 hour before arrival. She denies any fever, hematuria, vomiting, change in bowel habit, or sick contacts. She cannot recall her last menstrual period at this time. The patient is afebrile and her vitals are within normal limits as you begin your physical examination, which reveals a soft abdomen with mild diffuse tenderness to palpation without rebound. The patient has exquisite right flank pain. An initial urine dip is negative. Given the information you have so far, which of the following is the most probable diagnosis?

a. Appendicitis
b. PID
c. Ectopic pregnancy
d. Ureteral stone
e. Diverticulitis

434. A 23-year-old G_1P_0 presents to the ED with vaginal spotting that began earlier in the day. She denies any abdominal pain, trauma, dysuria, or back pain. Her initial vital signs include a HR of 90 beats per minute, BP of 125/60 mm Hg, a RR of 14 breaths per minute with an O_2 saturation of 99% on room air. Her pelvic examination is significant for a scant amount of blood in the posterior vaginal vault and a closed os. The patient has no tenderness upon bimanual examination. She states that she is 6 weeks pregnant. Given this patient's presentation, which of the following ancillary tests must be performed?

a. Complete blood count
b. Basic metabolic panel
c. Coagulation panel
d. Type and screen
e. Urinalysis

435. A 36-year-old G_4P_{2103} presents to the ED with vaginal spotting for the past 2 days. She also reports occasional abdominal cramping and low back pain. The patient states that she is 4 months pregnant. She denies any other past medical history or gynecological problems. Her initial vital signs include a HR of 89 beats per minute, BP of 144/70 mm Hg, RR of 15 breaths per minute with an O_2 saturation of 98% on room air. Her pelvic examination reveals a closed os. Upon ultrasound examination, an intrauterine pregnancy is visualized; however a fetal HR is not detected. Given this patient's symptoms and physical examination, which of the following is the most appropriate diagnosis?

a. Threatened abortion
b. Complete abortion
c. Missed abortion
d. Inevitable abortion
e. Incomplete abortion

436. A 22-year-old woman presents to the ED with vaginal bleeding that began earlier in the day. She reports that her last menstrual period was 3 weeks ago. She denies any metromenorrhagia in the past. Upon physical examination, her cervical os is closed with clots in the posterior vaginal vault. There is no adnexal or cervical motion tenderness. She has mild abdominal cramps but no localizing pain. Her pregnancy test is negative. Given this patient's clinical presentation, what is the most likely diagnosis?

a. Threatened abortion
b. Normal menstrual flow
c. Ectopic pregnancy
d. Dysfunctional uterine bleeding
e. PID

437. A 26-year-old G_1P_{1001} presents to the ED with vaginal spotting for the last 3 days with occasional left-sided pelvic pain. Her physical examination includes a closed cervical os, scant blood within the vaginal vault with left adnexal tenderness. Given this patient's history and physical examination, you suspect an ectopic pregnancy. In addition to a quantitative β-hCG, which of the following laboratory tests may prove helpful in the evaluation of this patient?

a. Estrogen level
b. Follicle-stimulating hormone (FSH) level
c. Thyrotropin (TSH) level
d. Progesterone level
e. Complete blood count

438. A 30-year-old woman with no prior pregnancies presents to the ED with diffuse pelvic pain and vaginal spotting. The following transvaginal ultrasound is performed and shown below. What is the minimum β-hCG level needed to obtain this sonographic image?

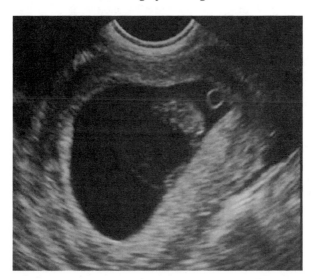

(Reproduced, with permission, from Knoop KJ, Stack LB, Storrow AB. Atlas of Emergency Medicine. New York, NY: McGraw-Hill, 2002: 645.) (Courtesy of Michael J. Lambert, MD, RDMS))

a. 1000
b. 950
c. 1500
d. 4000
e. 6500

439. A 32-year-old G_2P_{1001} presents to the ED with severe abdominal pain and vaginal bleeding. She reports that she is currently in her third trimester and that she has been diagnosed and treated for preeclampsia. Her vitals are significant for a BP of 195/100 mm Hg. Upon physical examination, her abdomen is distended and hard to the touch. Given this patient's history and physical examination, what emergent intervention is most appropriate?

a. Ultrasound
b. Pelvic examination
c. Tocolytics
d. Blood transfusion
e. Maternal/fetal monitoring with possible delivery

440. A 33-year-old G_3P_{2002} presents to the ED complaining of vaginal bleeding that started earlier in the day. She has gone through two pads over the last 12 hours. She describes mild lower abdominal pain. Her BP is 105/75 mm Hg, HR is 78 beats per minute, temperature is 98.9°F, and RR is 14 breaths per minute. Pelvic exam reveals clotted blood in the vaginal vault with a closed cervical os. Transvaginal ultrasound documents an intrauterine pregnancy. Which of the following is the correct diagnosis?

a. An embryonic gestation
b. Complete abortion
c. Incomplete abortion
d. Inevitable abortion
e. Threatened abortion

441. A 28-year-old G_2P_{0010} presents to the ED stating that she is pregnant and has vaginal spotting of blood. Pelvic exam reveals blood in the vaginal vault, but no active bleed, and a closed internal os. Transvaginal ultrasound reveals an intrauterine pregnancy consistent with a gestational age of 11 weeks. Her BP is 130/75 mm Hg, HR is 82 beats per minute, temperature is 99.1°F, and RR is 16 breaths per minute. Laboratory results reveal a WBC 10,500/μL, hematocrit 40%, platelets 225/μL. She is blood type B negative. Which of the following is the most appropriate intervention prior to discharging the patient from the ED?

a. Administer 50 μg of Anti-D Immune Globulin
b. Administer 2 g of magnesium sulfate to prevent eclampsia
c. Administer penicillin G to prevent chorioamionitis
d. Administer ferrous sulfate to prevent anemia
e. Administer packed red blood cells to increase blood volume

Vaginal Bleeding

Answers

420. The answer is c. (*Rosen, pp 228–229.*) A *beta human chorionic gonadotropin (β-hCG)* should be one of the first ancillary tests considered in a patient presenting with vaginal bleeding regardless of their sexual, contraceptive, and menstrual history. In addition to the initial and timely urine qualitative test, a follow-up serum quantitative β-hCG is warranted if positive. Patients that present with these symptoms and a positive β-hCG need follow-up for repeat testing to check trending levels. Determining if a patient is pregnant may also help distinguish if, for example, the emergent cause of this patient's bleeding is an ectopic pregnancy versus a pathological cervical lesion.

Although a type and screen (**a**) may be necessary in patients with severe vaginal bleeding that causes hemodynamic instability, this patient is currently stable. A type and screen is indicated, however, if this patient is pregnant to determine Rh status. A coagulation panel (**b**) may be considered later in determining if the vaginal bleeding is induced by conditions such as Von Willebrand's disease, a relatively common cause of menorrhagia. A complete blood count (**d**) may also be helpful in distinguishing such conditions as idiopathic thrombocytopenia purpura. Remember the most important question to answer initially is if this patient is pregnant.

421. The answer is d. (*Rosen, pp 226–231.*) This patient has a significant risk factor for having an *ectopic pregnancy*. Tubal ligations raise the likelihood of having an ectopic pregnancy by providing an outlet for improper implantation of an embryo into the abdominal cavity or somewhere outside of the uterus. Implantation most commonly occurs in the fallopian tubes, 95% of the time. Again, a β-hCG is crucial in the beginning stages in the work-up of this patient. In a normal pregnancy, the β-hCG doubles every 2 days and typically only increases by 2/3 in ectopic pregnancies. Progesterone levels also differ and may be helpful. A transvaginal ultrasound is also warranted to determine the size and location of the ectopic and any associated free fluid indicating rupture. β-hCG levels dictate whether a transvaginal (>1500) or transabdominal (>6500) approach should be used. Smaller, nonruptured ectopics may be treated with methotrexate. However, this patient is hemodynamically compromised and has most likely ruptured. Surgical intervention is warranted in these cases. Patients with ectopic pregnancies may also present with back or flank pain, syncope or peritonitis in cases with significant abdominal hemorrhage. Risk factors also include previous ectopics, intrauterine devices, PID, sexually transmitted diseases (STDs), in vitro fertilization and recent elective abortion. The incidence of a coexisting heterotopic pregnancy is about 1/30,000 but increases to 1/8000 in women on fertility drugs.

Both gastrointestinal and gynecological conditions should be included in the differential diagnosis of women presenting with abdominal pain, and appendicitis (**a**) is often at the top of the list. However, its probability is lowered by the associated vaginal bleeding. PID (**b**) often presents with gradual pelvic pain and discharge with other systemic signs of an infectious etiology, such as fever. Placenta previa (**c**) usually presents with *painless* vaginal bleeding in the second trimester. Abruptio placentae (**e**) also presents in the second or third trimester and is *painful*.

422. The answer is a. (*Rosen, pp 230–231.*) *Uterine rupture* presents as uterine pain without contraction and vaginal bleeding. It is most prevalent in women who have had a previous cesarean section, recent cocaine or prostaglandin use. *Cocaine* causes extreme vasoconstriction that compromises blood flow to the uterus and fetus causing friable and necrotic tissue, which is prone to rupture. This is an obstetrical emergency that necessitates surgical intervention for stabilization of both mother and child.

Normal contractions (**b**) may be seen at this time as well, however, they are more commonly seen with a lowered fundal height as the fetus advances down the vaginal canal. Placenta accreta (**c**) is usually *painless* and associated with brisk, bright-red vaginal bleeding. It is caused by an indistinct placental cleavage plane and seen in the delivery of the placenta itself. Vaginal bleeding may be seen with ruptured membranes as in vasa previa. (**d**), however this is relatively *painless* and rarely seen in the ED setting. Ruptured ovarian cysts (**e**) should still be considered in the pregnant patient and although this may also be painful, it is rarely severe and other more life-threatening causes should be higher up on the differential diagnosis. The distinguishing characteristic in this patient is her cocaine use.

423. The answer is b. (*Rosen, pp 230–231.*) *Placenta previa* is the most probable etiology for this patient's *vaginal bleeding* given that it is *not painful*. Bleeding is rarely severe and the physical examination is usually unremarkable except for a gravid uterus and bright-red blood in the vaginal vault.

Manual and speculum pelvic examination should not be done until placenta previa can be ruled out with an ultrasound, which is often diagnostic. Transvaginal ultrasound can be done due to the wide angle of the probe and low probability of penetrating the cervical os. Vaginal examination may then be performed with awareness that surgical intervention may be necessary to control bleeding. It is also important to note the stage of pregnancy given that first-trimester pregnancies more commonly include spontaneous abortions and ectopics that may present with vaginal spotting.

It is important to emphasize the importance of the patient's presentation with regard to *painful* or *painless* vaginal bleeding. Although other factors may alter pain, in general, it is a useful tool in helping to differentiate the diagnosis. Abruptio placentae (c), uterine rupture (d) and ovarian torsion (e) are painful etiologies of vaginal bleeding. Ectopic pregnancy (a) is usually more painful after it ruptures but may present as painless vaginal bleeding in the first trimester.

424. The answer is e. (*Rosen, pp 226–229.*) This is *sexual abuse* until proven otherwise. Any type of vaginal bleeding of acute onset in an otherwise well child without any past medical history needs to be further evaluated for signs of abuse. A sexual assault examiner may assist in the proper examination and documentation of a child that presents to the ED. Vaginal or anal tears, bleeding diatheses, and mucosal trauma should all be visualized with the aid of colposcopy. Children may need conscious sedation as necessary to complete the examination.

Cervical dysplasia (b) is uncommon in children as are cervical polyps (c) and cervicitis (d) except in those children with a prior history of sexual abuse where an infectious etiology was transmitted. Polyps are generally seen in older women presenting with postcoital vaginal bleeding. Anovulatory bleeding (a) is also seen in postmenopausal populations. These patients should also be further evaluated with an endometrial biopsy to rule out hyperplasia or carcinoma.

425. The answer is c. (*Rosen, pp 230–231.*) Postpartum bleeding is classified as early, within 24–48 hours of delivery, or late, up to 1–2 weeks. Causes of early postpartum bleeding include *uterine atony* (most common cause), genital tract trauma, retained products of conception, and uterine inversion. Late bleeding episodes may be caused by endometritis or retained products of conception. Uterine atony is common after prolonged labor and oxytocin administration. Physical examination will reveal a soft uterus and blood in the vaginal vault. Treatment consists of bimanual massage and intravenous oxytocin to stimulate uterine contractions. Ergot alkaloids may be given in refractory cases.

Although genital tract trauma (a) is a possible cause of early postpartum bleeding, this patient's physical examination did not reveal any lacerations or mucosal trauma. As explained above, endometritis (b) is a later manifestation and accompanied with foul-smelling lochia in addition to a tender, swollen uterus. This patient is afebrile and did not exhibit any systemic signs of infection. Ectopic pregnancy (d) is extremely unlikely given this patient's recent history of giving birth. Uterine artery rupture (e) is also unlikely and most commonly occurs at time of delivery followed by a period of extreme hemodynamic instability.

426. The answer is d. (*Rosen, p 2482.*) Postpartum bleeding is classified as early, within 24–48 hours of delivery, or late, up to 1–2 weeks. Causes of early postpartum bleeding include uterine atony, genital tract trauma, retained products of conception, and uterine inversion. Late bleeding episodes may be caused by *endometritis* or retained products of conception. Patients with endometritis most often present with *fever, vaginal discharge, general malaise, and vaginal bleeding*. Upon pelvic examination, the uterus will be soft and tender to the touch. The majority of infections are caused by normal vaginal flora such as anaerobes, enterococci, and streptococci. Patients who do not respond to initial antibiotic therapy may warrant broader spectrum coverage and need to be further evaluated for a pelvic abscess or pelvic thrombophlebitis.

Uterine atony (a) and uterine inversion (c) are earlier causes of postpartum bleeding. Although retained products of conception (b) is a possibility in this patient, her presentation is more likely to be infectious. Tubo-ovarian torsion (e) is unlikely given that the patient's physical examination did not reveal any peritoneal signs. This patient's clinical picture is consistent with an infectious etiology. If a gynecological process is not found, other causes of infection must be ruled out including appendicitis.

427. The answer is b. (*Rosen, pp 2419–2420.*) Patients presenting with a *molar pregnancy* typically have severe nausea and vomiting, a uterus larger than expected for dates, intermittent vaginal bleeding, or passage of grape-like contents and hypertension. Risk factors include a previous history of molar pregnancy, and very young or advanced maternal ages. Typically, laboratory results reveal anemia on a complete blood count, β-hCG higher than expected, and an ultrasound that shows intrauterine echogenic material. Treatment includes dilation and curettage with future monitoring and evaluation for the development of *choriocarcinoma*.

Ectopic pregnancy (a) can be ruled out with the ultrasound evaluation. Ovarian torsion (b) can also be ruled out given the sonogram which would show good Doppler flow to both ovaries. Abruptio placentae (d) is unlikely given the early stage of this pregnancy. Hyperemesis gravidarum (e) is a syndrome of intractable nausea and vomiting that occurs early in pregnancy, but is generally not associated with significant changes in vital signs or abnormal findings on ultrasound.

428. The answer is c. (*Rosen, pp 2413–2416.*) *Inevitable abortions* are diagnosed in *first-trimester bleeding* with an *open cervical os* but *no passage of fetal products*. Determining whether the internal os is open is often misleading and confused with the normally distended external os. It is defined as open when one can place more than a fingertip within the cervix. In these cases, dilation and curettage with full evacuation of the pregnancy is warranted. Rh immunization may also be needed depending on the status of the patient; therefore, a type and screen should be obtained. First-trimester vaginal bleeding occurs in about 40% of pregnancies with approximately half of them eventually resulting in spontaneous miscarriage.

A threatened abortion (a) is defined by first-trimester vaginal bleeding, a closed cervical os, and no passage of fetal tissue by history or exam. A β-hCG and ultrasound are needed to confirm an intrauterine pregnancy and help rule out an ectopic pregnancy. Often times, it will be too early in the pregnancy to see either on ultrasound evaluation. These patients should be given close follow-up for a repeat β-hCG and ultrasound within 24–48 hours. Patients need to be given bleeding precautions upon discharge from the ED, given that they are in stable condition. This includes bed rest for 24 hours and the avoidance of intercourse, tampons, and douching until the bleeding stops. Complete abortions (b) are defined by the complete passage of fetal products and placenta. These patients require supportive management, dilation, and curettage for removal of all potentially retained products of conception and Rh prophylaxis. Incomplete abortions (d) are defined by the partial passage of fetal products with an open cervical os. Dilation and curettage and Rh prophylaxis are also warranted. A missed abortion (e) is the retention of nonviable fetal products for some time after the abortion occurred. This may progress to spontaneous abortion with expulsion or may require a dilation and curettage for removal.

429. The answer is e. (*Rosen, pp 2413–2416.*) Given that this patient has a *closed cervical os* with *no history of passing tissue*, it is most likely a *threatened abortion*. This patient will need further ultrasound and β-hCG evaluation in

1–2 days to follow the pregnancy. Progesterone levels can also aid in distinguishing an ectopic pregnancy. Proper bleeding precautions should also be given and an Rh status determined.

Placenta previa (**a**) is unlikely given the early stage of pregnancy. An inevitable abortion (**b**) involves an open cervical os. In a complete abortion (**c**), a closed cervical os may be observed but there is also a history of the passage of fetal tissue. A septic abortion (**d**) is defined as a uterine infection during any time of an abortion. Patients present with vaginal bleeding and cramping pain with fever and purulent cervical discharge. Prompt evacuation is warranted in these cases along with the initiation of antibiotic and Rh prophylaxis.

430. The answer is b. (*Rosen, pp 219–224.*) This patient exhibits signs of hyperandrogenism and anovulation as evidenced by her history of irregular, heavy periods and being treated with oral contraceptives. Her physical examination is consistent with hirsutism, which is a result of increased serum testosterone. Many of these patients are also obese. For these reasons, *polycystic ovarian syndrome* is the most probable reason for this patient's symptoms.

Intrauterine and ectopic pregnancy (**a** and **c**) should always be ruled out with a β-hCG. Follicular cysts (**d**) are very common and usually occur within the first 2 weeks of the menstrual cycle. Pain is secondary to stretching of the capsule and cyst rupture. Follicular cysts usually resolve within 1–3 months and do not result in bleeding. Corpus luteum cysts (**e**) occur in the last 2 weeks of the menstrual cycle and are less common. Bleeding into the capsule may occur but these cysts usually regress at the end of the menstrual cycle. In general, cysts are usually asymptomatic unless they are complicated by rupture, torsion, or hemorrhage. Ultrasound is the preferred mode of imaging.

431. The answer is d. (*Rosen, pp 219–224.*) *Endometriosis* is defined by the presence of endometrial glands and tissue outside of the lining of the uterus. This tissue may be present on the ovaries, fallopian tubes, bladder, rectum, appendix, or other gastrointestinal tissue. There are many different hypotheses as to how this ectopic tissue forms, the most commonly accepted being "retrograde menstruation." Pain most commonly occurs before or at the beginning of menses. Other symptoms that indicate ectopic endometrial implantation and activation include dyspareunia and problems with defecation. Clinical suspicions can only be confirmed with direct visualization through *laparoscopy*. Treatment includes analgesia for acute episodes and hormonal therapy to suppress the normal menstrual cycle so that purely the endometrial tissue may be sloughed during menses.

Surgical intervention is taken for those cases that are truly refractory to these treatments.

Ureteral colic (**a**) is unlikely given the lack of flank tenderness, dysuria, and prior history of stones. Obtaining a urinalysis will be complicated by the presence of menstrual blood. Again, pregnancy (**b**) and therefore ectopics (**c**) should always be ruled out with a quick and easy β-hCG. The probability of appendicitis (**e**) is low given that this patient's abdominal examination is unremarkable.

432. The answer is a. (*Rosen, pp 219–224.*) The menstrual cycle consists of a follicular phase and a luteal phase. The follicular, or proliferative, phase begins on the first day of menses and continues until ovulation whereupon the luteal, or secretory, phase begins. During the follicular phase, endometrial glands form under the influences of estrogen, primarily estradiol. In the luteal phase, estrogen is still present but progesterone takes over and is mainly responsible for endometrial secretion and prepares the lining of the uterus for implantation. The luteal phase is characterized by an elevated body temperature and stromal edema. When implantation does not occur, menses ensues as a result of falling hormonal levels, which cause coiling and constrict the endometrial arteries. An elevated β-hCG maintains the corpus luteum. *Dysfunctional uterine bleeding (DUB)* is any abnormality in the regular bleeding pattern of the menstrual cycle and anovulation is the usual cause. This is the ovaries' failure to secrete an ovum, which thereby prevents luteinization from occurring. Without progesterone, the endometrium proliferates. This can lead to endometrial hyperplasia, which increases the risk for carcinoma. Other causes of symptoms of DUB include uterine fibroids, uterine polyps, genital tract trauma, exogenous estrogens, endocrine axis dysfunction, and bleeding disorders. Menopause occurs on average at the age of 51.5 years. Given that this woman is close to this age, this could also be perimenopausal symptoms. Hormone levels may be checked to see if they are falling. However, endometrial carcinoma may present in a similar way and needs to be ruled out with an *endometrial biopsy.*

Hormonal therapy (**b**) should not be used in this patient given that she is older and this can increase her chances of endometrial hyperplasia. Dilation and curettage (**d**) is not warranted given that she does not have a diagnosis yet. Any surgical intervention, (**c and e**) should be held until a biopsy is performed.

433. The answer is c. (*Rosen, pp 226–231.*) It is very important to stress the possibility that any fertile female is pregnant until proven otherwise.

Obtaining a urine β-hCG along with an ultrasound could save your patient's life, as other essential tests and consults are being acquired. In this case of a *ruptured ectopic pregnancy*, the presentation is atypical but it may be said that it is essentially typical of ectopics. These are, by very nature, implantations that can occur anywhere in the abdominal cavity. It is therefore imperative to keep this life-threatening diagnosis at the top of your differential.

Appendicitis (**a**) is unlikely given this patient's examination and temperature. This patient does not have any of the signs for PID (**b**) or any changes in bowel habits that would suggest diverticulitis (**e**). This clinical scenario is challenging in the sense that the ectopic pregnancy mimics a very painful albeit not life-threatening illness like a ureteral stone (**d**). It is important to take into account negative tests, as in the urine dip, as well as positive ones to narrow in on the diagnosis. These can be tricky, as some stones are obstructing and do cause hematuria.

434. The answer is d. (*Rosen, pp 228–229.*) In any patient who is *pregnant* with *vaginal bleeding,* it is imperative to obtain a type and screen in order to identify the *Rh status* of the patient. Rhesus isoimmunization is an immunologic disorder that affects Rh-negative mothers of Rh-positive fetuses. Any transplacental maternal exposure to fetal Rh-positive blood cells can initiate this, whether its origin is traumatic or not. Initial exposure leads to primary sensitization and the production of antibodies. In subsequent pregnancies, these maternal antibodies can then cross the placenta and attack the fetal Rh-positive blood cells. Prevention can be accomplished by giving Rhogam to all mothers who are Rh-negative. Administration of the immune globulin can be given prophylactically at 28 weeks or at the time of maternal exposure.

435. The answer is c. (*Rosen, pp 2413–2416.*) This patient presents with *vaginal bleeding* and a **closed os**, which narrows the diagnosis to either a threatened, complete, or missed abortion. The ultrasound examination reveals an *intrauterine pregnancy* that is still present *without a fetal heart rate,* which confirms the *missed abortion.* A dilation and curettage and Rh prophylaxis is warranted to prevent further infection and coagulopathy.

436. The answer is b. (*Rosen, pp 219–224.*) It is important to remember that sometimes patients come to the ED with benign or normal conditions in which education and counsel are the treatments of choice.

In this case, it is true that her menstrual flow is early but a one-time occurrence does not give the diagnoses of dysfunctional uterine bleeding (**d**) or endometriosis. If this patient had a history of bleeding before the day of her presentation, a complete abortion would have to be investigated. Given her negative β-hCG, an ectopic pregnancy (**c**) or threatened abortion (**a**) can be ruled out. PID (**e**) presents with fever, abdominal pain, purulent vaginal discharge, and a positive STD history, not vaginal bleeding.

437. The answer is d. *(Rosen, pp 228–229.)* *Progesterone levels* may be helpful in distinguishing ectopic pregnancies. A level of <5 ng/mL is highly suggestive of an ectopic pregnancy, given that the uterus may not be able to carry the pregnancy. Higher levels indicate that embryo implantation inside of the uterus is more likely.

Estrogen levels (**a**) and FSH (**b**) may prove helpful in distinguishing menopausal symptoms or aiding infertile women. TSH levels (**c**) are useful when reaching a diagnosis in women with irregular menstrual flow. A complete blood count (**e**) is not warranted given that this patient is not hemorrhaging. A type and screen should be performed to determine Rh status.

438. The answer is c. *(Rosen, pp 226–231.)* Given that this is a transvaginal ultrasound, the threshold for visualizing a pregnancy is lower than the transabdominal approach (>6500).

439. The answer is e. *(Rosen, pp 230–231.)* There is a high probability that this patient is suffering from a uterine rupture or abruptio placentae. *Monitoring* should be instilled immediately with *preparation for delivery.* Emergent obstetrical consultation is warranted for repair and possible Cesarean-section. Risk factors include trauma, hypertension, recreational drug use, smoking, multiparity, and advanced maternal age.

Ultrasound (**a**) is not useful in these cases, given that this is mainly a clinical diagnosis. Tocolytics (**c**) should not be given to prevent delivery, as this is often the treatment of choice. In cases of hemodynamic compromise due to excessive blood loss, blood transfusions (**d**) are indicated. A type and crossmatch should be done in this case in preparation for such an intervention. A brief external look to examine for vaginal bleeding may be done, but a complete pelvic examination (**b**) is not warranted as it may worsen bleeding.

440. The answer is e. *(Rosen, pp 2413–2415.)* In *threatened abortion,* the patient has vaginal bleeding with a closed internal os in the first 20 weeks of gestation. The risk of miscarriage is approximately 35–50%, depending on the patient population and severity of symptoms.

(**a**) Anembryonic gestation is the term used for what was described as a missed abortion, which referred to clinical failure of uterine growth over time. It is now known that fetal death occurs weeks before symptoms of spontaneous abortion and ultrasound is able to diagnose fetal death. **(b)** Completed abortion occurs when the uterus has expelled all of the fetal and placental material, the os is closed, and the uterus is contracted. This diagnosis should only be made after a dilation and curettage with pathologic confirmation of gestational products or by a conversion of β-hCG to 0, which may take up to 4 weeks. **(c)** Incomplete abortion is a term used to describe products of conception that are present at the os or vaginal canal. **(d)** Inevitable abortion is the term used to describe vaginal bleeding with an open internal os but no products of conception visualized.

441. The answer is a. (*Rosen, p 2415.*) *Rh isoimmunization* occurs when a Rh-negative female is exposed to Rh-positive blood during pregnancy or delivery. Initial exposure leads to primary sensitization with production of immunoglobulin M antibodies. A patient with a threatened abortion, who has Rh negative blood, is at increased risk for Rh isoimmunization and therefore should receive *anti-D Immune Globulin*. A 50 μg dose is used during the first trimester and a 300 μg dose after the first trimester.

(b) Eclampsia is a syndrome of hypertension, proteinuria, generalized edema, and seizures that usually occurs after the second trimester in pregnancy. **(c)** Chorioamionitis is an infection of the chorioamniotic membrane. Pregnant patients after 16 weeks present with fever and uterine tenderness. **(d)** Ferrous sulfate is used as a supplement to help treat anemia. This patient is not anemic. **(e)** This patient does not require a blood transfusion; her blood pressure is normal and her hematocrit is normal.

Eye Pain and Visual Change

Questions

442. A 24-year-old woman presents to the emergency department (ED) complaining of right eye pain and blurry vision since waking up this morning. She states that the pain began after taking out contact lenses that were in her eyes for over 1 week. Her blood pressure (BP) is 120/75 mm Hg, heart rate (HR) is 75 beats per minute, temperature is 99.1°F, and respiratory rate (RR) is 16 breaths per minute. Her right and left eye visual acuity is 20/60 and 20/20, respectively. Her conjunctivae are injected. The slit lamp exam reveals a large area of fluorescein uptake over the visual axis. Which of the following is the most appropriate therapy?

a. Call the ophthalmology consult for an emergent corneal transplant
b. Prescribe a systemic analgesic for pain control and advise the patient to not wear her contact lenses for the next week
c. Prescribe ciprofloxacin eye drops, oral analgesia, update tetanus prophylaxis, and arrange for ophthalmology follow-up
d. Prescribe oral amoxicillin, a topical anesthetic such as tetracaine and have patient follow-up with an ophthalmologist
e. Prescribe ciprofloxacin eye drops and have patient strictly wear an eye patch until her pain resolves

443. A 60-year-old woman presents to the ED complaining of pain in her right eye and burning sensation over half of her forehead and scalp. On physical exam, you notice a patch of grouped vesicles on an erythematous base located in a dermatomal distribution on her scalp and forehead. There are also a few vesicles located at the tip of the patient's nose. Her visual acuity is 20/20 bilaterally, heart is without murmurs, lungs are clear, abdomen is soft, and there are no gross findings on neurologic examination. Which of the following is the most concerning complication of this patient's clinical presentation?

a. Central nervous system (CNS) involvement leading to meningitis
b. Ophthalmic involvement leading to anterior uveitis or corneal scarring
c. Cardiac involvement leading to endocarditis
d. Permanent scarring of her face
e. Nasopalantine involvement leading to epistaxis

444. A 31-year-old nurse in your hospital has noticed a lesion in her left eye. She denies change in vision, pain, fevers, or discharge. A picture of her eye is shown below. Which of the following is the most likely diagnosis?

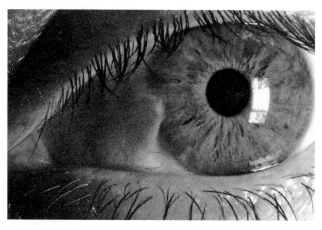

(Reproduced, with permission, from Knoop KJ, Stack LB, Storrow AB. Atlas of Emergency Medicine. *New York, NY: McGraw-Hill, 2002: 43.)*

a. Hordeolum
b. Chalazion
c. Dacrocystitis
d. Pinguecula
e. Pterygium

445. A 72-year old man presents with right eye pain for 1 day. The patient has a history of diabetes, hypertension, and "some type of eye problem." He does not recall the name of his eye problem or the name of his ophthalmic medication. However, he does remember that the eye drop has a yellow cap. Which class of ophthalmic medication is the patient taking?

a. Antibiotic
b. β-Blocker
c. Mydriatic/cycloplegic agent
d. Miotic
e. Anesthetic

446. A 35-year-old woman presents with a right-sided red eye for 3 days. She denies pain and notes that she has watery discharge from the eye. She has been coughing and congested for the past 5 days. On exam, the patient has a temperature of 98.4°F, HR of 72 beats per minute, BP of 110/70 mm Hg, and respiration rate of 14 breaths per minute. Her visual acuity is 20/20. On inspection, the conjunctiva is erythematous with minimal chemosis and clear discharge. The slit lamp, fluorescein, and fundoscopic exams are otherwise unremarkable. The patient has a nontender, preauricular lymph node and enlarged tonsils, without exudates. What is the most likely diagnosis?

a. Gonococcal conjunctivitis
b. Bacterial conjunctivitis
c. Viral conjunctivitis
d. Allergic conjunctivitis
e. Pseudomonal conjunctivitis

447. A 24-year old girl presents to the ED at 4 AM with severe left eye pain that woke her from sleep. She wears soft contact lenses and does not routinely take them out to sleep. She is in severe pain and wearing sunglasses in the exam room. You give her a drop of proparacaine to treat her pain prior to your exam. On exam, her vision is at baseline and she has no afferent pupillary defect. There is some perilimbic conjunctival erythema. On fluorescein exam, a linear area on the left side of the cornea is highlighted when cobalt blue light is applied. No underlying white infiltrate is visualized. No white cells or flare are visualized in the anterior chamber. What is the most appropriate treatment for this condition?

a. Immediate ophthalmology consult
b. Tobramycin ophthalmic ointment
c. Erythromycin ophthalmic ointment
d. Eye patch
e. Proparacaine ophthalmic drops

448. A 45-year-old woman presents with right eye pain and redness for 1 day. She has photophobia and watery discharge from the eye. She does not wear glasses or contact lenses and has no prior eye problems. On exam, the patient's visual acuity is 20/20 in the left eye and 20/70 in the right eye. She has conjunctival injection around the cornea and clear watery discharge. On slit lamp exam, the lids, lashes, and anterior chamber are normal. When fluorescein is applied, a branching, white-colored epithelial defect is seen. The remainder of the head exam is normal and the patient has no cutaneous lesions. Which of the following is the most appropriate treatment for this patient?

a. Admission for intravenous (IV) antibiotics
b. Admission for IV antiviral agents
c. Topical steroids
d. Topical antiviral medication
e. Immediate ophthalmology consultation

449. A 65-year-old woman with a history of hypertension, polymyalgia rheumatica, and coronary artery disease presents to the ED with right-sided headache. She also complains of pain in her mouth after eating half her meal. She denies change in vision or diplopia. On exam, her temperature is 96.7°F, BP 150/94 mm Hg, HR 84 beats per minute, and respirations 16 breaths per minute. Her corrected vision is 20/50 left eye and 20/100 right eye. Pupils are equal, round, and reactive to light. Extraocular eye movements are intact. Slit lamp exam is normal and fluorescein exam reveals no lesions. Intraocular pressure (IOP) in the left eye is 13 and 14 in the right eye. The neurological exam is normal. Which of the following is the most appropriate next step in management?

a. Serum erythrocyte sedimentation rate (ESR)
b. Head computed tomography (CT)
c. Timolol ophthalmic drops
d. Mannitol IV
e. Steroids IV

450. A 9-year-old boy is brought in to the ED by his mother for a red eye. The patient complains of rhinorrhea and a nonproductive cough, but has no eye pain or discharge. He also has no associated ecchymosis, bony tenderness of the orbit, or pain on extraocular eye movement. His vision is normal, extraocular movements are intact, and IOP is 12. A picture of his eye is shown on the next page. What is the most appropriate management of this condition?

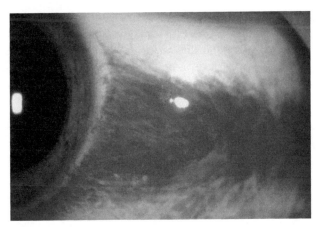

(Reproduced, with permission, from Riordan-Eva P, Asbury T, Whitcher JP. Vaughan & Asbury's General Ophthalmology. New York, NY: McGraw-Hill, 2004: 124.)

a. Call ophthalmology immediately
b. Administer 1% atropine
c. Elevate patient's head
d. Administer ophthalmic timolol
e. Reassurance only

451. A 28-year-old mechanic with no past medical history presents to the ED after a small amount of battery acid was splashed in his right eye. He is complaining of extreme pain and tearing from his eye. Which of the following is the most appropriate next step in management?

a. Call ophthalmology now
b. Check visual acuity
c. Check the pH of the tears
d. Irrigate with normal saline
e. Apply erythromycin ointment

452. A 45-year-old man lacerated his right forehead after an altercation in a local bar. Instead of seeking medical attention, the patient applied super glue to his wound. He successfully stopped the bleeding, but some of the glue got into his right eye and now he comes to the ED with difficulty opening his right eye. What is the most appropriate treatment of this patient?

a. Call ophthalmology immediately
b. Wash eye with acetone
c. Wash eye with normal saline
d. Use forceps to remove all the glue from the eye
e. Apply erythromycin ointment

453. The local sorority house recently installed a self-tanning station. Two days later three sorority girls present to the ED with bilateral eye pain, tearing, and photophobia. After ophthalmic anesthesia instillation, a complete eye exam is performed. Visual acuity is normal. Extraocular eye movements are intact and pupils are equal, round, and reactive to light. IOP is normal. Slit lamp exam is normal, but fluorescein exam under cobalt blue light illuminates small dots throughout the cornea. What is the most likely diagnosis?

a. Ultraviolet keratitis
b. Anterior uveitis
c. Herpes simplex keratitis
d. Allergic conjunctivitis
e. Corneal ulcer

454. A 12-year-old girl presents to the ED for left eye pain and swelling for 2 days. The patient has had cough, congestion, and rhinorrhea for the last week that is improving. On exam, her temperature is 100.8°F, HR 115 beats per minute, RR 12 breaths per minute, and BP 110/70 mm Hg. On eye exam, there is purple-red swelling of both upper and lower eyelids with injection of the conjunctiva. Pupils are equal and reactive to light. There is restricted lateral gaze. Visual acuity is 20/70 in the left eye and 20/25 in the right eye. The rest of the physical exam is normal. What is the most appropriate next step in management?

a. Administer diphenhydramine
b. Administer amoxicillin/clavulanate
c. Administer vancomycin IV
d. CT scan of orbits and sinuses
e. Administer artificial tears

455. A 60-year-old man with a history of hypertension and migraine headaches presents to the ED with a headache. He describes left-sided headache and eye pain that is associated with nausea and vomiting. The patient has a long history of migraines, but says his migraines do not usually include eye pain. On exam, his temperature is 97.6°F, HR 84 beats per minute, RR 12 breaths per minute, and BP 134/80 mm Hg. His neurological exam is normal. His left eye is mid-dilated and nonreactive. His cornea is cloudy. His corrected visual acuity is 20/50 in the left eye and 20/20 in the right eye. What is the most appropriate next step in management?

a. Administer hydromorphone
b. Head CT scan
c. Check IOP
d. Check ESR
e. Discharge patient

456. A 22-year-old presents to the ED for left eye pain. He was in an altercation yesterday and was punched in the left eye. On exam, his left eye is ecchymotic and the eyelids are swollen shut. He has tenderness over the infraorbital rim, but no step-offs. You use an eyelid speculum to examine his eye. His pupils are equal and reactive to light. His visual acuity is normal. On testing extraocular movements, you find he is unable to look upward with his left eye. He also complains of diplopia when looking upward. Fundoscopic exam is normal. What is the most likely diagnosis?

a. Orbital blowout fracture
b. Ruptured globe
c. Retinal detachment
d. Cranial nerve III palsy
e. Traumatic retrobulbar hematoma

457. You are examining the pupils of a patient. On inspection, the pupils are 3 mm and equal bilaterally. You shine a flashlight into the right pupil and both pupils constrict to 1 mm. You then shine the flashlight into the left pupil and both pupils slightly dilate. What is this condition called?

a. Aniscoria
b. Argyll Robertson pupil
c. Afferent pupillary defect
d. Horner's syndrome
e. Normal pupil reaction

458. A 65-year-old man with a history of diabetes, hypertension, coronary artery disease, and atrial fibrillation presents with loss of vision in his left eye since he awoke 6 hours ago. The patient denies fever, eye pain, or eye discharge. On physical exam of the left eye, vision is limited to counting fingers. His pupil is 3 mm and reactive. Extraocular movements are intact. Slit-lamp exam is also normal. The dilated fundoscopic exam is shown below. Which of the following is the most likely diagnosis?

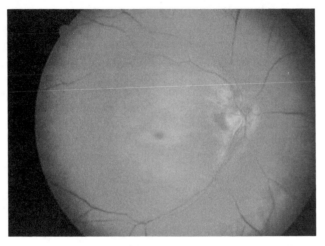

(Reproduced, with permission, from Knoop KJ, Stack LB, Storrow AB. Atlas of Emergency Medicine. New York, NY: McGraw-Hill, 2002: 82.)

a. Retinal detachment
b. Central retinal artery occlusion
c. Central retinal vein occlusion
d. Vitreous hemorrhage
e. Acute angle closure glaucoma

Eye Pain and Visual Change

Answers

442. The answer is c. (*Rosen, pp 752–754.*) The patient most likely sustained a *corneal abrasion* from prolonged *contact lens* use. Epithelial defects of the cornea are diagnosed by slit lamp exam by observing *fluorescein uptake* in the area of the defect. Treatment usually consists of cycloplegia, and topical or oral pain medications. Contact lens patients should be treated with topical antibiotics with *antipseudomonal* coverage. Patients should not wear their contact lens until complete healing of the corneal epithelium. All patients should follow-up with an ophthalmologist.

(**a**) Corneal abrasions usually heal well with appropriate care and do not require a transplant. (**d**) Amoxicillin is not an appropriate antibiotic because it is not topical and not antipseudomonal. In addition, tetracaine, if used frequently, can decompose the cornea and cause permanent damage. (**e**) Eye patching should be avoided, particularly with injuries involving contact lens. Data suggest that eye patching confers no benefit in healing small, uncomplicated corneal abrasions and may provide a better environment for pseudomonas to proliferate.

443. The answer is b. (*Rosen, pp 1656–1657.*) The patient has *herpes zoster,* or *shingles,* an infection caused by the *varicella-zoster virus.* The patient's rash most likely involves the *ophthalmic division* of the *trigeminal nerve.* In addition, the vesicles found on the tip of the patient's nose correlate strongly with viral involvement of the eye. *Hutchinson's sign* is used to denote vesicles on the tip of a patient's nose in the setting of herpes zoster. When there is ocular involvement the infection is called *herpes zoster ophthalmicus. Ocular complications* occur in 20–70% of the cases involving the ophthalmic division of the trigeminal nerve. Severity varies from mild conjunctivitis to panophthalmitis. In addition, the patient is at risk for anterior uveitis, secondary glaucoma, and corneal scarring.

(**a**) Complications of zoster include CNS involvement that can lead to meningoencephalitis, myelitis, and peripheral neuropathy, however, the patient's current neurologic exam is unremarkable. (**c**) Although zoster can disseminate to the visceral organs, like the brain, no cases of endocarditis have ever been reported. (d) The rash of zoster usually heals within a month and do not leave a permanent scar. (e) Epistaxis is not a complication of zoster.

444. The answer is e. *(Knoop, pp 43–44.)* This patient has a *pterygium*, a triangle-shaped growth of tissue from the bulbar conjunctiva to the periphery of the cornea. It is more common on the nasal side of the cornea and may affect one or both eyes. Pterygiums are associated with exposure to wind, dust, and sunlight. Most cases are asymptomatic and can be followed by an ophthalmologist. In cases where the pterygium grows into the visual axis or restricts extraocular motion, surgical excision is indicated.

Pinguecula (d) is a yellow-whitish, fatty lesion of the bulbar conjunctiva that may be on either side of the cornea, but is more commonly seen on the nasal side. Dacrocystits (c) is an inflammation of the lacrimal sac that is characterized by pain, swelling, and erythema of the lacrimal sac on the extreme nasal aspect of the lower lid. Pressure on the lacrimal sac in a patient with dacrocystitis may express pus. Hordeolum (a) or stye is an acute infection and abscess of the glands within the eyelids. Chalazions (b) are granulomatous inflammations of meibomian glands in the eyelids. In contrast to the erythematous, edematous, and painful hordeolums, chalazions are usually hard and nontender swellings.

445. The answer is b. *(Vaughan & Asbury's General Ophthalmology 16/ed chapter 3)* Ophthalmic medications are *color-coded*. While this question may seem esoteric, it can be clinically useful to know the colors of eye medications. In this case, knowing that yellow caps are *β-blockers* suggests that this patient may be currently treated for glaucoma. Medication color knowledge can also help you rapidly locate a specific medication from a large group of eye medications.

Antibiotics (a) are usually tan, mydriatics, and cycloplegics (c) are red, miotics (d) are green, and anesthetics (e) are white. Mydriatics and cycloplegics are medications that cause ciliary muscle paralysis and pupil dilation. Miotics are medications that cause pupillary constriction.

446. The answer is c. *(Tintinalli, pp 1452–1453.)* This patient has classic *viral conjunctivitis* that is associated with a viral upper respiratory infection. Patients with viral conjunctivitis typically have *reddened conjunctiva* and *watery discharge*. Preauricular adenopathy is also associated with viral etiology. Treatment includes cool compresses and an antihistamine/α-adrenergic combination medication—naphazoline/pheniramine—for symptomatic care.

Patients with bacterial conjunctivitis (**b**) have thick mucopurulent discharge and often wake-up with their eyelids stuck together. These patients are treated with broad-spectrum antibiotics. Bacterial and viral conjunctivitis do not always present classically and they can be difficult to distinguish clinically. Many physicians will therefore treat conjunctivitis patients with antibiotic eye drops until they can be reexamined by an ophthalmologist. Patients who wear contact lenses are at risk for pseudomonal conjunctivitis (**e**). They should be treated with an antibiotic that covers *Pseudomonas*, such as a fluoroquinolone or aminoglycoside. It is very important to always consider gonococcal conjunctivitis (**a**) in sexually active individuals, because this infection can cause permanent visual loss if not rapidly identified and treated. Patients with gonococcal conjunctivitis have a severe conjunctivitis with copious mucopurulent drainage and erythematous conjunctiva. Inpatient IV antibiotics should be started while waiting for results of ocular Gram stain and culture. Allergic conjunctivitis (**d**) presents with watery discharge and eye redness, but itching is the most prominent symptom. Cyclical exacerbations associated with allergen exposure may be clues to the diagnosis of allergic conjunctivitis.

447. The answer is b. (*Tintinalli, p 1455.*) This patient has a *corneal abrasion* from prolonged contact lens use. The abrasion *lights* up after fluorescein staining and cobalt blue illumination of the cornea. Contact lens wearers with abrasions are at high risk for *Pseudomonas* infection and should be treated with Tobramycin ophthalmic ointment (**b**) or fluoroquinolone drops. It is critical to distinguish an abrasion from a corneal ulcer. Ulcers are deeper infections of the cornea that develop from corneal epithelial defects (i.e., abrasions). Contact lens wearers are also at high risk for corneal ulcers. The hallmark of a corneal ulcer is a shaggy, white infiltrate within the corneal epithelial defect.

(**c**) Uncomplicated corneal abrasions may be treated with erythromycin ointment. Corneal ulcers are treated aggressively with anti-Pseudomonal antibiotics and immediate ophthalmology consultation (**a**). Some ophthalmologists will see the patient in the ED to perform corneal Gram stain and cultures; while other ophthalmologists will examine the patient in 12 hours in the office setting. Eye patches (**d**) are controversial, but may be used for uncomplicated corneal abrasions. Patches should not be given to patients at risk for fungal infections or pseudomonal infections as they are at risk for rapid corneal melting and perforation. Topical anesthetic agents, such as proparacaine (**e**), may be helpful to facilitate the exam in the ED, but should never be dispensed to patients. Repeated use of these agents can cause corneal injury and vision loss.

448. The answer is d. (*Tintinalli, pp 1453–1454.*) This patient has a *corneal epithelial disease* caused by the *Herpes simplex virus*. The hallmark of this disease is the branching or *dendritic* ulcer. Patients may also present without corneal involvement, but will have typical herpetic skin lesions in the eyelids and conjunctiva. Patients should be treated with topical antivirals, such as trifluridine, with topical antibiotics added to prevent secondary bacterial infection.

IV antibiotics (**a**) are not indicated for herpes simplex keratitis. Corticosteroids (**c**) must be avoided as steroids may enhance viral replication and worsen infection. Patients should follow-up with ophthalmology in 1–2 days. If there is evidence for herpes zoster opthalmicus, an infection involving the trigeminal nerve with ocular involvement, then ophthalmology should be consulted immediately (**e**) and the patient should be admitted for IV antivirals (**b**).

449. The answer is e. (*Tintinalli, pp 1461–1462.*) IV *steroids* should be started immediately when there is a high clinical suspicion for *temporal arteritis*. Temporal arteritis, also known as "giant cell arteritis," is a systemic vasculitis affecting the optic nerve arterial supply that can result in blindness and spread to the unaffected eye. Typical patients are women over the age of 50. There is also an association with polymyalgia rheumatica. Patients classically present with headache, anorexia, jaw claudication, fever, temporal artery tenderness to palpation, afferent pupillary defect, and visual deficits.

An elevated ESR (>100 mm/s) (**a**) is suggestive of temporal arteritis, but only a temporal artery biopsy is specific for the diagnosis. Confirmatory biopsy should be performed within 1 week of initiating steroids. Glaucoma also presents with headache and vision changes; however, this patient's IOPs are within normal limits (10–21 mm Hg). This patient therefore does not need medications to reduce the IOP, such as timolol (**c**) or mannitol (**d**). Up to one-third of patients with temporal arteritis can have associated transient ischemic attacks and strokes. Performing a head CT (**b**) is a consideration, but should be performed after steroid treatment is initiated.

450. The answer is e. (*Tintinalli, pp 1455, 1457–1458.*) This patient has *subconjunctival hemorrhage* caused by conjunctival vessel rupture from coughing. This common emergency department complaint can result spontaneously or from valsalva induced pressure spikes (such as coughing or bearing down), trauma, and hypertension.

Patients can be reassured that subconjunctival hemorrhages spontaneously resolve in 1–2 weeks (**e**). Subconjunctival hemorrhage is sometimes confused with hyphema or blood in the anterior chamber. Hyphemas can be traumatic from a ruptured iris vessel or spontaneous, usually associated with sickle-cell disease. Bleeding within the anterior chamber can cause elevated IOP and must be treated aggressively with β-blockers (**d**) and mannitol. Carbonic anhydrase inhibitors (Diamox) should be avoided in sickle-cell patients as these medications lower anterior chamber pH, ultimately enhancing RBC sickling and increasing IOP. Pupillary activity stretches the iris vessels and exacerbates bleeding with hyphema; therefore, mydriatic agents such as atropine (**b**) are used to keep the pupil dilated. The head of the bed can be elevated (**c**) to minimize elevations of IOP. Many ophthalmologists will admit all patients with hyphemas. This is because 30% of hyphemas rebleed in 3–5 days, resulting in dangerously high elevations in IOP necessitating surgical therapy. Some ophthalmologists will follow patients with hyphemas less than one-third of the anterior chamber as outpatients. However, ophthalmology should be urgently consulted while the patient is in the ED and individual decisions can be discussed (**a**).

451. The answer is d. (*Tintinalli, pp 1458–1459.*) Chemical injuries to the eye must be *irrigated* with a minimum of 1–2 L of normal saline as soon as they arrive in the ED. Topical anesthesia and the use of a Morgan Lens (a special device to provide large volume irrigation to the eye) can help facilitate this procedure.

(**b**) Irreversible eye damage can occur if irrigation is withheld for a physical exam and visual acuity testing. Checking the pH of the tears (**c**) helps determine the effectiveness of irrigation, but should be checked after irrigation has begun. When the ocular pH returns to 7.5–8.0, irrigation can be stopped and a complete eye examination should be performed. Remember to check visual acuity and pay special attention to corneal clouding or corneal epithelial defects. (**e**) Patients with epithelial defects or corneal clouding should receive an ophthalmic antibiotic. Patients without corneal or anterior chamber involvement only need erythromycin ointment. The ophthalmologist (**a**) should be notified, after initial stabilization, of all patients with chemical injury to the eye and follow-up should be arranged within 12–24 hours in consultation with the ophthalmologist.

452. The answer is e. (*Tintinalli, p 1459.*) Fortunately, super glue or crazy glue (cyanoacrylate) exposure to the eye is usually not permanently damaging to the eye. Corneal irritation can occur from the hard, irregularly shaped glue. To prevent this abrasive effect, large amounts of erythromycin ointment should be applied to the eye and eyelids as a lubricant. Large clumps of glue can be removed manually.

Instrumentation to remove all glue products (d) is not necessary in the ED. The glue will loosen over time and be easier to remove in several days. Washing the eye with normal saline (c) will not be helpful unless there are large free clumps that will be washed away. (b) While applying acetone may help remove cyanoacrylate from clothing and surfaces, acetone (or any other chemical) should never be infused into the eye. (a) These patients should follow-up with ophthalmology in 1–2 days.

453. The answer is a. (*Tintinalli, p 1459.*) These girls forgot to wear eye protection while using the sun-tanning lights and have *ultraviolet keratitis.* History of exposure to sun-tanning lamps, welding, or the sun suggests the diagnosis and fluorescein staining showing *superficial punctate keratitis* confirms the diagnosis. Treatment consists of analgesia, cycloplegics to reduce ciliary spasm and pain, erythromycin ointment, and ophthalmology follow-up in 1–2 days. Fortunately, most patients with ultraviolet keratitis make a full recovery with supportive care alone.

Iritis or anterior uveitis (b) can also cause eye redness and pain. It is an intraocular inflammation of the anterior uveal tract with numerous possible infectious and inflammatory etiologies. Iritis is diagnosed by history and visualization of cells and flare in the anterior chamber on slit lamp examination. Consistent with an infectious or inflammatory etiology, cells represent leukocytes floating in the aqueous humor and flare represents a hazy protein accumulation. Herpes simplex keratitis (c) has the hallmark dendritic epithelial defect on fluorescein examination. Patients with allergic conjunctivitis (d) present with ocular discharge, itching, and dry eyes. While a punctate keratitis may be seen on fluorescein examination, a history of exquisite ocular pain is not consistent with allergic conjunctivitis. Corneal ulcers (e) may present with erythema and ocular pain, but show white, hazy infiltrates on fluorescein exam.

454. The answer is c. (*Tintinalli, pp 1454–1455.*) This patient has *orbital cellulitis,* an infection deep to the orbital septum. The patient had a recent upper respiratory infection and sinusitis which likely resulted in orbital extension of the infection. *Staphylococcus aureus* and *Haemophilus influenzae* are common etiologies, and mucormycosis must be considered in diabetics and immunocompromised patients. Distinctive clinical findings of orbital cellulitis are eye pain, fever, *impaired eye motility,* decreased visual acuity, and proptosis. Patients should be treated with IV antibiotics, such as cefuroxime, a combination of penicillin and nafcillin, or vancomycin and admitted to the hospital. In this case, the diagnosis is clear from the history and physical exam and treatment should be started promptly. Orbital cellulitis must be differentiated from preseptal cellulitis and allergic reactions. Preseptal cellulitis is a superficial cellulitis that does not penetrate the orbital septum. Patients present with swollen, red eyelids, but no vision change, pupil changes, or changes in eye motility.

Orbital and sinus CT scans (d) may be performed after antibiotics are started to rule out an abscess. CT scans are also useful when the diagnosis of orbital cellulitis is in consideration but not clinically clear. Patients over the age of 5 with preseptal cellulitis may be treated with amoxicillin/clavulanate orally (b) and close follow-up with their regular doctor. Children less than 5 years old are at risk for systemic bacteremia and should be admitted for IV antibiotics. Patients with allergic reactions have swelling and erythema of the eyelids, but no fever or tenderness to palpation. These patients may be treated with artificial tears (e) and antihistamines, such as (a) diphenhydramine.

455. The answer is c. (*Tintinalli, pp 1459, 1461–1462.*) This patient has *acute angle-closure glaucoma,* when the aqueous humor production in the posterior chamber of the eye is unable to drain through the anterior chamber and the resultant obstruction causes *increased IOP.* On exam, patients with increased IOP have a mid-dilated, nonreactive pupil with *corneal clouding* and decreased vision. The diagnosis is clenched by checking the IOP with a tonopen or tonometer. Normal IOP is 10–21 mm Hg. Patients with increased IOP should be treated with medications to decrease production of aqueous humor. Checking IOP is a simple, rapid test that should be performed on all patients with headache and orbital pain. If this test is negative, other causes of headache and eye pain should be investigated.

This patient is not experiencing his typical migraine headache and he has abnormalities on his physical exam. Discharging the patient without further investigation is therefore inappropriate (e). Pain control is appropriate for this patient, but given his nausea and vomiting, he is not likely to tolerate oral hydromorphone (a). Checking an ESR (d) is helpful if you suspect temporal arteritis. Head CT scan (b) can be considered in the workup of an atypical headache, but simpler tests, such as tonometry, should be performed first.

456. The answer is a. (*Tintinalli, pp 1457–1464, 1587–1588. Vassallo, pp 251–256.*) This patient has an *orbital blowout fracture* of the inferior wall causing *entrapment of the inferior rectus muscle* and *restricted eye motility* with diplopia. A CT scan with thin cuts through the orbits can confirm the diagnosis. Patients with this injury are generally started on oral antibiotics due to the risk of infection with sinus wall fractures and may follow-up with the institution's appropriate surgical service in 3–10 days. These injuries are associated with other eye problems and a careful eye exam must be performed to rule out abrasions, lacerations, foreign bodies, hyphema, iritis, retinal detachment, and lens dislocation.

The patient has no evidence of a retinal detachment (**c**) given his normal visual acuity and fundoscopic exam. However, even with a normal exam in the ED, patients with orbital blowout fractures should be referred to an ophthalmologist for a repeat exam to rule out a traumatic retinal detachment. Ruptured globes (**b**) are more common with penetrating trauma and clues to this diagnosis are shallow anterior chamber, hyphema, irregular pupil, significant decrease in vision. If a ruptured globe is suspected, a hard eye shield should be applied and ophthalmology consulted. Do not check IOP in patients with suspected ruptured globes as this can worsen the injury. Cranial nerve III palsy (**d**) presents with problems with medial gaze, upward gaze, downward gaze as well as ptosis. This patient only has difficulty with upward gaze suggesting that cranial nerve III is intact. Traumatic retrobulbar hemorrhage (**e**) is a displacement of the globe and septum anteriorly caused by bleeding into the orbit. Since the globe has limited capacity for expansion, continued bleeding puts pressure on ocular structures. Optic nerve compression leads to decreased visual acuity and continued globe pressure leads to proptosis. Patients with a traumatic history and clinical signs suggestive of retrobulbar hemorrhage require emergency orbital decompression via lateral cantholysis.

457. The answer is c. (*Knoop, p 67. Tintinalli, pp 1451, 1463.*) This patient has an *afferent pupillary defect (APD)*, also known as a *Marcus Gunn pupil*. In patients with an APD, light shined into the affected pupil causes a small dilation with no constriction. APD is due to a lesion in the anterior visual pathway of the retina, optic nerve, or optic chiasm preventing reception of the light in the affected eye. Neither pupil constricts since constriction is centrally mediated in the midbrain. APDs are sensitive for disease, but not specific. The differential diagnosis for an APD includes central retinal artery or vein occlusion, optic nerve disorders such as optic neuritis, tumor or glaucoma, and lesions in the optic chiasm or tract.

Anisocoria (**a**) is unequal pupil size. Under normal room lighting, normal pupils may be 1–2 mm different in size. An Argyll-Robertson pupil (**b**) constricts during accommodation (as expected), but does not constrict in response to light. This is usually seen in both eyes and is associated with neurosyphilis. Horner's syndrome (**d**) is decreased sympathetic innervation of the eye from interruption of the sympathetic chain at any point from the brainstem to the sympathetic plexus around the carotid artery. Clinically, patients with Horner's syndrome have ptosis, miosis, and anhydrosis. (**e**) Normal pupil response to light is pupil constriction followed by a small amount of dilatation.

458. The answer is b. (*Tintinalli, pp 1460–1462.*) The differential diagnosis for acute painless loss of vision includes retinal detachment, central retinal artery and vein occlusions, vitreous hemorrhage, and transient ischemic attack. An ophthalmologist should be called immediately when entertaining these diagnoses because a thorough fundoscopic exam and prompt treatment is essential. On fundoscopic exam, the patient has a *macular cherry red spot* with *a pale retina* and less pronounced arteries. This is diagnostic of *central retinal artery occlusion*. Occlusion of the central retinal blood supply is commonly caused by emboli, thrombi, vasculitis, or trauma. Treatment aims to dislodge the clot from the main artery to one of its branches and includes digital massage, vasodilation, and lowering IOP.

Acute angle-closure glaucoma (**e**) usually causes painful loss of vision. Central retinal vein occlusion (**c**) presents similarly to retinal artery occlusion but is caused by thrombosis of the central retinal vein from stasis, edema, and hemorrhage. Fundoscopic exam shows diffuse retinal hemorrhages and optic disc edema, also called the "blood and thunder" fundus. Treatment involves aspirin and prompt ophthalmology referral. Retinal detachment (**a**) occurs when vitreous fluid accumulates behind a retinal tear displacing the retina. On fundoscopy, the retina will be hanging in the vitreous. Clinically, retinal detachment may be heralded by blurry vision or floaters followed by painless vision loss. Vitreous hemorrhage (**d**) is bleeding within the posterior chamber. On fundoscopic exam, these patients have blood obstructing the view of the fundus. There are many causes of vitreous hemorrhage, including diabetic retinopathy, retinal detachment, trauma, and age-related macular degeneration.

Endocrine Emergencies

Questions

459. A 30-year-old man with type 1 diabetes presents to the emergency department (ED). His blood pressure (BP) is 100/70 mm Hg and heart rate (HR) is 140 beats per minute. His blood glucose is 750 mg/dL, potassium level is 5.9 mEq/L, bicarbonate is 5 mEq/L, arterial pH 7.1. His urine is positive for ketones. Which of the following is the best initial therapy for this patient?

a. Give normal saline as a 2 L bolus then administer 20 units of regular insulin subcutaneously
b. Bolus 2 amps of bicarbonate and administer 10 units of insulin intravenously
c. Give him 5 mg of metoprolol to slow down his heart, start intravenous (IV) hydration and then give 10 units of regular insulin intravenously
d. Give normal saline in 2 L bolus and then administer 10 units of insulin intravenously followed by an insulin drip and continued hydration
e. Give normal saline in 2 L bolus with 20 mEq/L KCl in each bag

460. A 39-year-old woman is brought into the ED by her family who states that she has had 4 days of diarrhea and has now started acting "crazy" with mood swings and confusion. The family states that she usually takes a medication for a problem with her neck. Her BP is 130/45 mm Hg, HR is 140 beats per minute, temperature is 101.5°F, and her respiratory rate (RR) is 22 breaths per minute. An electrocardiogram (ECG) reveals atrial fibrillation with a normal QRS complex. After you address the airway, breathing, and circulation (ABCs), which of the following is the most appropriate next step in management?

a. Administer 2 amps of bicarbonate to treat for tricyclic antidepressant overdose
b. Administer chlordiazepoxide, thiamine, and folate
c. Administer ceftriaxone and prepare for a lumbar puncture
d. Administer propranolol, propylthiouracil (PTU), then wait an hour to give Lugol's iodine solution
e. Administer ciprofloxacin and give a 2 L bolus of normal saline for treatment of dehydration secondary to infectious diarrhea

- HypoTN
- lethargic
- ECG ↓ amplitude

461. A 65-year-old woman is brought into the ED by her family who states that she has been weak, lethargic, and saying "crazy things" over the last 2 days. Her family also states that her medical history is significant only for a disease of her thyroid. Her BP is 120/90 mm Hg, HR is 51 beats per minute, temperature is 94°F rectally, and her RR is 12 breaths per minute. On exam, the patient is overweight, her skin is dry, and you notice periorbital nonpitting edema. On neurologic exam, the patient does not respond to stimulation. Which of the following is the most likely diagnosis?

a. Apathetic thyrotoxicosis
b. Myxedema coma
c. Graves' disease
d. Acute stroke
e. Schizophrenia

462. A 74-year-old woman who is a known diabetic is brought to the ED by emergency medical service (EMS) with altered mental status. The home health aide states that the patient ran out of her medications 4 days ago. Her BP is 130/85 mm Hg, HR is 110 beats per minute, temperature is 99.8°F, and her RR is 18 breaths per minute. On exam, she cannot follow commands but responds to stimuli. Laboratory results reveal white blood cell (WBC) count of 14,000/μL, hematocrit 49%, platelets 325/μL, sodium 128 mEq/L, potassium 3.0 mEq/L, chloride 95 mEq/L, bicarbonate 22 mEq/L, blood urea nitrogen (BUN) 40 mg/dL, creatinine 1.8 mg/dL, and glucose 850 mg/dL. Urinalysis shows 3+ glucose, 1+ protein, no blood or ketones. After addressing the ABCs, which of the following is the most appropriate next step in management?

a. Begin fluid resuscitation with a 2–3 L bolus of normal saline then administer 10 units of regular insulin intravenously
b. Begin fluid resuscitation with a 2–3 L bolus of normal saline then administer 10 units of regular insulin intravenously, begin phenytoin for seizure prophylaxis
c. Administer 10 units of regular insulin intravenously then begin fluid resuscitation with a 2–3 L bolus of normal saline
d. Order a CT scan of the brain, if negative for acute stroke, begin fluid resuscitation with a 2–3 L bolus of normal saline
e. Arrange for urgent hemodialysis

463. A 21-year-old man presents to the ED. He has a known history of type 1 diabetes. He is hypotensive with BP of 95/65 mm Hg, tachycardic at 120 beats per minute, and tachypneic at 30 breaths per minute. Laboratory results reveal a WBC 20,000/μL, hematocrit 45%, platelets 225/μL, sodium 131 mEq/L, potassium 5.3 mEq/L, chloride 95 mEq/L, bicarbonate

5 mEq/L, BUN 20 mg/dL, creatinine 0.9 mg/dL, and glucose 425 mg/dL. Arterial blood gas reveals a pH of 7.2. Urinalysis reveals glucosuria and ketosis. There is a fruity odor to his breath. Which of the following provides the strongest evidence for the diagnosis?

a. Hypotension, tachycardia, and tachypnea
b. Glucose of 425 mg/dL, ketosis, and leukocytosis
c. Glucose of 425 mg/dL, ketosis, pH 7.2, and bicarbonate of 5 mEq/L
d. Glucose of 425 mg/dL, hypotension, and fruity odor to breath
e. Glucosuria, hypotension, and leukocytosis

464. A 21-year-old man presents to the ED complaining of abdominal pain, nausea, and vomiting for 1 day and increased weakness for the last 2–3 days. He states that he is using the bathroom to urinate frequently and is drinking large amounts of water. He has no previous medical problems and is not taking any medications. His BP is 110/72 mm Hg, HR is 119 beats per minute, temperature is 98.8°F, and RR is 14 breaths per minute. On exam he appears mildly confused, is pale, diaphoretic, and has unusually deep respirations and a fruity odor to his breath. Which of the following is the next best step?

a. Check fingerstick glucose
b. Administer antiemetics
c. Administer analgesics
d. Send basic metabolic panel
e. Obtain abdominal radiograph

465. A 32-year-old man is brought to the ED by EMS for confusion. EMS reports that the patient was at a local pharmacy filing his prescriptions when the pharmacist noticed the patient sweating and having difficulty answering questions. In the ED, the patient's BP is 130/68 mm Hg, HR is 120 beats per minute, temperature is 98.9°F, and RR is 12 breaths per minute. The patient is unable to explain what happened. His fingerstick glucose is 410 mg/dL and his urine is positive for ketones. An electrolyte panel reveals Na^+ 131 mEq/L, K^+ 4 mEq/L, Cl^- 91 mEq/L, and Ca^{2+} 11 mEq/L. Which of the following electrolytes are most important to supplement during the management of his medical condition?

a. Sodium, potassium, and calcium
b. Sodium
c. Potassium
d. Calcium
e. Sodium and calcium

466. A 36-year-old immigrant woman is brought to the ED from her workplace. She was found to be agitated and behaving bizarrely. The patient's past medical history and medications are unknown. Her BP is 162/92 mm Hg, HR is 140 beats per minute, temperature is 101.8°F, and RR is 18 breaths per minute. On exam, the patient is delirious, tremulous, and has a large goiter. Which of the following is the most appropriate management of this patient?

a. Administer dantrolene
b. Administer acetaminophen and broad coverage antibiotics
c. Protect airway, administer iodine
d. Administer diazepam
e. Protect airway, administer acetaminophen, propranolol, and PTU

467. A 75-year-old woman is brought to the ED by EMS after she had a witnessed seizure on the street. A bystander reports that the patient fell to the ground, had tonic-clonic activity, and was drooling. Her BP is 162/85 mm Hg, HR is 95 beats per minute, temperature is 99.4°F, and RR is 16 breaths per minute. On exam the patient is unresponsive and has a bleeding superficial scalp laceration. Which of the following electrolyte disturbances is *least likely* to cause a seizure?

a. Hypoglycemia
b. Hyperglycemia
c. Hyponatremia
d. Hypernatremia
e. Hypokalemia

468. A 53-year-old woman is brought to the ED by her husband, who states that she is feeling very weak over the last 2 days, is nauseated, and vomiting at least three times. The husband states that his wife was taking a high dose medication for her joint pain but ran out of her pills last week. Her vital signs are a BP of 90/50 mm Hg, HR 87 beats per minute, RR 16 breaths per minute, and temperature 98.1°F. You place her on the monitor, begin IV fluids, and send her blood to the lab. Thirty minutes later the metabolic panel results are back and reveal the following:

Na^+	126 mEq/L
K^+	5 mEq/L
Cl^-	99 mEq/L
HCO_3	21 mEq/L
BUN	24 mg/dL

Cr	1.6 mg/dL
Gluc	69 mg/dL
Ca^+	11 mEq/L

What is the most likely diagnosis?

a. Myxedema coma
b. Thyroid storm
c. Hyperaldosteronism
d. Adrenal insufficiency
e. Diabetic ketoacidosis (DKA)

469. A 44-year-old agitated woman is brought to the ED by her husband. He states that she has had fevers to 101°F and a productive cough at home for the last 3 days. Today she became labile, agitated, and complained of abdominal pain. She was recently diagnosed with Graves' disease and started on PTU. Her BP is 156/87 mm Hg, HR is 145 beats per minute, temperature is 102.4°F, and RR is 20 breaths per minute. On exam, the patient is agitated, confused, and has rales on auscultation bilaterally. Which of the following is the most likely diagnosis?

a. Pheochromocytoma
b. Cocaine ingestion
c. Heat stroke
d. Thyroid storm
e. Neuroleptic malignant syndrome

Endocrine Emergencies

Answers

459. The answer is d. (*Rosen, pp 1750–1754.*) The mainstay of treatment for *DKA* is *aggressive fluid resuscitation* and *insulin* therapy. The patient should receive 2 L of normal saline within 2 hours of presentation followed by 4–6 L over the next 8–12 hours depending on the patient's fluid status. In DKA, the average adult has a water deficit of 5–10 L. After fluid administration, regular insulin is administered usually first as a 10 unit bolus intravenously and then at a rate of 0.1 unit/kg/h. Insulin must be administered for ketosis and acidosis to resolve.

(**a**) Intramuscular and subcutaneous insulin administration is avoided in DKA as absorption may be erratic secondary to volume depletion and poor perfusion. (**b**) Currently, no study shows a benefit of using bicarbonate in DKA. Bicarbonate administration can cause worsening hypokalemia, paradoxical CNS acidosis, impaired oxyhemoglobin dissociation, hypertonicity, and sodium over load. (**c**) Metoprolol, a β-blocker, is not indicated in DKA. The tachycardia in DKA is secondary to volume depletion and acidosis. Correcting the underlying cause will treat the tachycardia. (**e**) Potassium replacement may be necessary later in therapy due to an overall loss of potassium, but should not be included in the initial fluid boluses. Rapid administration of potassium has potential to precipitate fatal dysrhythmias.

460. The answer is d. (*Rosen, pp 1770–1774.*) *Thyroid storm* is a *medical emergency* that will lead to death if not treated in time. The manifestations of thyroid storm include temperature greater than 100°F, tachycardia out of proportion to fever, widened pulse pressure, and dysfunction of the CNS (e.g., confusion, agitation), cardiovascular system (e.g., high-output congestive heart failure, atrial fibrillation), or gastrointestinal (GI) system (e.g., diarrhea, abdominal pain). Thyroid storm is a *clinical diagnosis* since no confirmatory tests are immediately available. The most important factor in reducing mortality is blocking peripheral adrenergic hyperactivity with *propranolol*, a β-blocker. *PTU* is used to inhibit new hormone synthesis in the thyroid and has a small effect on inhibiting peripheral conversion of T_4 to T_3. *Iodine* is administered to block hormone release from the thyroid but should be given 1 hour after PTU to prevent organification of the iodine.

(a) Tricyclic antidepressant overdose can present with altered mental status and tachycardia. Bicarbonate is administered for a widened QRS on ECG. (b) Chlordiazepoxide is given to patients to prevent alcohol withdrawal, which can also present with confusion and tachycardia. (c) Ceftriaxone is commonly used to treat meningitis, which can present with confusion, tachycardia, and fever. (e) The patient's diarrhea is not due to an infectious etiology and therefore ciprofloxacin is not required. She may require fluid resuscitation, but for now her BP is stable.

461. The answer is b. *(Rosen, pp 1774–1778.) Myxedema coma* is a syndrome that represents *extreme hypothyroidism*. It is a life-threatening condition that has a mortality of up to 50%. Signs and symptoms of hypothyroidism are usually present including dry skin, delayed deep tendon reflexes, coarse hair, and generalized nonpitting edema. Myxedema coma, however, is better characterized by profound *lethargy or coma* and *hypothermia*. Hypothermia is present in approximately 80% of patients. In addition, patients may present with respiratory depression and sinus bradycardia.

(a) Apathetic thyrotoxicosis is an atypical presentation of hyperthyroidism seen commonly in the elderly but noted in all ages. Signs and symptoms are few and subtle. Patients usually have multinodular goiter. The diagnosis should be considered in elderly patients with chronic weight loss, proximal muscle weakness, depressed affect, new-onset atrial fibrillation, or congestive heart failure. (c) Graves' disease is secondary to autoimmune stimulation of thyrotropin (TSH) receptors leading to elevated levels of thyroid hormones. (d) An acute stroke should not cause periorbital edema and hypothermia. (e) Schizophrenia may be mistakenly diagnosed in patients with thyroid abnormalities. It is not a correct diagnosis in this scenario when the patient is unconscious and hypothermic.

462. The answer is a. *(Rosen, pp 1755–1757.) Hyperglycemic hyperosmolar nonketotic coma (HHNC)* is a syndrome representing marked *hyperglycemia* (serum glucose > 600 mg/dL), *hyperosmolarity* (plasma osmolarity >350 mOsm/L), considerable *dehydration* (9 L in 70-kg patient), and *decreased mental functioning* that may progress to coma. HHNC may be the initial presentation of previously unrecognized diabetes in an adult with *type 2 diabetes mellitus (DM)*. Elderly diabetics are at greater risk for this illness. Osmotic diuresis is even more pronounced than in DKA. Rapid correction of hyperosmolar state may lead to cerebral edema. Unlike DKA, acidosis and ketosis are usually absent or minimal. The mainstay to treatment is fluid resuscitation, insulin administration, electrolyte repletion, and searching for an underlying precipitant.

(**b**) Phenytoin is contraindicated for seizures in HHNC because it is often ineffective and may impair endogenous insulin release. (**c**) Fluid resuscitation is the mainstay of treatment and should always be administered prior to insulin. (**d**) Although the patient may ultimately receive a CT scan, fluid resuscitation is priority due to the profound dehydration in these patients. (**e**) If a patient has functioning kidneys, hemodialysis is not necessary. However, if the patient has end-stage renal disease, then hemodialysis may be necessary to treat over hydration.

463. The answer is c. (*Rosen, pp 1750–1754.*) The triad of *hyperglycemia, ketosis,* and *acidosis* is diagnostic for *DKA.* All abnormalities in DKA are connected and are based on insulin deficiency. When hyperglycemia surpasses the renal threshold for resorption, glucose is excreted in the urine. This causes an osmotic diuresis which in combination with decreased oral intake and vomiting leads to dehydration and electrolyte abnormalities. Cells, unable to receive glucose from the circulation, switch to starvation mode by increasing proteolysis. The liver starts producing ketoacids subsequently causing acidemia. The acidotic patient increases RR in an attempt to blow-off excess CO_2 and bicarbonate is used up in the process.

(**a**) Hypotension, tachycardia, and tachypnea are commonly seen in DKA but are not specific for the condition. (**b**) Leukocytosis is seen in many other conditions other than DKA. (**d**) Although a fruity odor to breath may suggest acetone, a product of ketone production, it is not reliably present and difficult to distinguish. (**e**) Glucosuria is present with hyperglycemia. Ketones are required for DKA.

464. The answer is a. (*Tintinalli, p 1287.*) You should be suspicious for *DKA* as the initial presentation of DM in this patient. Glucose levels are elevated, typically greater than 200 mg/dL. DKA is an acute, life-threatening disorder occurring in patients with *insulin insufficiency* (more common in type 1 diabetes) and results in *hyperglycemia, ketosis, and acidosis* from osmotic diuresis leading to dehydration and acidosis. This patient exhibits classic signs and symptoms of DKA, such as tachycardia, GI distress, polyuria, polydipsia, fatigue, and confusion. Very deep breathing (*Kussmaul's respirations*) reflects respiratory compensation for metabolic acidosis. *Fruity breath odor* in this patient is the result of acetoacetate acid conversion to acetone, which is eliminated during respiration.

Administering antiemetics and analgesics (**b and c**) will temporarily treat the symptoms without addressing the underlying problem. A basic metabolic panel (**d**) is necessary to check for electrolyte abnormalities. Abdominal radiographs (**e**) might be appropriate if you suspect abdominal pathology. In this case, GI distress is a symptom of a metabolic disturbance.

465. The answer is c. *(Tintinalli, p 1291.) Potassium* is the most important electrolyte to follow in DKA therapy. Renal losses and vomiting in DKA cause profound *total body potassium deficit.* The measured potassium levels, however, are often *falsely normal or elevated* due to acidosis and total body fluid deficit. Acidemia causes extracellular shift of potassium in exchange for hydrogen ions. With initiation of DKA therapy, potassium levels will quickly fall to true levels causing *significant hypokalemia,* if not closely monitored and replaced.

Although sodium and calcium levels (**a, b, d and e**) should be monitored, they are not affected as much as potassium. Hyperglycemia-related osmotic diuresis leads to renal losses of sodium chloride in urine. The measured sodium level is artificially lowered further by the hyperglycemia. For every 100 mg of glucose over 100 mg/dL, 1.6 mEq should be added to the measured serum sodium level. In treating DKA, normal saline infusion replaces lost sodium. Hypertonic saline should not be used for sodium replacement in DKA. Osmotic diuresis also causes renal losses of calcium, magnesium, and phosphorus. Initially their levels might be elevated due to hemoconcentration. These electrolytes should be monitored and restored appropriately during treatment.

466. The answer is e. *(Tintinalli, p 1312.)* This patient presents in a *hyperadrenergic state, altered mental status, and a large goiter,* placing the diagnosis of *thyroid storm* on top of the differential. The patient is likely to have undiagnosed hyperthyroidism. This is a clinical diagnosis and has to be treated empirically and rapidly since mortality is high despite treatment. The management of thyroid storm involves supportive care (airway protection, oxygenation, IV hydration) and specific therapy to treat adrenergic symptoms and to decrease synthesis and release of thyroid hormone. *β-Adrenergic blockers* are given to reverse adrenergic hyperactivity. *PTU* blocks de novo synthesis of thyroid hormone. *Iodine* blocks release of the preformed hormone but can be given only after PTU has taken effect otherwise it will promote further hormone production.

Dantrolene (**a**) is used in the management of malignant hyperthermia and neuroleptic malignant syndrome. Administering acetaminophen and

broad coverage antibiotics (**b**) or diazepam (**e**) will not address the underlying etiology of the patient's illness. Iodine (**c**) should not be administered
prior to PTU.

467. The answer is e. (*Tintinalli, pp 169, 171, 1284, 1287, 1307.*) *Hypokalemia*
presents with *muscle weakness* and characteristic *ECG changes*, such as flat
T waves and U waves, and is not associated with seizures or altered mental
status.

Glucose level can be rapidly obtained from a fingerstick glucose check.
Hypoglycemia (**a**) is a known reversibly cause of seizures and is corrected
with administration of dextrose. Significant hyperglycemia (**b**) occurs in
DKA (glucose usually is 200–800 mg/dL) or nonketotic hyperosmolar crisis
(glucose usually is more than 800 mg/dL) and is treated with IV fluids and
insulin. Hyper and hyponatremia are known causes of seizures.

468. The answer is d. (*Rosen, pp 1779–1782.*) *Adrenal cortical insufficiency*
is an uncommon, potentially life-threatening condition that if recognized
early, is readily treatable. The most common cause of adrenal insufficiency
is hypothalamic-pituitary-adrenal axis suppression from *long-term exogenous glucocorticoid administration*. This patient abruptly stopped her high-
dose steroids. The clinical presentation of adrenal insufficiency is vague but
typically includes weakness, fatigue, nausea, vomiting, *hypotension,* and
hypoglycemia. Electrolyte abnormalities are common. *Hyponatremia* and
hyperkalemia are present in more than two-thirds of cases. Management
includes supportive care with administration of glucocorticoids and electrolyte correction.

(**a and b**) Myxedema coma is a syndrome of extreme hypothyroidism,
whereas thyroid storm is extreme hyperthyroidism. (**c**) Hyperaldosteronism is characterized by hypertension and hypokalemia. (**e**) DKA typically
presents with elevated glucose, an anion-gap metabolic acidosis, and
ketone production.

469. The answer is d. (*Tintinalli, p 1312.*) This patient presents with a
rare but life-threatening hypermetabolic state of *thyroid storm*. It occurs in
patients with known or undiagnosed hyperthyroidism and is usually triggered by infection, trauma, myocardial infarction, stroke, or noncompliance
with antihyperthyroid medications. Thyroid storm is a clinical diagnosis.
The signs and symptoms of this disorder reflect an overactive sympathetic
system and include fever, tachycardia out of the proportion to the fever, GI
symptoms, and altered mental status. Patients may also develop high-output

heart failure. The clue to the diagnosis in this case is the patient's known hyperthyroidism.

Pheochromocytoma (a) presents with a similar hyperadrenergic state due to a catecholamine-secreting tumor but does not result in altered mentation. The hallmark of this disease is hypertension associated with headache, palpitations, and diaphoresis. Cocaine (b) acts as a CNS stimulant by blocking reuptake of excitatory neurotransmitters norepinephrine, dopamine, and serotonin. It is, however, less likely than thyroid storm in this patient given her underlying hyperthyroidism and pulmonary infection. Heat stroke (c) should be suspected in patients with core body temperature > 40°C (104°F) and altered mental status. Neuroleptic malignant syndrome (e) is a rare life-threatening reaction to a medication with dopamine receptor antagonism. Such medications include neuroleptics such as haloperidol, clozapine, and risperidone, lithium and many antiemetics such as prochlorperazine, promethazine, and metoclopramide. The syndrome presents as fever, altered mental status, and muscular rigidity.

Psychosocial Disorders

Questions

470. A 31-year-old woman presents to the emergency department (ED) 20 minutes after the sudden onset of chest pain, palpitations, shortness of breath, and numbness of her mouth, fingers, and toes. She tells you that it feels like she has a lump in her throat. Her medical history includes multiple visits to the ED over a period of 6 months with a similar presentation. Her only medication is an oral contraceptive. She occasionally drinks a glass of wine after a busy day of work when she feels stressed. She tells you that her mom takes medication for anxiety. Her blood pressure (BP) is 125/75 mm Hg, heart rate (HR) 88 beats per minute, and O_2 saturation 99% on room air. An electrocardiogram (ECG) shows a sinus rhythm. Her symptoms resolve while in the ED. Which of the following is the most likely diagnosis?

a. Paroxysmal atrial tachycardia
b. Hyperthyroidism
c. Major depressive disorder
d. Panic disorder
e. Posttraumatic stress disorder

471. A 23-year-old woman is brought to the ED for vision loss in her left eye that began shortly after waking up in the morning. She states that she is very depressed since her father was diagnosed with terminal cancer. She was supposed to visit her father today in the hospital but is now in your ED because of her vision loss. Your physical exam is unremarkable. An evaluation by the ophthalmologist is also normal. A head computed tomography (CT) scan is normal. Which of the following is the most likely diagnosis?

a. Somatization disorder
b. Conversion disorder
c. Hypochondriasis
d. Retinal detachment
e. Anxiety disorder

472. Which of the following clinical presentations requires hospitalization?

a. A 37-year-old man with paranoid schizophrenia who has been off his medications for a week and is hearing voices with no apparent violence in his thought content
b. A 19-year-old woman who ingested 10 multivitamin pills after an argument with her boyfriend
c. A 39-year-old man with no previous psychiatric history presents with pressured speech, no sleep for 4 days, and is feeling "great"
d. A 22-year-old woman who is having visual hallucinations after ingesting d-lysergic acid diethylamide (LSD)
e. A 43-year-old homeless man with a history of schizophrenia who was recently discharged from the psychiatric ward being managed on antipsychotic medications

473. A 35-year-old woman is eating dinner at a restaurant. Approximately 1 hour after finishing the main course of lamb, red wine, and a fine selection of cheese, the patient experiences a severe occipital headache, diaphoresis, mydriasis, neck stiffness, and palpitations. Which of the following medications is this patient most likely taking?

a. Paroxetine
b. Alprazolam
c. Tranylcypromine
d. Citalopram
e. Amitriptyline

474. You walk into the examining room to interview a patient. He refused giving vital signs at the triage station until he saw a doctor because he was afraid that the nurse would inject poison into him. He appears agitated and starts raising his voice as soon as you are in the room. You ask him in a calm voice if you could help him and he replies by shouting obscenities and throwing a box of gloves at you. You start to walk towards him but he says he will kill you if you get any closer. Which of the following is the most appropriate next step in management?

a. Tell the patient he is being uncooperative and is to leave the ED immediately
b. Have the nurse go into the room alone to try to calm the patient
c. Let the patient sit in the room for another hour and see if he calms down
d. Ask the nurse to prepare an injection of lorazepam that you will give to sedate the patient
e. Alert hospital security that there is a violent patient and prepare to place the patient in physical restraints

475. A 42-year-old man with a history of schizophrenia is brought into the ED by a friend who states that the patient has not taken his medication for over 2 weeks and is now behaving bizarrely. His BP is 130/70 mm Hg, HR 89 beats per minute, respiratory rate (RR) 15 breaths per minute, and O_2 saturation 99% on room air. On exam he appears agitated and is shouting, "the aliens are about to get me." He is cooperative enough that you decide to use pharmacologic sedation. Which of the following is the most appropriate choice for sedating this patient?

a. Haloperidol and lorazepam
b. Etomidate and succinylcholine
c. Chlorpromazine and lorazepam
d. Ketamine and lorazepam
e. Clozapine

476. A 48-year-old man is brought to the ED by family members who state that the patient has remained home-bound for weeks, sleeping for many hours, and appears disheveled. The patient states that he is "fine" and denies any medical symptoms. Initial vitals include a HR of 77 beats per minute, a BP of 118/55 mm Hg, and a RR of 12 breaths per minute with an O_2 saturation of 97% on room air. The patient is afebrile with an unremarkable physical examination. He denies any chest discomfort, difficulty breathing, constipation, cold intolerance, weakness, weight changes, or pain. The patient reports that he has had difficulty concentrating, a decreased appetite, and excessive sleeping patterns. The family reports that this has happened before, but that his symptoms self-resolved and were not nearly as severe. Given this patient's presentation, which of the following is the most likely etiology of this patient's symptoms?

a. Hypothyroidism
b. Major depressive episode
c. Diabetes mellitus
d. Subdural hematoma
e. Cushing's syndrome

477. A 32-year-old woman presents to the ED after an aggressive outburst at work where her behavior was deemed a threat to others. Her coworkers state that she is normally very dependable, kind, and gracious but that over the course of the week they noticed that she was especially reserved and at times found her conversing with herself. Her initial vitals include a HR of 89 beats per minute, a RR of 15 breaths per minute, and a BP of 130/75 mm Hg with an O_2 saturation of 99% on room air. She tells you that she was recently started on a new medication. Which of the following types of medications may be responsible for this patient's behavior?

a. β-Blockers
b. Oral contraceptives
c. Corticosteroids
d. Nonsteroidal anti-inflammatory drugs (NSAIDs)
e. Calcium-channel blockers

478. A 23-year-old woman is brought to the ED by police officials who state that they found the patient in the middle of a busy intersection screaming. Upon arrival, you see a disheveled woman who is yelling, "You can't get away with this! I'm the Queen of England!" She does not allow for the triage nurse to obtain her vitals, but you can see a young woman who is of normal habitus without any signs of trauma. Her speech is pressured, she is easily distracted by the commotion of the ED and begins to answer your questions but then continues to describe grandiose ideas about her social status. Given this patient's acute presentation, what is the most likely etiology of her symptoms?

a. Hypothyroid disorder
b. Manic episode
c. Benzodiazepine overdose
d. Anticonvulsant overdose
e. Barbiturate overdose

479. A mother brings her 7-year-old daughter to the ED with a reported illness of 3 days where the child has been weak and not eating her usual amount. The mother also reports that she noticed her daughter's urine to be of a reddish color and that her stools have been smaller in caliber. She brings a specimen of her daughter's urine with her. She reports that her daughter has been hospitalized multiple times before for similar reasons and dehydration. Upon physical examination, the patient is without distress, quiet, and states that she feels tired. Her chest is clear to auscultation, her abdomen is benign and her neurological exam nonfocal. A urinalysis performed fails to show any blood or myoglobin in the child's urine. Which of the following should be included in the differential diagnosis of this child?

a. Malingering
b. Factitious disorder
c. Munchausen's syndrome
d. Munchausen's syndrome by proxy
e. Conversion disorder

480. A 42-year-old woman presents to the ED with acute paralysis of her left lower extremity. She denies any trauma, past medical or surgical history. She denies any medication or illicit drug use. Upon physical examination, she denies sensation in a nondermatomal pattern, has intact pulses bilaterally and no signs of trauma. Upon asking the patient to move her legs, she moves the right extremity while unknowingly stabilizing balance with her left. Which of the following conditions may be responsible for the presentation of this patient?

a. Malingering
b. Factitious disorder
c. Munchausen's syndrome
d. Munchausen's syndrome by proxy
e. Conversion disorder

481. A 62-year-old man presents to the ED after he was found talking to himself by witnesses on a nearby street. Upon arrival, the patient appears confused and is actively hallucinating. His initial vitals include an irregular HR of 80–110 beats per minute, a RR of 14 breaths per minute, a BP of 160/80 mm Hg with a O_2 saturation of 97% on room air. An ECG indicates atrial fibrillation. The patient can be redirected but states that he is distracted by colorful, floating images in the room. Given this patient's presentation, what is the most likely etiology of his symptoms?

a. Acute psychotic disorder
b. Malingering
c. Conversion disorder
d. Digoxin overdose
e. Antidepressant overdose

482. An 18-year-old man presents to the ED after telling a school counselor that he wanted to harm himself. His physical examination is unremarkable without any signs of trauma. He reports occasional excessive alcohol use. He states that his parents recently separated and that he has been living with either parent on a rotating schedule. Overall, he feels supported by family and friends but continues to feel hopeless despite this. Which of the following factors in this patient is most likely to increase his risk of an actual suicidal attempt?

a. Sex
b. Age
c. Hopelessness
d. Alcohol use
e. Parent separation

483. A thin 16-year-old girl is brought in the ED after collapsing at home. Her initial vitals include a HR of 110 beats per minute, BP of 80/55 mm Hg, and a RR of 18 breaths per minute with an O_2 saturation of 98% on room air. Upon physical examination, you note a cachectic female in mild distress. Her chest is clear to auscultation; her sunken-in abdomen is soft and nontender. Upon inspecting her extremities, you notice small areas of erythema over the dorsum of her right hand distally. Given this patient's presentation and physical examination, which of the following etiologies must be further explored in this patient?

a. Bulimia
b. Gastroenteritis
c. Malingering
d. Factitious disorder
e. Suicidality

484. A 55-year-old woman presents to the ED after a reported syncopal event. Her initial vitals include a HR of 105 beats per minute, a RR of 16 breaths per minute, a BP of 125/60 mm Hg, and an O_2 saturation of 98% on room air. Her ECG is shown on the next page. Which of the following substances is responsible for this patient's ECG findings?

Referred by: Unco

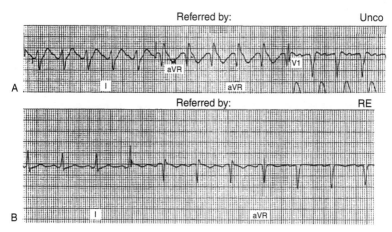

Referred by: RE

(Reproduced, with permission, from Tintinalli J, Kelen G, and Stapczynski J. Emergency Medicine A Comprehensive Study Guide. New York, NY: McGraw-Hill, 2004: 1031.)

a. Benzodiazepine
b. Alcohol
c. Tricyclic antidepressant
d. Insulin
e. Valproic acid

485. A 28-year-old presents to the ED with depressive symptoms and feelings of hopelessness. She denies any active suicidal ideation, but has had increasing feelings of guilt over the last few weeks. The patient denies any past medical history except for giving birth 8 weeks ago. Her initial vitals are within normal limits. Given this patient's presentation, which of the following etiologies is most likely?

a. Dysthymic disorder
b. Bipolar disorder
c. Postpartum depression
d. Major depressive disorder
e. Cyclothymic disorder

Psychosocial Disorders

Answers

470. The answer is d. (*Tintinalli, pp 1826–1827.*) A person with *panic attacks* will often present to multiple EDs and be discharged after a workup is normal. A panic attack is a discrete period of intense fear or discomfort in which four or more of the following symptoms develop acutely and peak within 10 minutes: accelerated HR, palpitations, pounding heart, diaphoresis, trembling or shaking, sensation of shortness of breath or a choking feeling, chest pain, nausea, dizziness, lightheadedness, parethesias, fear of dying, chills, or hot flushes.

(**a**) Paroxysmal atrial tachycardia is a conduction defect of the heart characterized by random episodes of tachycardia. This disorder is seen on an ECG. The above patient's ECG is normal. (**b**) Hyperthyroidism can mimic a panic attack, but there is usually greater autonomic hyperactivity. In addition, thyroid hormone levels are increased. (**c**) There are no symptoms of depression described in the patient's presentation. Nonetheless, panic attacks can occur with major depressive disorder. (**e**) The diagnosis of posttraumatic stress disorder cannot be made with the patient's history.

471. The answer is b. (*Tintinalli, pp 1830–1831.*) The diagnosis of *conversion disorder* is made by fulfilling the following five criteria:

- A symptom is expressed as a change or loss of physical function
- Recent psychological stressor or conflict
- The patient unconsciously produces the symptom
- The symptom cannot be explained by any known organic etiology
- The symptom is not limited to pain or sexual dysfunction

Conversions disorders generally involve neurologic or orthopedic manifestations. The disorder usually presents as a *single symptom* with a *sudden onset* related to a *severe stress.* In this case, the stress is the diagnosis of terminal cancer in the patient's father. Classic symptoms of conversion disorder include paralysis, aphonia, seizures, coordination disturbances, blindness, tunnel vision, and numbness. The diagnosis cannot be made until all possible organic etiologies are ruled out. Treatment involves identifying the stressor and addressing the issue.

(a) Somatization disorder involves patients with many complaints with no organic cause. (c) Hypochondriasis involves the preoccupation of serious illness despite appropriate medical evaluation and reassurance. (d) Retinal detachment can cause unilateral vision loss and generally presents with progressively worsening vision loss with patients complaining of "floaters." (e) Anxiety disorders involve excessive fear and apprehension that dominates the psychological life of a person.

472. The answer is c. (*Tintinalli, p 1810.*) This patient presents with a first manic episode. It is necessary to admit these patients in order to prevent behavior that is impulsive and dangerous. A full manic syndrome is one of the most striking and distinctive conditions in clinical practice. The main disturbance in mood is one of elation or irritability.

(a) This man is not a threat to him or others and can be treated as an outpatient. (b) This is a suicidal gesture and the patient should be evaluated by a psychiatrist. She may be able to be managed as an outpatient if reliable family and social support systems are in place and appropriate psychiatric follow-up is arranged. (d) This patient can be safely discharged once her visual hallucinations resolve. (e) This man is appropriately treated.

473. The answer is c. (*Tintinalli, p 1041.*) *Tranylcypromine is a monoamine oxidase inhibitor (MAOI)* that is used in the treatment of depression. Patients who take this medication should avoid eating or drinking foods that contain *tyramine* (similar structure to amphetamine). Tyramine is found in many foods such as aged cheese, wine, certain fish, meats, and sauerkraut. The combination of a MAOI and tyramine can lead to a *sympathomimetic reaction* called a *tyramine reaction.* It occurs within 15–90 minutes of ingestion of tyramine. The hallmark symptoms include headache, hypertension, diaphoresis, mydriasis, neck stiffness, pallor, neuromuscular excitation, palpitations, and chest pain. Most symptoms gradually resolve over 6 hours; however deaths have been reported secondary to intracranial hemorrhage and myocardial infarction. Patients who take a MAOI should be instructed to avoid all tyramine-containing foods.

All of the other answer choices do not cause a tyramine reaction—it is limited only to MAOIs. (a and d) are a serotonin reuptake inhibitors, (b) is a benzodiazepine, (e) is a tricyclic antidepressant.

474. The answer is e. (*Tintinalli, p 1812.*) *Violent behavior requires immediate restraint.* Hospital security and the police are best trained to subdue violent patients with the least chance of staff or patient injury. Patients who are threatening or who demonstrate violent behavior should be disrobed, gowned, and searched for weapons. Patients whose behavior suggests the potential for violence should be approached cautiously with adequate security force nearby. The physician should stand in a location that neither threatens the patient nor blocks the exit of the patient or the physician from the room. Physical restraints are frequently required for the violent or severely agitated psychotic, delirious, or intoxicated patient who is a danger to themselves or others. Pharmacologic restraints (haloperidol, lorazepam) are also useful in obtaining behavior control and should be considered once the initial evaluation has been completed.

(a) The patient should not be allowed to leave the hospital prior to a medical and psychiatric evaluation. (b) No staff member should be alone with a patient who is violent or threatens violence. (c) Although using calming techniques are useful to assuage many patients, it is important not to delay the medical evaluation and prolong detection of a life-threatening process. (d) Giving the patient a sedating medication is useful however you should try to first medically evaluate the patient. In addition, you should not enter the patient's room alone with a needle in your hand.

475. The answer is a. (*Tintinalli, pp 1816–1817.*) Rapid tranquilization is a method of pharmacologic management of acute agitation or psychosis using high-potency neuroleptics and benzodiazepines. The most common regimen used is the combination of *haloperidol* and *lorazepam,* which can be administered via parenteral, intramuscular, or oral routes. There is a synergistic effect between the two medications. Moreover, the benzodiazepine may prevent the potential extrapyramidal affects that occasionally occur with neuroleptic use.

(b) Etomidate and succinylcholine are used for rapid sequence intubation, which is not indicated in this patient. (c) Chlorpromazine is a low-potency antipsychotic that may cause significant hypotension and is rarely used in the ED setting. (d) Ketamine is a dissociative agent that is not typically used in psychotic patients. (e) Clozapine is an atypical antipsychotic that is used in schizophrenics when other neuroleptics are ineffective. It is not an agent of choice for acute sedation or psychosis.

476. The answer is b. (*Rosen, pp 1549–1583.*) A *major depressive episode* is characterized by two or more of the following symptoms over a 2 week period: loss of interest in usual activities, depressed or irritable mood, changes in weight or appetite, insomnia or hypersomnia, psychomotor agitation or retardation, loss of energy, difficulty concentrating, recurrent thoughts of death, and suicidal ideation. This particular patient has three of these symptoms, including excessive sleeping patterns, difficulty concentrating, and a decreased appetite. The danger is that the patient's feelings may be so intensely painful that suicide may be seen as the only way to cope. Some patients may also complain of generalized physical pain, without any clear medical diagnosis able to be made. The cardinal symptom of depression is a *sad or dysphoric mood*.

Hypothyroidism (**a**) and Cushing's syndrome (**e**) may also be exhibited in patients that appear to be depressed. A simple thyroid stimulating hormone and cortisol level may be drawn to differentiate a medical etiology for these symptoms. Hyperthyroidism also presents as generalized sluggishness, difficulty concentrating, constipation, cold intolerance, hair loss of the distal one-third of both eyebrows, dysphagia, and myalgias. Fingerstick glucose should also be performed to evaluate for diabetes mellitus (**c**), which may present as sluggishness, paresthesias, and general malaise. It is also important to keep in mind traumatic causes to this patient's symptoms, given that he lives alone without witnesses to report a fall that may result in a subdural hematoma (**d**). Intracerebral bleeding may present with sluggishness, especially in subdurals where there is a relatively slower bleed of the bridging veins.

477. The answer is c. (*Rosen, pp 1549–1583.*) *Steroid psychosis* is described as a constellation of psychiatric symptoms within the first 5 days of treatment with a corticosteroid. Studies indicate that the amount needed to produce this effect is greater than 40 mg of prednisone, or its equivalent, prescribed daily. Symptoms include emotional lability, anxiety, distractibility, pressured speech, sensory flooding, insomnia, depression, agitation, auditory and visual hallucinations, intermittent memory impairment, mutism, disturbances of body image, and delusions and hypomania. It is important to note that previous history of psychological difficulties does not predict the development of steroid psychosis. Symptoms can be very severe and should be taken into account when prescribing this medication to patients. Three percent of patients with steroid psychosis commit suicide.

The most common side effect of β-blockers (**a**) is a depressed mood, due to its sympatholytic effects, however these are generally mild and do not require treatment. Oral contraceptives (**b**), although hormonal in nature, are not thought to produce psychiatric symptoms. Calcium-channel blockers (**e**) and NSAIDs (**d**) have not shown to cause psychosis.

478. The answer is b. (*Rosen, pp 1549–1583.*) This is a typical *manic episode* of which an elevated mood, grandiosity, flight of ideas, distractibility, and psychomotor agitation are its cardinal features. Other medical conditions such as hyperthyroidism, antidepressant, or stimulant abuse may cause similar symptoms and must be ruled out with laboratory testing. Certain frontal lobe release syndromes that impair executive functioning must also be investigated as a cause of this patient's symptoms. These patients are usually combative, display impaired judgment and impulsivity and may need to be chemically or physically restrained.

Hypothyroid disorder (**a**), benzodiazepines (**c**), anticonvulsants (**d**), and barbiturates (**e**) may all cause depressive symptoms.

479. The answer is d. (*Rosen, pp 1549–1583.*) Given that this is an apparent illness or health-related abnormality produced by a parent or caregiver upon another, the *by proxy* title is given. This is a psychiatric illness defined by the Diagnostic and Statistical Manual of Mental Disorders (DSM-IV) as an apparent illness concocted by a caregiver upon a child who presents for medical aid multiple times without ever being given a true diagnosis. There is a failure by the perpetrator to acknowledge the true etiology and a cessation of symptoms in the child once they are separated from the perpetrator. Simulated illness, without producing direct harm upon the child, is commonly seen. As seen in this example, placing tincture in the child's urine to mimic blood. Sadly, produced illness in which the child is harmed is most commonly seen (50% of cases). The most common presentations include bleeding, seizures, vomiting, diarrhea, fever, and rash. Ninety-eight percent of perpetrators are biological mothers from all socioeconomic backgrounds. Many have a background in health professions or have features of *Munchausen's syndrome* in themselves. Most of these mothers have had an abusive experience early in life and use the health care system as a means to satisfy personal nurturing demands. They are said to gain a sense of purpose and meaning when their child is in the hospital, as well as an outlet for pity and comfort. These children may display incidental characteristics that cannot be linked to the presenting complaints. These children may also suffer from learning difficulties or clinical depression due to many hospitalizations that are incurred upon them.

Malingering (**a**) is frequently found in connection with antisocial personality disorder. These patients are often vague about prior hospitalizations or treatments. In contrast to those with a factitious disorder (**b**), these patients prefer to counterfeit mental illness given the difficulty in objectively verifying or disproving the etiology of the patient's reported symptoms. Amnesia, paranoia, depression, and suicidal ideation are commonly seen. The idea of an external gain motivates these individuals to fabricate medical symptoms. Conversely, factitious disorders are characterized by symptoms or signs that are intentionally produced or feigned by the patient in the absence of external incentives. Munchausen's syndrome **(c)** is one of the most dramatic of the factitious disorders. Its name is derived from a Baron Karl F. von Munchausen who amused his friends with fantastic and incredible tales about his personal life. Conversion disorder **(e)** is a rare disorder that is characterized by the abrupt, dramatic onset of a single symptom. It typically presents as some nonpainful neurologic disorder for which there is no objective data for.

480. The answer is e. (*Rosen, pp 1549–1583.*) *Conversion disorder,* also known as *hysterical neurosis,* is a rare disorder that is characterized by the abrupt, dramatic onset of a single symptom. It typically presents as some nonpainful neurologic disorder for which there is no objective data for. It is also not under the patient's voluntary control and results from an underlying need for attention or comfort. The most common presentations to the ED include *pseudoneurologic* symptoms which may include pseudoseizures, syncope, coma, or paralysis. Most patients are women of lower socioeconomic status. Symptoms are acute, but may wax and wane in response to stressors in the person's life. The history may show similar symptoms in the past and psychiatric illness in up to 30% of patients. Patients generally describe their symptoms with a lack of appropriate concern (la belle indifference).

481. The answer is d. (*Rosen, pp 1549–1583.*) This patient is experiencing a *visual hallucination,* most typical of a medical rather than psychiatric etiology. *Digoxin* is a common precipitant of these symptoms and may begin with yellow-blue changes in vision, known as Van Gogh vision. Digoxin directly binds the Na-K ATPase which increases sodium and calcium levels, increasing the contractility of the heart. Hallucinations are often an early symptom of digoxin overdose. Treatment for this includes a protein fragment that binds this medication.

(a) Auditory hallucinations are usually seen in psychiatric illness or an acute psychotic episode. Antidepressants **(e)** typically do not produce changes in vision or hallucinations. His symptoms are also not typical of malingering **(b)**, given that he was not brought in of his own accord without secondary gain, or of conversion disorder **(c)**.

482. The answer is c. (*Rosen, pp 1549–1583.*) In the psychiatric literature, there exists a "SADPERSONS" scale that enumerates risk factors. Two points are given for factors that are considered higher risk. These include depression or *hopelessness,* rational thinking loss, organized or serious attempt, and stated future intent. Lower risk factors, given one point, are male sex, age < 19 or > 45, previous attempts or psychiatric care, excessive alcohol or drug use, separation, divorce or widowed status, and no social supports. Firearms in the household, family violence, abuse, and chronic illness also increase risk.

Sex (male)	1
Age (< 19 or > 45)	1
Depression or hopelessness	2
Previous attempts/ psychiatric care	1
Excessive alcohol or drug use	1
Rational thinking loss	2
Separated, divorced, or widowed	1
Organized or serious attempt	2
No social support	1
Stated future attempt	2

483. The answer is a. *(Rosen, pp 1549–1583.)* The physical examination in this patient reveals hand abrasions, indicative of self-purging. Her general appearance suggests either inadequate food intake or excessive calorie burning. *Bulimics* generally consume an adequate amount of food, albeit low-calorie, but purge their intake with the goal of weight loss. Other eating disorders, such anorexia nervosa, can take the form of starvation, diuretic or laxative use, or excessive exercise. These patients generally suffer from a false visualization of their body, believing that their physical form weighs more than what it does in reality. Social pressures, history of abuse or violence, and other eating disorders may factor in to this patient's presentation.

Gastroenteritis (**b**) is unlikely given the lack of history or symptoms. Suicidality (**e**) should be examined in all patients, as their actions may represent a form of occult or hidden self-harm. This patient does not exhibit signs of malingering (**c**) or factitious disorder (**d**).

484. The answer is c. *(Rosen, pp 1549–1583.)* *Tricyclic antidepressants (TCAs)* are responsible for more drug-related deaths than any other prescription medication. This ECG shows QRS interval prolongation, a common finding with this medication. The mechanism of toxicity is multifold and includes blocking the reuptake of dopamine, serotonin, and norepinephrine.

It also binds to the GABA receptor, thereby lowering seizure threshold. Sodium-channel blockade produces the widened QRS interval. There are also anticholinergic and antihistamine effects. Sodium bicarbonate is a first line intervention for dysrhythmias, acting as alkalizing binder for the acidic TCA. This treatment has been shown to improve conduction and contractility with the goal of preserving a narrow QRS.

Benzodiazepines (**a**), ethanol (**b**), insulin (**d**) and valproic acid have not been shown to exhibit any ECG abnormalities.

485. The answer is c. (*Rosen, pp 1549–1583.*) This patient recently gave birth and presents with symptoms of hopelessness and guilt in the subsequent weeks, typical of symptoms seen in this postpartum period. Over half of mothers report depressed mood after childbirth, also known as the "baby blues." This may be linked to rapid decreases in estrogen and progesterone immediately after childbirth. About 40% mothers reports that these symptoms last a few days with about half of those having continuing symptoms into weeks. About 2% express suicidal ideation. *Postpartum depression* is more prevalent in those who are unemployed, do not have help with childcare or have a mood disorder. Treatment varies from cognitive management to antidepressants.

Dysthymic disorder (**a**) is described as a long-standing, fluctuating, low-grade depression with times of acute episodes. Affected individuals are able to carry out daily routines but gain little pleasure from leisure activities. Cyclothymic disorder (**e**) is characterized by a life of mood swings, with insufficient severity to meet bipolar disorder criteria. (**b**) The patient does not exhibit a lifetime history to be given a diagnosis of either of these or the severe mood swings of bipolar disorder. (**d**) This patient also does not meet the criteria for a major depressive episode.

Wound Care

Questions

486. A 34-year-old firefighter presents to the emergency department (ED) after getting trapped in a burning house and sustaining buns to various parts of his body as seen below. You examine the patient and notice that the injuries are circumferential to his right arm. You are not able to Doppler a radial pulse. What is the most appropriate next step in the management of this patient's injury?

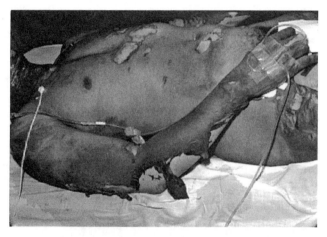

(Reproduced, with permission, from Tierney LM, McPhee SJ, Papadakis MA. Current Medical Diagnosis & Treatment. New York, NY: McGraw-Hill, 2006.) (Courtesy of B Moelleken.))

a. Immediate transfer to a burn center for definitive treatment
b. Decompressive escharotomy of the right upper extremity
c. Vascular surgery consultation and upper extremity angiogram
d. Conservative management with aggressive fluid resuscitation
e. Initiation of antibiotic therapy and tetanus prophylaxis, if indicated

487. A 40-year-old woman presents to the ED with a laceration sustained during a fall while ice-skating. She has a 3.5 cm superficial laceration above her right eyebrow running parallel to it. The wound is otherwise not visibly soiled and you see no foreign body in it. Muscle is intact below the wound so you do not anticipate needing deep sutures. You elect to use a commercially available tissue adhesive to close the wound for its ease of use and relative rapidity. The patient is up to date with her tetanus. Which of the following statements is true regarding the use of tissue adhesive to close a wound?

a. In a clean, superficial wound, irrigation can be skipped if tissue adhesive is used
b. The patient can be seated upright for what is a relatively short procedure
c. Wound apposition is not as important as epidermis will grow across the adhesive
d. Vital structures such as the eye must be covered
e. If the wound opens, the patient should be instructed to let it heal by secondary intention

488. A 26-year-old chef presents to your ED after lacerating his left third digit over the ventral aspect of the third phalanx. The wound is transverse, deep, does not cross a joint, and all tendons and sensory structures appear to be intact. Which of the following methods will provide appropriate anesthesia for irrigation, debridement, and closure?

a. Local infiltration through the wound margins with 3 cc of 2% lidocaine with epinephrine
b. Topical application of lidocaine-epinephrine-tetracaine(LET) for 20 minutes underneath a biocclusive dressing
c. A proximal radial nerve block with 5 cc of 2% lidocaine
d. A digital block at the base of the proximal phalanx with 3 cc of 1% lidocaine
e. Application of a penrose drain tourniquet and then irrigation over the wound with 5 cc 2% lidocaine

489. A 3-year-old girl presents to your ED after falling while running and hitting her head on the ground. Her mother states she cried immediately and has been upset but consolable since the accident, which occurred almost 2 hours ago. There is a vertical laceration over the middle of her forehead that crosses her hairline. The patient is crying and is difficult to control in the ED. What is the most appropriate method for closure of the wound?

a. 6-0 nonabsorbable nylon suture in an interrupted fashion
b. Staple closure
c. Commercially available glue such as Dermabond
d. 3-0 braided absorbable suture
e. Steri-strip adhesive bandages

490. A 52-year-old construction worker presents to the ED after puncturing his palm with a nail. He states his last tetanus toxoid immunization was 14 years ago and he remembers the next day the injection site was red, painful, and swollen. He states he received a complete tetanus immunization series when he was younger. Which of the following is true regarding tetanus immunization in this patient?

a. He does not need tetanus immunization if he was immunized as a child and again in adulthood
b. Local reaction to previous immunization is a risk for anaphylaxis in the future
c. He should receive tetanus immune globulin only
d. He should receive tetanus toxoid and tetanus immune globulin
e. He should receive tetanus toxoid only

491. A 25-year-old man who was recently assaulted presents to the ED with a laceration to the inside of his mouth after being hit across the face by a book. The laceration is 4 cm long in the transverse plane on the inside of his lip and involves only mucosa. He states his teeth catch on it and it is extremely painful. What is the most appropriate suture for closure of the wound?

a. Nonabsorbable nylon suture
b. Chromic gut suture
c. Wire suture
d. Polydiaxanone suture
e. Prolene suture

492. A 27-year-old man was in an altercation and presents to you with the laceration shown below. There are no dental fractures and his tetanus immunization is up to date. What are the most appropriate next steps in management?

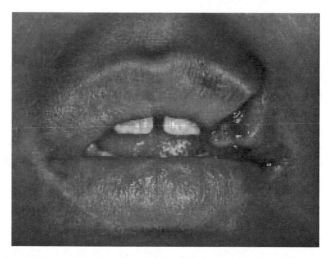

(Reproduced, with permission, from Knoop KJ, Stack LB, Storrow AB. Atlas of Emergency Medicine. *New York, NY: McGraw-Hill, 2002: 162.)*

a. Infraorbital nerve block and initiation of closure by approximating the vermilion border
b. Infiltration of local anesthesia into the lip and then approximation of the vermilion border
c. Infraorbital nerve block and closure of mucosal defects prior to the vermilion border
d. Infiltration of the lip with local anesthesia, closure of dermis and mucosal defects, and then approximation of the vermilion border
e. Closure with a commercially available tissue adhesive and steri-strips to avoid distorting tissue architecture

493. A 10-year-old boy is cut on the forearm with a knife that dropped out of a cabinet. The laceration is superficial and the closure uncomplicated. What is the appropriate time for the boy to return for suture removal?

a. 3–5 days
b. 7–10 days
c. 10–14 days
d. 14–21 days
e. When the wound does not begin to separate with gentle traction

494. A 32-year-old woman presents to the ED after being bitten on the palm of her hand by her own cat. The cat is vaccinated for rabies and otherwise behaving normally. Which of the following is true of cat bites?

a. Infection is rare and usually presents as a delayed sequelae 1–2 weeks later
b. Cat bites are usually superficial
c. Amoxicillin-clavulanate is recommended to cover *Pasteurella multocida*
d. Clindamycin is recommended to cover *Eikenella* species
e. After irrigation, prompt closure with a single stitch will prevent abscess formation

495. An 18-year-old man who weighs 100 kg presents to the ED with a cutaneous abscess on his left buttock. You wish to provide anesthesia using local infiltration with 1% lidocaine. The patient states he had an allergic reaction to lidocaine previously. Which of the following is true of lidocaine?

a. If a patient is allergic to benzocaine, they are likely allergic to lidocaine, as well
b. Hypersensitivity reactions are common to local anesthetic agents
c. The maximum safe dose of lidocaine is 12 mg/kg, or 1.2 g in this patient
d. It is more likely the patient had a reaction to a preservative than the lidocaine
e. Lidocaine has minimal systemic toxic effects

496. A 40-year-old-woman presents to the ED with a 6 cm linear, superficial laceration on the lateral aspect of her left leg sustained when she stepped through a glass coffee table. Preparation of the wound is best accomplished with which of the following?

a. Soaking the wound in 1 L of lukewarm water for 20 minutes
b. Soaking the wound in 10% betadine solution for 20 minutes
c. High-pressure irrigation with 600 cc normal saline
d. Scrubbing the wound with an alcohol soaked sponge
e. Careful irrigation with normal saline and a bulb syringe

497. A 33-year-old man presents to the ED with a laceration on his left arm after falling from his motorcycle. His jacket and pants are covered in bits of glass. You believe there may be glass in his laceration. Which of the following is true of imaging for foreign bodies?

a. Plain radiographs can frequently locate glass
b. Ultrasound is the study of choice in extremity injuries
c. CT scan is now considered first-line as it is readily available and more sensitive for foreign bodies
d. If the patient has no foreign body sensation, it is unlikely that there is need for imaging
e. Normal plain radiographs rule out clinically significant foreign bodies

498. A 14-year-old girl presents to your ED after burning her right forearm when hot cocoa spilled on it while camping. There burned area is approximately 12 cm long a 4 cm wide. There is blistering, slight charring, and the base of hair follicles is visualized. What type of burn is this?

a. First-degree
b. Second-degree superficial partial thickness
c. Second-degree deep partial thickness
d. Third-degree
e. Fourth-degree

499. A 23-year-old man presents to the ED complaining of a wound to his left lower extremity. He states he was pulling branches out of a flooded creek in his backyard when he punctured his left calf. He states his legs were in the water when the wound occurred. On exam, the wound is a 1 cm diameter puncture wound that penetrates several centimeters deep with surrounding erythema. You clean and irrigate the wound without evidence for a foreign body. What is the next most appropriate step in managing the wound?

a. Closure of the wound with nonabsorbable ethilon suture
b. Dressing the wound and treat with a fluoroquinolone as an outpatient
c. Outpatient treatment with an antifungal
d. X-ray to rule out foreign body
e. Irrigation with an iodine based solution into the deep part of the wound

500. A 78-year-old man presents to the ED complaining of a wound to the lateral aspect of his right arm. He states the wound occurred when he was trying to carry a bag through a door and caught the extremity on a sharp object. On exam, there is a 6 cm crescent-shaped laceration in the shape of a thin flap. You do not think it has a robust blood supply or that it will hold sutures well. The patient has a medical history of chronic obstructive pulmonary disease (COPD) for which he is chronically taking prednisone. What is the most appropriate management of this wound?

a. Resection of the skin flap and allowing the underlying tissue to heal with a covered dressing
b. Staple closure
c. Horizontal mattress nonabsorbable sutures in an interrupted fashion
d. Application of adhesive tape perpendicular to the wound with reinforcing strips laid parallel
e. Bandaging the skin with the flap in place as is

Wound Care

Answers

486. The answer is b. (*Hollander & Singer, pp 184–185. Tintinalli, pp 1220–1223.*) The patient has a *circumferential third-degree burn* to his right upper extremity. If pulses *are absent or diminished* in the setting of a circumferential extremity burn, *escharotomy* performed by a surgeon is indicated. If there is a full thickness and circumferential burn to the chest, escharotomy should be performed to decompress the chest wall for improved ventilation. Sedation is indicated for this procedure.

Transfer to a burn center (**a**) is certainly indicated for this patient, but not prior to the initial resuscitation and decompression. Burn centers have experience managing the complex fluid requirements and electrolyte shifts that burn victims exhibit. They are also equipped for advanced techniques in wound care. Indications for transfer to a burn center include any third-degree burn, burns to greater than 10% body surface area, burn location (face, hand feet, genitalia, or over a major joint), burns to children in a hospital not equipped for pediatric care, concomitant inhalation injury, and trauma. Escharotomy should not be delayed (**c**) for vascular surgery consultation. Angiography is unlikely to be useful in the setting of an acute burn. The arterial compromise in this case is caused by surrounding edema in a confined space. Definitive therapy is aimed at decreasing pressure in the surrounding compartments. Burn victims require significant fluid resuscitation (**d**) as their care progresses in the ED. Antibiotics and tetanus (**e**) should be administered but after the initial resuscitation.

487. The answer is d. (*Hollander & Singer, pp 90–96.*) *Tissue adhesives* (i.e., Dermabond) represent a fast and effective way to close certain lacerations. However, clinicians need to be vigilant in the other aspects of wound management and only use it for appropriate wounds. Tissue adhesive can be used for superficial wounds not subject to significant tension. Vital structures such as the eye must be kept safe from potential exposure to tissue adhesive as corneal injury can result from accidental exposure.

Irrigation (**a**) is necessary regardless of the method of closure. Similarly, the presence of a foreign body should also be evaluated. Although it is tempting to allow the patient to remain seated (**b**), the potential for runoff into the eye is very high, which can cause corneal injury. The patient should remain supine for the procedure with the length of the wound parallel to the floor. Application of petrolatum jelly in a thin ring around the wound will help to prevent runoff. Apposition (c) of wound edges is more important when using tissue adhesives. Adhesive should only come in contact with the epidermis. If the wound is inappropriately apposed, exposure of the dermis to the adhesive can result in inflammation and blistering, worsening the cosmetic result. Inappropriate opposition with dermis exposure also allows the adhesive to function like a foreign body, causing wound dehiscence. If a wound dehisces (e), the patient should be instructed to return to the ED for evaluation of delayed closure with suture.

488. The answer is d. (*Rosen, pp 741–743.*) Application of a *lidocaine digital block* at the base of the finger will block the digital nerves, allowing for appropriate anesthesia. The needle is inserted into the web space on either side and anesthesia is deposited anteriorly and posteriorly. This is repeated on the opposite side of the affected digit. Alternatively, local infiltration with lidocaine without epinephrine may provide adequate anesthesia.

Local infiltration with 3 cc 2% lidocaine with epinephrine (a) is incorrect as epinephrine is contraindicated in areas of end organ circulation (tip of nose, glans penis, scrotum, ears, nose, and fingers). LET (b) contains epinephrine and is also contraindicated. In addition, it is unlikely to provide adequate anesthesia for a deep wound. A radial nerve block (c) would not provide anesthesia to the palmar aspect of the hand. A penrose tourniquet (e) is sometimes used to decrease bleeding during repair, however, irrigating a wound with anesthetic will not provide adequate anesthesia.

489. The answer is a. (*Rosen, pp 741–745.*) This wound involves the face and the scalp. Therefore, cosmesis and tensile strength are both important. *Nylon suture* has minimal tissue reactivity and is unlikely to break. If the wound is deep, a layer of absorbable suture can be placed first to approximate deeper tissues; paying careful attention to facial structures that might be encountered such as the parotid gland or the facial nerve.

(b) Staples should not be used on the face. (c) Commercially available tissue adhesives such as Dermabond can be used for superficial lacerations that are not under tension, but would be difficult to place across the hairline. (d) Absorbable suture causes tissue reaction resulting in poor cosmesis and 3-0 is too large for the face. (e) Steri-strips are unlikely to provide the required tensile strength and would likely be removed by a 3-year-old.

490. The answer is e. *(Rosen, pp 749–751, 1791–1793.)* More than 10 years have passed since the patient's last tetanus immunization, so repeat *vaccination* is indicated with *tetanus toxoid.* If the patient had completed a primary series of immunizations and had a known booster vaccination within the last 10 years, no vaccination would have been necessary.

(**a**) Primary immunization results in antibody formation but does not persist indefinitely. Local reactions (**b**) can include pain, swelling, or erythema and can be dramatic but do not preclude future immunization. Patients may also complain of low-grade fever, pleurisy, and fatigue in the days after immunization. Tetanus immune globulin (**c**) alone is indicated if the patient has had an anaphylactic reaction to toxoid in the past. A patient should receive toxoid and immune globulin (**d**), at separate sites, only when immunization status is uncertain.

491. The answer is b. *(Rosen, pp 746–747.)* Closure in the oral cavity requires that a suture be absorbable and have an acceptable knot mass, therefore *chromic gut* is the best choice. It falls away within several days in the rapidly healing oral cavity.

(**a**) Nylon suture is not absorbable and is therefore inappropriate. It is used for closure of dermis. (**c**) Wire suture has very low tissue reactivity but is painful and is rarely used in the ED except occasionally by experienced practitioners or surgeons for tendon closure. (**d**) Polydiaxanone suture (PDS) is an absorbable monofilament that is difficult to tie and has a large knot mass. (**e**) Prolene is a nonabsorbable suture that is also difficult to tie with a large knot mass.

492. The answer is a. *(Hollander & Singer, pp 35–37. Knoop, p 162.)* This is a laceration of the face *crossing the vermilion border of the lip.* The goal of repair in these cases is approximation of the vermilion border with less than 2 mm of displacement. Reapproximation with significant displacement is cosmetically unappealing. In order to accomplish satisfactory closure, anesthesia should not distort tissue anatomy. In cases of upper lip laceration, infraorbital nerve blocks can be used to provide anesthesia to the midface and upper lip. Repair should then focus on approximating the border prior to closing the other aspects of the wound. The first stitch should bring the vermillion border together as illustrated on the next page.

Infiltration with local anesthesia into the area itself (**b & d**) will distort the tissue anatomy and may make proper alignment unreliable. It should only be used if the patient fails nerve block. Initial alignment of the dermis

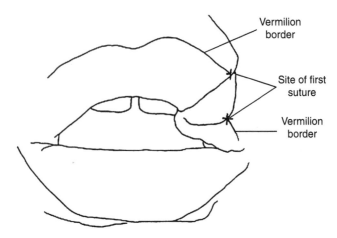

(Reproduced, with permission, from Knoop KJ, Stack LB, Storrow AB. Atlas of Emergency Medicine. *New York, NY: McGraw-Hill, 2002: 162.)*

or mucosal aspects of the laceration (**c & d**) may make approximation of the vermilion border difficult. Tissue adhesive and steri-strips (**e**) should not be used to close the lip as it is subject to pulling forces of facial movement. Wound separation in this case could result in a cosmetically unappealing outcome.

493. The answer is c. *(Rosen, p 749.)* Lacerations of an extremity can be removed as early as *10 days or as late as 14 days* depending on tension and viability of the wound edges. If the laceration is over a joint and subject to tension, it is important to keep the sutures in place for closer to 14 days.

(**a**) Facial lacerations should be removed within 3–5 days as the face heals quickly and "tram track" scars are prevented by prompt removal. (**b**) 7–10 days is an appropriate time frame for removal of scalp and trunk lacerations which are not under severe tension and are less visible. (**d**) Generally, there is no suture placed by an emergency physician that is removed later than 14 days. (**e**) Testing to see if the wound withstands traction may be tempting but is not recommended because partially healed wounds can easily be separated.

494. The answer is c. *(Rosen, pp 748–749.)* The most common organism to cause infection in *cat bites* is *P. multocida,* which is sensitive to penicillin. The infection is often polymicrobial and includes *staphylococcal* and *streptococcal* species, which may be β-lactamase resistant. Therefore, amoxicillin-clavulanate is indicated.

(a) Cat bites carry a high infection rate and typically occur shortly after the bite. (b) They tend to be deep and difficult to irrigate. (d) *Eikenella* is more often associated with human bites or "fight bites," and is often resistant to clindamycin. (e) Contaminated wounds on the hand, particularly punctures and animal bites, typically should not be closed primarily due to the risk of infection.

495. The answer is d. *(Rosen, pp 2572–2574.)* Many patients with true *allergic reactions* to lidocaine or other local anesthetics have reacted instead to the *preservative methylparaben*. This preservative is not contained in cardiac lidocaine or in single use vials.

(a) Patients who have an allergy to one of the ester group of local anesthetics (procaine, tetracaine, benzocaine) have not been described to have cross reactivity to those with an amide group (lidocaine, bupivacaine). (b) Allergy or reaction to either is uncommon and often represents vagal or emotional reaction to the experience or pain and discomfort from the injection. (c) The maximum safe dose of lidocaine is 3–5 mg/kg or up to 7 mg/kg when epinephrine is added and it is applied locally. (e) Lidocaine has many systemic toxic effects including headache, seizures, tinnitus, and cardiac arrhythmias.

496. The answer is c. *(Rosen, pp 742–744.)* *High-pressure irrigation* is the most effective method for cleaning open wounds not contaminated with large amounts of dirt or debris. Five to seven per square inch (PSI) is recommended and can be achieved using a 19 gauge catheter and a large (60 cc) syringe. Normal saline is the solution of choice. A rule of thumb is to use 100 cc for every 1 cm of laceration.

(a) Soaking the wound in water provides no mechanical debridement. (b) 10% betadine is tissue toxic to open wounds, as is chlorhexadine. Both are reserved for preparing skin prior to procedures and should not be used on exposed tissue. (d) Similarly, alcohol is directly tissue toxic and has no role in wound preparation. (e) Irrigation with a bulb syringe will not achieve high enough pressures to provide mechanical debridement.

497. The answer is a. *(Rosen, pp 740–741.)* Plain radiographs are often effective in locating glass, which is radiopaque and will often be visible provided it is >1 mm thick.

(b) Ultrasound can help find radiolucent objects but its use is not standard and false negatives may occur due to air, debris, or pus in a wound. (c) CT scan identifies foreign bodies with greater sensitivity but its cost and exposure to radiation warrant plain films first. If plain films are negative, yet a high clinical suspicion exists, follow-up with CT is recommended. (d) Foreign body sensation is useful in pinpointing a potential foreign body. Its absence does not rule it out, particularly in areas that may be insensate, or in patients who are unconscious. (e) Plain radiographs do not rule out clinically significant foreign bodies as they only visualize radiopaque materials. Further imaging may be needed.

498. The answer is c. *(Rosen, pp 501–513.)* The burn is a scald burn that caused a *deep partial thickness second-degree burn.* Second-degree burns are defined by damage of the epidermis and dermis with involvement *of the skin appendages.* Deep partial thickness burns are partially blanched and deep parts of the follicles may be visible with many burst blisters. Two-point discrimination may be impaired. The distinction is important because superficial second-degree burns heal with few problems while deeper burns can cause contraction and are at greater risk for infection.

(a) First-degree burns are superficial and involve only the epidermis. They are often caused by sun exposure and heal without scarring. (b) Superficial second-degree burns have mostly intact blistering, are red and painful. There is little thermal damage to the pain receptors. (d) Third-degree burns involve the dermis and the underlying tissue. They are painless, charred in appearance, and usually require skin grafting. (e) Fourth-degree burns involve fascia, muscle, bone, or other structures. They require complex repair. Third- and fourth-degree burns are caused by flame, scald injury, electrical injury, or chemical injury.

499. The answer is b. *(Hollander & Singer, pp 196–197.)* The patient sustained a wound with *stagnant freshwater* exposure. Coverage with empiric antibiotics is indicated in this setting to prevent suppurative complications. In addition to normal gram positive organisms, *Pseudomonas* and *Aeromonas species* are organisms that are likely to cause infection. Empiric coverage with a first-generation cephalosporin does not cover these species effectively.

Puncture wounds should not be closed (a) except under very special circumstances. They should be allowed to heal by secondary intention. Creation of a dead space in the soft tissue coupled with bacterial inoculation is a setup for a wound infection. If the wound is in an area that is cosmetically important (i.e., the face), then closure after irrigation can be considered with close follow-up. Antifungals (c) have no role in this patient. Evaluation with a radiograph (d) is unlikely to show a foreign body in this setting. The puncture wound was likely caused by the sharp end of a wooden branch. Wood splinters are radiolucent and will not be visible on plain radiograph. Irrigation with an iodine based solution (e) is likely to cause more harm than benefit. Iodine based solutions are tissue toxic. Their role is in sterilizing skin of its local flora but they should never be used to clean the inside of a wound.

500. The answer is d. *(Hollander & Singer, pp 65–67.) Tissue adhesive tapes* can be used to close superficial lacerations that are not subject to a great deal of tension. The advantage over sutures is their low cost, rapid closure, no damage to the host's defenses, lack of tissue ischemia, and they do not require removal. On the other hand, they can easily be removed, must be kept dry, and adhere poorly to oily skin. Indications for their use include linear, superficial lacerations with little to no tension; avulsion flaps, poor vascular supply, skin that is thin due to age or concomitant corticosteroid use, difficulty with follow-up, or if the wound is going to be covered by a cast or splint.

(a) There is rarely a reason to resect an avulsion flap. Even if the flap has a poor vascular supply, it functions as a biological dressing that has no tissue reactivity. Staple closure (b) is indicated in wounds with excellent vascular supply with low to moderate tension in areas that do not require careful opposition. Scalp lacerations that do not require closure of galea are ideally closed with staples. Closure with mattress style suture (c) is indicated for wounds in areas of high tension. They require good skin integrity on both sides of the laceration and would likely provide no benefit to this devascularized tissue flap. For small avulsion flaps, leaving them in place (e) is appropriate provided you do not anticipate significant patient discomfort due to movement of the flap.

Bibliography

2005 American Heart Association Guidelines for Cardiopulmonary Resuscitation and Emergency Cardiovascular Care. *Circulation.* 2005:112.

American College of Surgeons: Advanced Trauma Life Support Program for Doctors. Seventh edition. Chicago, 2004.

Aminoff MJ, Simon RR, Greenberg D. *Clinical Neurology.* 6th ed. New York, NY, McGraw-Hill; 2005.

Braunwald E, Fauci AS, Kasper DL, et al (eds). *Harrison's Principles of Internal Medicine.* 15th ed. New York, NY, McGraw-Hill; 2001.

Burnette LB. Cocaine Toxicity. *eMedicine Journal* 2006. Available at: http://www.emedicine.com/emerg/topic102.htm. Accessed on January 1, 2007.

Capobianco D, Dodick D. Diagnosis and treatment of cluster headache. *Semin Neurol.* 2006(26):242–259.

Center for Disease Control Treatment Guidelines 2006, Sexually Transmitted Diseases.

Centor RM, Witherspoon JM, Dalton HP, et al. The diagnosis of strep throat in adults in the emergency room. *Med Decis Making.* 1981;1:239–246.

Chauhan V. Synchronized Electrical Cardioversion, *eMedicine Journal* 2006. Available at: http://www.emedicine.com/med/topic2968.htm. Accessed on January 1, 2007.

Cohen J, Powderly W. *Infectious Diseases e-dition: Text with Continually Updated Online Reference.* 2nd ed. St Louis, Mosby; 2003.

Evans RW. Post-traumatic headaches. *Neurol Clin.* 2004;22(1):237–249.

Feied C. Pulmonary Embolism. *eMedicine Journal* 2006. Available at: http://www.emedicine.com/emerg/topic490.htm

Flowers LK. Costochondritis. *eMedicine Journal* 2005. Available at: http://www.emedicine.com/emerg/topic116.htm

Goetz CG. *Textbook of Clinical Neurology.* 2nd ed. Philadelphia, PA, Saunders; 2003.

Goldfrank L, Flomenbaum N, Lewin N, et al. *Goldfrank's Toxicologic Emergencies.* 7th ed. New York, NY, McGraw-Hill; 2002.

Goldman L, Ausiello D. *Cecil Textbook of Medicine.* 22nd ed. Philadelphia, PA, Saunders; 2003.

Hamilton GC, Sanders AB, Strange GR, et al. *Emergency Medicine: An Approach to Clinical Problem-Solving.* 2nd ed. Philadelphia, PA, Saunders; 2003.

Kao L, Nanagas KA. Carbon monoxide poisoning. *Emerg Med Clin North Am.* 2004;22(4):985–1018.

Knoop KJ, Stack LB, Storrow AB. *Atlas of Emergency Medicine.* 2nd ed. New York, NY, McGraw-Hill; 2002.

Manno EM. Subarachnoid Hemorrhage. *Neurology Clinics of North America.* 2004(22):347–366.

Marx JA, Hockberger RS, Walls RM, et al (eds). *Rosen's Emergency Medicine Concepts and Clinical Practice.* 5th ed. St Louis, Mosby; 2002.

McIntyre KE. Subclavian Steal Syndrome, *eMedicine Journal* 2006. Available at: http://www.emedicine.com/med/topic2771.htm

Mycek MJ, Harvey RA, Champe PC. *Pharmacology.* 2nd ed. Philadelphia, PA Lippincott Williams & Wilkins; 2000.

Paller AS, Mancini AJ. *Hurwitz Clinical Pediatric Dermatology e-dition: Text with Continually Updated Online Reference.* 3rd ed. Philadelphia, PA, Saunders; 2003.

Riordan-Eva P, Asbury T, Whitcher JP. *Vaughan & Asbury's General Ophthalmology.* 16th ed. New York, NY, McGraw-Hill; 2003.

Riviello RJ. Evaluating and treating sexual assault in the emergency department. *Emerg Med Rep.* Sept 5, 2005;26(19).

Roberts JR, Hedges JR. *Clinical Procedures in Emergency Medicine.* 4th ed. Philadelphia, PA, Saunders, 2004.

Scaletta TA, Schaider JJ. *Emergent Management of Trauma.* 2nd ed. New York, NY, McGraw-Hill; 2001.

Scheinfeld N. Teratology and Drug Use during Pregnancy. *eMedicine Journal* 2006. Available at: http://www.emedicine.com/med/topic3242.htm. Accessed on January 1, 2007.

Selwyn A. Coronary Artery Vasospasm. *eMedicine Journal* 2005. Available at: http:// www.emedicine.com/med/topic447.htm. Accessed on January 1, 2007.

Simon RR, Koenigsknecht SJ. *Emergency Orthopedics—The Extremities.* 4th ed. New York, NY, McGraw-Hill; 2001.

Singer AJ, Hollander JE. *Lacerations and Acute Wounds.* 1st ed. Philadelphia, PA, F.A. Davis Company; 2003.

Sovari AA. Long QT Syndrome. *eMedicine Journal* 2007. Available at: http://www.emedicine.com/med/topic1983.htm

Tierney LM, McPhee SJ, Papadakis MA. *Current Medical Diagnosis and Treatment.* 45th ed. New York, NY, McGraw-Hill; 2006.

Tintinalli JE. *Emergency Medicine: A Comprehensive Study Guide.* 6th ed. New York, NY, McGraw-Hill; 2004.

Townsend CM, Beauchamp RD, Evers BM, et al. *Sabiston Textbook of Surgery.* 17th ed. Philadelphia, PA, Saunders; 2004.

van den Berghe G, et al, Intensive insulin therapy in the critically ill patients, *NEJM.* Nov 8, 2001;345(19):1359–1367.

Wiesenfarth J. Aortic Dissection. *eMedicine Journal* 2005. Available at: http://www.emedicine.com/emerg/topic28.htm

Workowski KA, Berman SM. *Sexually Transmitted Diseases Treatment Guidelines.* Center for Disease Control Morbidity and Mortality Weekly Report. 2006; 55(11)

Index